Chronic Venous Insufficiency

Springer
London
Berlin
Heidelberg
New York
Barcelona
Hong Kong
Milan
Paris
Santa Clara
Singapore
Tokyo

Jeffrey L. Ballard and John J. Bergan (Eds)

Chronic Venous Insufficiency

Diagnosis and Treatment

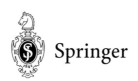 Springer

Jeffrey L. Ballard, MD, FACS
Loma Linda University Medical Center, Division of Vascular Surgery, 11175 Campus St,
RM#21123, Loma Linda, California, CA 92354, USA

John J. Bergan, MD FACS
North Coast Surgeons, 9850 Genessee Avenue, Suite 560, La Jolla, California, CA 92037, USA

ISBN 1-85233-172-0 Springer-Verlag London Berlin Heidelberg

British Library Cataloguing in Publication Data
Chronic venous insufficiency : diagnosis and treatment
    1. Venous insufficiency – Diagnosis   2. Venous insufficiency –
Treatment
    I. Ballard, Jeffrey L.   II. Bergan, John J.
    616.1′4
    ISBN 1852331720

Library of Congress Cataloging-in-Publication Data
Chronic venous insufficiency: diagnosis and treatment / John J. Bergan and
    Jeffrey L. Ballard (eds).
        p.   cm.
    Includes bibliographical references and index.
    ISBN 1-85233-172-0 (alk. paper)
    1. Venous insufficiency – Surgery Atlases.   2. Leg – Blood-vessels –
Diseases Atlases.   3. Venous insufficiency – Pathophysiology
Atlases.   I. Ballard, Jeffrey L., 1960– .   II. Bergan, John J., 1927– .
    [DNLM: 1. Venous Insufficiency – diagnosis.   2. Venous
Insufficiency – surgery.   WG 600 V4647 1999]
RC700.V45V46 1999
616.1′4–dc21
DNLM/DLC
For Library of Congress   99-22604

Typeset by EXPO Holdings, Malaysia
Printed and bound at Kyodo Printing Company (S'pore) PTE Ltd, Singapore
28/3830-543210 Printed on acid-free paper SPIN 10636691

To Tami for her remarkable patience, love and understanding,
To Lauren and Katelyn for their comic relief and inspiration,
To JMM who provided the key opportunity,

and

In La Jolla, to EB and RB who gave continuing good cheer.

Preface

Painful varicose veins, severe skin changes and recurrent ulceration manifest lower extremity chronic venous insufficiency. It is estimated to afflict 5% of the population over age 80 and a significant proportion, probably greater than 1%, of Western populations under age 65. Although these conditions command medical attention, in fact they are largely neglected by physicians and often relegated to nursing care in outpatient clinics. However, several events have now changed this pattern of care. The first is the recognition that chronic venous insufficiency is not dominated by the postphlebitic state and that these conditions can be ameliorated or even cured by intervention. The second is a growing realization that such interventions can be carried out in a minimally invasive and often outpatient basis.

This volume organizes severe chronic venous insufficiency into several categories separated into basic considerations and treatment alternatives. These, in turn, lead to the development of guidelines for care. While the volume is not entitled "Guidelines", in fact it is designed to provide criteria so that universities can use them for teaching and outpatient clinics and private offices can use them for care. A review of the table of contents shows that sclerotherapy, often used in the past, has given way to ambulatory phlebectomy and direct surgical intervention on the axial greater and lesser saphenous veins. Reconstructive venous surgery by bypass has been replaced by interventional radiologic techniques. Further, the abandoned Linton perforator vein procedure has been resurrected as an endoscopic intervention, which can be carried out on an outpatient basis.

Thus, recent developments in the treatment of chronic venous insufficiency are chronicled in this text. If it stimulates interest in veins and venous insufficiency and eager students continue to view this area of vascular surgery as open territory for research then it will have achieved one of our goals. If it improves the diagnosis and ultimate treatment of those afflicted with this malady then it has succeeded in the editors' primary purpose.

Jeffrey L. Ballard, MD, FACS   *John J. Bergan, MD, FACS*

Contents

Contributors

Jeffrey L. Ballard, MD, FACS
Associate Professor of Surgery
Loma Linda University Medical Center
Loma Linda, California, USA

John J. Bergan, MD, FACS, FRC, (Hon), Eng
Professor of Surgery
Loma Linda University Medical Center
La Jolla, California, USA

Clinical Professor of Surgery
University of California, San Diego
San Diego, California, USA

Clinical Professor of Surgery
Uniformed Services University of the Health
    Sciences
Bethesda, Maryland, USA

Professor of Surgery Emeritus
Northwestern University Medical School
Chicago, Illinois, USA

Michael D. Dake, MD
Division Chief
Cardiovascular/Interventional Radiology
Stanford University Medical School
Stanford, California, USA

Simon G. Darke, MS, FRCS
Consultant Vascular Surgeon
Royal Bournemouth Hospital
Bournemouth, Dorset, UK

Raymond M. Dunn, MD
Associate Professor of Surgery
University of Massachusetts Medical School
Worchester, Massachusetts, USA

Máté Dzsinich, PhD, DSc
2nd Department of Pathology
Semmelweis University of Medicine
Budapest, Hungary

Bo Eklof, MD, PhD
Clinical Professor of Surgery
University of Hawaii, John A. Burns School of
    Medicine
Honolulu, Hawaii, USA

Christina E. Gazak, MFA
The University of Utah, School of Medicine
Salt Lake City, Utah, USA

Peter Gloviczki, MD
Professor of Surgery
Mayo Clinic and Foundation
Mayo Medical School
Rochester, Minnesota, USA

J. Jérôme Guex, MD
Angiologist
Nice, France

Russell D. Hull, MBBS, MSc
Professor of Medicine
Division of Hematology
Calgary, Alberta, Canada

Anna Kádár, MD, PhD, DSc
2nd Department of Pathology
Semmelweis University of Medicine
Budapest, Hungary

Robert L. Kistner, MD
Clinical Professor of Surgery
University of Hawaii, John A. Burns School of
    Medicine
Honolulu, Hawaii, USA

Peter F. Lawrence, MD
Professor and Vice Chair of Surgery
Associate Dean for Program Development
Vice President for Specialty Services
University of California, Irvine
Irvine, California, USA

Elna M. Masuda, MD
Clinical Assistant Professor of Surgery
University of Hawaii, John J. Burns School of
  Medicine
Honolulu, Hawaii, USA

Géza Mózes, MD, PhD
2nd Department of Pathology
Semmelweis University of Medicine
Budapest, Hungary

Jay Murray, MD
Division of Vascular Surgery
Naval Medical Center
San Diego, California, USA

Graham F. Pineo, MD
Professor of Medicine
University of Calgary
Calgary, Alberta, Canada

Albert-Adrien Ramelet, MD
Specialiste FMH en dermatologie et en
  angiologie
Lausanne, France

JDS Reid, MD, FRCS(C)
Clinical Associate Professor
University of British Columbia
Department of Surgery
St Paul's Hospital
Vancouver
British Columbia, Canada

Jeffrey Rhodes, MD
Division of Vascular Surgery
Mayo Clinic and Foundation
Rochester, Minnesota, USA

Michael J. Rohrer, MD
Associate Professor of Surgery
University of Massachusetts Medical School
Worchester, Massachusetts, USA

Joseph G. Sladen, MD, FACS(C)
Former Clinical Professor of Surgery
St Paul's Hospital
University of British Columbia
Vancouver
British Columbia, Canada

606, 1160 Burrand Street
Vancouver
British Columbia, Canada V6Z 2E8

Steven Sparks, MD
Assistant Professor of Surgery
University of California, San Diego
San Diego, California, USA

Patricia E. Thorpe, MD
Associate Professor of Radiology & Surgery
Creighton University
Omaha, Nebraska, USA

Suresh Vedantham, MD
Cardiovascular/Interventional Radiology
Stanford University Medical Center
Stanford, California, USA

Adam J. Veradakis, MD
Resident
University of Massachusetts Medical School
Worchester, Massachusetts, USA

Robert A. Weiss, MD
Assistant Professor, Department of Dermatology
Johns Hopkins University, School of Medicine
Baltimore, Maryland, USA

Danian Yang, MD, PhD
Research Fellow
Straub Clinic and Hospital
Honolulu, Hawaii, USA

Section A

BASIC CONSIDERATIONS

Epidemiology of Chronic Venous Insufficiency

1

Peter F. Lawrence and Christine E. Gazak

Overview

Epidemiological studies can provide information on the spectrum and frequency of venous disease in a population and help physicians better understand its scope and incidence. Such information not only contributes to the recognition of mechanisms that cause the clinical sequelae of venous disease; it also assists in the development of screening and treatment strategies. To better understand the impact of venous disease on productivity in the form of lost work days, medical costs, and its cost to society in general, we must assess the prevalence and incidence of venous disease in the general population and be able to identify subgroups who have or who are likely to develop venous disease.

Although the first major study of venous disease took place in the US National Health Survey of 1935–36,[1] no recent study on prevalence in the USA has been conducted, and the incidence of venous disease (its occurrence in a population longitudinally through time) has yet to be thoroughly explored in the Western world. However, studies on rates of increase in specific populations have been performed in New Guinea and other areas of the world[2] that have become Westernized in recent years and subject to changes in health status. Prevalence of venous disease (the cross-sectional measurement of the number of cases in a population at one point in time) has been calculated extensively in Europe and Israel. Consequently, most information about epidemiology of venous disease comes from Europe,[3] where population demographics such as occupation, environment and lifestyle differ in many ways from the USA.

Chronic venous disease in the lower extremities is one of the most common conditions in adults in the industrialized world and affects an estimated 40% of the US population.[4] Chronic venous insufficiency with ulceration affects up to 2% of the population in Western countries, a prevalence comparable to that of diabetes. The cost to healthcare systems is massive: 4.6 million US work-days are missed per year due to venous disease,[4] and in the United Kingdom an estimated 10–30% of nursing time and £600 million (US $1 billion) – 2% of the national healthcare budget – is spent per year on the management of leg ulcers alone.[5]

One in five patients with chronic venous insufficiency suffers leg ulceration at any one time, and many individuals endure recurrent episodes of ulceration. The disease becomes more prevalent with advancing age (Fig. 1.1), so it is likely that more patients will be treated as the average population age increases. Chronic venous insufficiency with active leg ulceration occurs in roughly 0.2% of the population.[6,7] Despite its increasing prevalence and high cost, venous disease, with the exception of venous thrombosis and pulmonary embolism, is appreciated by few physicians as a significant health care problem since it is rarely limb- or life-threatening.

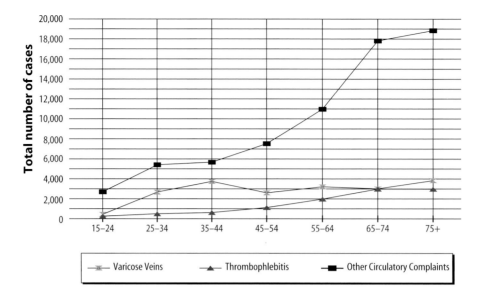

Fig. 1.1. Total US hospitalizations for varicose veins, thrombophlebitis, and chronic venous insufficiency distributed in age-specific groups.

Lack of severity is one explanation for the paucity of data on venous disease. Although venous disease has a high frequency in the US, it is a matter of debate whether the diagnosis of a nonmorbid venous complaint is a relevant illness or simply a normal variation in the population at large. This is much like the diagnosis of fibrocystic disease in a female patient. In addition, widespread screening of the disease is extremely rare. Screening tools, such as ultrasound, can be costly and impractical for an entire population, and lower-cost screening methods, such as the physical examination, are often neglected by the physician who perceives venous disease as an insignificant problem or a "vanity complaint."

Definitions of Venous Disease

Another difficulty in calculating venous disease rates lies in the definition of its scope. There is a broad spectrum of venous complaints, ranging from minor cosmetic blemishes (telangiectasias or spider-webs) to chronic venous ulcers and deep venous thrombosis, all of which are often grouped in the same category of diseases. To provide precise evaluation of venous disease, it is important to clearly delineate between types of venous complaints.

Varicose veins, the most common venous complaint, refer to any dilated, tortuous, elongated vein,

regardless of size. Three main classifications are: *trunk veins*, or varicose veins of the greater or lesser saphenous system and its named tributaries; *reticular veins*, subcutaneous veins that begin at the tributaries of trunk veins; and *telangiectasias* or *hyphen-webs* ("spider-veins"), which refer to intradermal varicose veins that are small and rarely symptomatic. Telangiectasias may or may not be included in papers describing the epidemiology of venous disease because of their relatively benign nature. Studies that include these veins in their analysis will report a much higher incidence and prevalence of varicose veins in the general population than those that do not.

Other than varicose veins, the most common venous disorders that bring patients to a physician are deep venous thrombosis (DVT), superficial thrombophlebitis and the sequelae of chronic venous insufficiency: edema, pigmentation, dermatitis and ulceration. These are usually diagnosed by physical examination and/or noninvasive testing.

Prevalence of Venous Disease

Because of the variety of definitions of varicose veins and the numerous methods used in assessing venous disease, exact prevalence is difficult to determine. One study conducted in a West London community[8] used self-report questionnaires to find the incidence and distribution of venous disease for that community. A random sample of 2,103 patients from three general practice sites were asked to complete a questionnaire on venous disease, including any previous self-report or physician diagnosis and usage of support hose. Of the 1,338 returned questionnaires, 31% reported having some form of venous disease. Twenty-five per cent reported varicose veins, 5% noted a history of phlebitis, 4% had a current or prior leg ulcer, 4% reported venous thrombosis and 1% reported a pulmonary embolism.

A Finnish study sought to assess the reliability of self-reporting of varicose veins.[9] A random sample of 166 patients who previously reported having varicose veins in a self-report questionnaire were examined by a surgeon to determine which variables in the questionnaire predicted misclassification; that is, the self-reported variables that were unreliable in correlating a given condition to a diagnosis of varicose veins. The researchers found that the only statistically significant variable associated with misclassification was a positive reporting of family history of varicose veins: those patients who reported a family history of varicose veins were more likely to assume they had varicose veins when they did not. Other self-reported variables such as height, weight, occupational status and age did not appear to correlate with misclassification.

Risk Factors for Varicose Veins

There are definite risk factors for varicose veins. Although disagreement about the significance of some of these factors exists, a convincing argument can be made that the combination of several conditions can reliably predict varicose veins. In a survey of 696 Czechoslovakian women employed at a large department store,[10] 421 were diagnosed with varicose veins. Women who were older, had at least one pregnancy, who stood at work or who were obese had a statistically higher prevalence of trunk varices than their thinner, younger, seated-worker counterparts. While factors such as differences in diet, economic status and genetic history must be taken into account, variables such as age and weight are considered significant predictors of varicose veins in other studies.[3] Below are the risk factors

reported in a number of studies, listed in decreasing importance:

1. *Age*: in virtually all studies, and as shown in Fig. 1.1, the prevalence of varicose veins increases with age in both men and women, independent of other risk factors. The relationship between age and varicose veins is unknown. However, it probably reflects a congenital weakness in the vein wall or valve cusp, which eventually weakens under lifestyle-related physical stress until valve incompetence and varicose veins occur.

2. *Sex*: the majority of epidemiological studies indicate that women have more varicose veins than men of comparable age. Although this difference has been reported from a 1:1 to a 10:1 ratio, most studies find that women have a three- to fourfold greater risk for varicose veins than men. While it is possible that women are more likely to notice varicose veins and self-report them, independent physical examinations have verified a higher incidence of varicose veins in women. Many potential explanations for this difference exist, but pregnancy appears to be the most frequent and important stress leading to a greater prevalence of varicose veins in women.

3. *Genetics*: epidemiological studies have reported a greater incidence of varicose veins in some countries than in others. A study comparing English and Egyptian cotton-mill workers found a greater incidence of varicose veins in the English population.[11] Another survey conducted in Jerusalem found that migrant men born in North Africa had significantly lower rates of varicose veins than their immigrant counterparts born in Europe, America and Israel.[12] These studies have been interpreted as proof of a hereditary etiology for varicose veins; an individual with a genetic predisposition will develop varicose veins more frequently when exposed to physical stresses such as pregnancy, obesity, etc.

4. *Occupation*: studies correlating occupation and risk for varicose veins have reported conflicting results. The previously mentioned Czech study found a correlation between prolonged standing and an increased risk for varicose veins. Another study examined chair sitting, with its resultant increase in venous pressure in calf veins, and found that in New Guinea, where women sat cross-legged on the ground and men sat on low stools or logs with their legs dangling, it was men who were more frequently diagnosed with varicose veins.

5. *Parity*: women with multiple pregnancies may be at increased risk for varicose veins, but the

etiology is unclear. Pregnancy-related varicose veins may be due to increased blood volume and venous pressure, or hormonal factors. In addition, previously developed varicose veins tend to increase in size with pregnancy. Stvrtinova[10] found a positive correlation between pregnancy and varicose veins, while other studies have found no significant relationship between pregnancy and varicose veins. With the current evidence, it seems that pregnancy increases the severity of varicose veins and may influence their development.

6. *Diet*: there is some evidence that a Western diet of refined foods and reduced fiber content leads to constipation, thereby resulting in increased intra-abdominal pressure and straining during bowel movement. Cleave[13] suggests that the increase in bowel pressure causes compression of the iliac veins, ultimately resulting in the development of varicose veins. Another theory by Burkitt[14] suggests the increased intra-abdominal pressure from straining during constipation (Valsalva maneuver) is transmitted to the veins of the legs. This eventually leads to dilation and valvular incompetence of the veins. A study separating diet from other ethnic, socio-economic or gender factors has not been conducted.

7. *Other factors*: many other factors with less supporting evidence have been suggested as causes for varicose veins, including obesity, heavy lifting and hematologic factors. Until further research provides substantiation for them, these factors can only be suggested as indirectly correlated to the increased likelihood of varicose veins.

Prevalence of Deep Venous Thrombosis and Chronic Venous Insufficiency

Venous thrombosis has been reported to occur in 1.6/1,000 persons in the general population, although subgroups of patients undergoing hip or knee prosthetic replacement have a higher incidence of DVT.[15] In contrast, the self-administered questionnaire to a west London community identified 6% of patients who had a prior episode of DVT, 6% who had been treated with anticoagulation, and 4% who had a prior or current leg ulcer, although the etiology of the leg ulcer was not deter-

mined. This variation may be due to a variety of factors, including discrepancies between hospital and self-reported data as well as differences in the populations studied. Overall, this reflects the need for more research in this area of venous disease.

Relationship between Valve Incompetence and Prior Venous Thrombosis

There has been considerable debate concerning the relationship between deep venous thrombosis and development of chronic venous insufficiency and/or ulcers. When DVT occurs, valve incompetence develops over time as the thrombosed segments recanalize. A study on the efficacy of compression stockings[16] reported that post-thrombotic syndrome develops in 60% of patients with DVT within 2 years of initial diagnosis. Markel et al.[17] studied patients with DVT longitudinally over time to determine the location and timing of valvular incompetence: at the onset of DVT, 17% of all deep valves were found to be incompetent, while after 12 months the percentage had grown to 69%. They also showed that valves in prior thrombosed segments are the ones that develop incompetence.

They also found, however, that 6% of patients with "normal" legs have deep valve incompetence in spite of no prior DVT. These patients have now been recognized to have primary valve incompetence, a congenital disorder that can lead to the same sequelae as the post-thrombotic leg. Therefore, while chronic venous insufficiency commonly develops from DVT, prior DVT is not necessary for chronic venous insufficiency to occur.

Venous Ulcers

Patients with chronic ulcers in the lower extremities often have chronic venous insufficiency as the cause. A Swedish epidemiologic study investigating the frequency and etiology of limb ulcers[6] found 827 ulcers in a rural and urban Swedish population

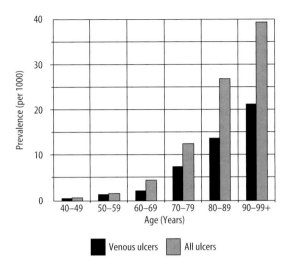

Fig. 1.2. Distribution of patients with venous ulcers as compared to all patients with nonvenous ulcers in an age-specific Swedish population.

Table 1.1. Venous complaints that have specific ICD-9 codes and may require hospitalization

Iliac vein thrombophlebitis (DVT)
Superficial thrombophlebitis of the lower extremities
Deep vein thrombophlebitis (DVT)
Upper extremity DVT
Unspecified phlebitis (superficial or deep)
Portal vein thrombosis
Budd–Chiari syndrome
Thrombophlebitis migrans
Thrombophlebitis of vena cava
Thrombophlebitis of other specified veins
Varicose vein of the leg (with ulcer)
Varicose vein of the leg (with inflammation)
Varicose vein of the leg (with both)
Varicose vein with inflammation and ulcer not mentioned
Compression of the vein (stenosis)
Venous insufficiency (unspecified)

of 270,800, for a prevalence of 0.16% and a male/female ratio of 1 : 1.9. Fifty four percent of the ulcers were due to venous disease, of which 60% had deep venous insufficiency and 40% had superficial or perforator vein incompetence.

The prevalence of venous ulcers increases with age, as it does in nonvenous ulcers (Fig. 1.2). The median age of initial venous ulcers in the Swedish study was 59 (vs. 73 for non venous ulcers). Fifty-four percent of patients had a venous ulcer for more than 1 year, while only 8% had a venous ulcer lasting less than 3 months. Recurrence of venous ulcers was found to be common (72%), particularly when there was deep venous involvement. The location of venous ulcers was usually the "gaiter" zone (95%), while nonvenous ulcers occurred most commonly in the foot. Interestingly, only 37% of patients with venous ulcers had a history of DVT. Therefore, many of these venous ulcers were either associated with primary valvular incompetence, incompetent superficial veins or possibly unrecognized DVT.

Venous Disease in Hospitalized Patients

Venous disease is a frequent cause for admission to the hospital, and is also identified in many more patients admitted to the hospital for other causes. In 1990, 99,903 patients were admitted to hospitals with a primary diagnosis of venous disease. Table 1.1 shows the diagnostic categories used in the study. In general categories, 67,098 of these patients were admitted for thrombophlebitis (presumably for anticoagulation), 8,647 for varicose veins (presumably requiring surgery), and 9,631 for chronic venous insufficiency (presumably for limb ulcer care and/or surgery). Over 270,000 US patients presented with venous disease as a secondary or other diagnosis. Roughly as many patients (98,000) are admitted to hospitals for a primary diagnosis of venous disease as are admitted for angioaccess procedures. Marked regional variations in the diagnosis of venous disease in hospitalized patients exist, possibly representing differences in population characteristics, admitting practices, or lifestyle (Fig. 1.3).

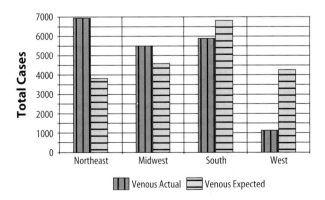

Fig. 1.3. Differences in US admitting practices for thrombophlebitis by region.

The observation that prevalence of venous disease in hospitalized patients increases with age is consistent with epidemiological studies of non-hospitalized venous patients. Studies have shown that some races are less likely to report venous disease, possibly reflecting differences in genetic susceptibility, lifestyle, occupation or admission patterns. US data from hospitalized patients in 1990 shows no statistically significant difference in venous disease by race.

Procedures on the venous system were performed in 59,901 patients, or two-thirds of all hospitalized patients presenting with the primary diagnosis of a venous complaint. Many of these procedures, such as those for varicose veins, were performed on an ambulatory basis. Fifty-one percent of all cases with a diagnosis of thrombophlebitis had one or more procedures performed, and presumably the thrombophlebitis was secondary to the procedure.

Morbidity and complications related to venous disease are common, but mortality is rare when a venous problem is the indication for admission. In-hospital morbidity and mortality is directly related to the magnitude of the surgical procedure, the age of the patient and the length of stay. Typically, varicose complaints, with or without ulcer, required a length of stay of 1 day or less, chronic venous insufficiency required a stay of 4 days or less, and thrombophlebitis required stays of up to 7 days, presumably for anticoagulation.

Summary

Venous disease is an extremely common condition, occurring in its milder forms in up to 40% of the adult population. It is more common in women, with increasing age, and with professions that require prolonged standing. More serious venous disease (DVT, venous ulcers, etc.) occurs in 0.4% of the population, and often is associated with hospitalization and surgical procedures.

References

1. US Department of Health, Education and Welfare. The magnitude of the chronic disease problem in the United States. National Health Survey 1935–1936, Preliminary Reports. 1938; Washington DC
2. Stanhope JM. Varicose veins in a population of lowland New Guinea. Int J Epidemiol 1975; 4:221–5
3. Callam MJ. Epidemiology of varicose veins. Br J Surg 1994; 81:167–73
4. Stanley JC, Barnes RW, Ernst CB. Vascular surgery in the United States: workforce issues. J Vasc Surg 1996; 23:172–81
5. Bosanquet N. Costs of venous ulcers: from maintenance therapy to investment programmes. Phlebology Suppl 1992; 1:44–6.
6. Ebbeskog B, Lindholm C, Ohman S. Leg and foot ulcer patients. Epidemiology and nursing care in an urban population in south Stockholm, Sweden. Scand J Prim Health Care 1996; 14(4): 238–43
7. Callam MJ, Ruckley CV, Harper DR, et al. Chronic ulceration of the leg: extent of the problem and provision of care. Br Med J 1985; 290:1855–6
8. Franks PJ, Wright DI, Moffatt CJ. Prevalence of venous disease: a community study in West London. Eur J Surg 1992; 158:143–7
9. Laurikka J. Misclassification in a questionnaire survey of varicose veins. J Clin Epidemiol 1995; 48:1175–8
10. Stvrtinova A, Kolesar J. Prevalence of varicose veins of the lower limbs in the women working at a department store. Int Angiol 1991; 10:2–5
11. Mekky S, Schilling RS, Walford J. Varicose veins in women cotton workers: an epidemiological study in England and Egypt. Br Med J 1969; 2:591–5
12. Amramson JH, Hopp C, Epstein LM. The epidemiology of varicose veins – a survey of western Jerusalem. J Epidemiol Comm Health 1981; 35:213–17
13. Cleave TL. Varicose veins – nature's error or man's? Lancet 1959; ii:172–5
14. Burkitt DP. Varicose veins, deep vein thrombosis, and hemorrhoids: epidemiology and suggested aetiology. Br Med J 1972; 2:556–61
15. Oishi CS, Grady-Benson JC, Otis SM et al. Total knee arthroplasty, as determined with duplex ultrasonography. J Bone Joint Surg Am 1994; 76(11):1658–63
16. Brandjes DPM, Buller HR, Heijboer H et al. Randomised trial of effect of compression stockings in patients with symptomatic proximal-vein thrombosis. Lancet 1997; 349:759–62
17. Markel A, Manzo RA, Bergelin RO et al. Valvular reflux after deep vein thrombosis: incidence and time of occurrence. J Vasc Surg 1992; 15(2):377–84

Risk Factors in Chronic Venous Insufficiency

2

Jeffrey L. Ballard and John J. Bergan

An estimated 10–35% of the adult population has some form of venous disease and chronic venous insufficiency (CVI) is the seventh leading cause of debilitating disease in the United States.[1,2] Aside from burdensome symptoms and unsightly varicose veins, skin changes and ultimately ulcerative sequelae exert a significant impact on health care expenditure.[3] Twenty-four million Americans have varicose veins, six million have skin changes due to chronic venous insufficiency (CVI) and 500,000 people have or have had a venous ulcer.[4] For much of the American working class, severe CVI is a significant cause of disability in the workplace.[5,6] Despite the widespread nature of this malady, knowledge of physiology and hemodynamics of the venous system is still a subject of considerable debate. Furthermore, risk factors associated with CVI are multiple, complex and lack epidemiological confirmation.

Some risk factors for the development of CVI such as age, genetic predisposition, sex, hormonal influences including pregnancy, menstrual cycle and lifestyle are mostly agreed upon.[7,8] Other factors such as obesity, dietary habits, tight undergarments, toilet posture, cigarette smoking and lack of exercise remain highly speculative.[8,9] Despite evidence-based research, direct relationships for all potential risk factors have not been factually validated.[10] Although some risk factors are statistically significantly seen more often in patients with CVI compared to controls, it has not been clearly established whether these pose a real risk for CVI or whether they are just a consequence of the disease process itself.[7,8]

Clearly, prospective studies with an epidemiological basis would substantiate risk factors for CVI. However, these are currently lacking and logistically may prove difficult to carryout due to inherent design problems. Fortunately, new diagnostic techniques have at least helped to improve both the study and treatment of chronic venous disease. These noninvasive techniques have demonstrated CVI to be associated with coexistent hemodynamic and physiologic abnormalities as well as certain risk factors. This intimate relationship between risk factors, venous hemodynamics and venous physiology will be discussed in this chapter.

Risk Factors in CVI

Physicians dating back to ancient Greece have treated chronic venous disease. Yet, its causal relationships remain poorly understood. Most epidemiological studies on this topic are cross-sectional surveys that suggest potential risk factors for CVI by describing their frequency in study populations. In one such study of 696 Czechoslovakian women employed in a department store, Stvrtinová and Kolesár found several factors that were associated with the incidence of varicose veins.[11] Older women with a history of at least one pregnancy who stood at work or were obese had a statistically higher incidence of varicosities than those who were younger, thinner and worked seated.[11] Similarly, other epidemiological studies have demonstrated age and weight to be significant risk factors for the development of CVI.[12–14]

Regardless of etiology, abnormal hemodynamic change converts venous physiology to pathophysiology and allows a constellation of symptoms and physical findings to progress.[15] Valvular incompetence plays a major role in this development of CVI.[12] Chronic changes are ultimately a manifestation of the effects of superficial, perforator and/or deep venous valvular incompetence. Degree of valvular incompetence in the deep or superficial venous compartments correlates with the presence of edema, skin changes and ulceration.[12,15,16] Physically, these changes range from annoying telangiectasias, reticular varicosities and painful varicose veins to hyperpigmentation atrophie blanche and healed or open ulceration. Symptoms may range from leg fatigue to disabling chronic pain, intractable ulceration or severe infection.[17]

Age

The aging population of western European countries correlates strongly with an increased prevalence of chronic venous disease.[18] Incidence of varicose veins is increased in both men and women in almost all epidemiological studies independent of other risk factors.[7,19] In a multivariate analysis of 474 patients, Capitao et al.[10] found increasing age to be the major risk factor associated with the development of CVI. In addition, several other risk factors such as body weight, environmental heat, sedentary lifestyle, heredity, high-dose estrogen, osteoarticular disease of the lower extremities, truncal varices, lymphedema and a history of thrombophlebitis independently correlated with severity of CVI.[10] In a remarkable survey (with an 87% response rate) of all 2,785 employees at the Volvo motor engine factory in Sweden, Nelzen et al.[20] noted an increased prevalence of venous ulceration with advancing age. The overall lifetime prevalence of nontraumatic open leg ulceration was 1.6%. This incidence ranged from 0.4% for those respondents between the ages of 30 and 49, to 1% in those 50–59 years old. These authors con-

cluded that prevalence of severe CVI was age related and that incidence of open leg ulceration in younger individuals exceeded previously reported figures.[21] A recent prospective dual case–control, multivariate analysis by Scott and colleagues, demonstrated that after adjusting for age many other independent factors were linked to more severe forms of CVI.[22] These were male sex, obesity, prior history of phlebitis and/or serious leg injury. A history of serious leg injury or phlebitis was associated with a 2.4-fold and 25.7-fold increased risk for CVI, respectively. Age-related factors not associated with CVI in this study included hypertension, heart disease, diabetes mellitus, increased parturition, number of medications, lifestyle and economic issues.[22]

Although the exact link between age and CVI is unknown, weakness in normally compliant and collapsible vein walls or valve cusps may contribute to this association. With advancing age, deregulation of venous tone by centrally located vasomotor centers, adrenergic nerve fibers and localized paracrine activity may also lead to vein wall weakness. Clarke et al.[23] studied venous valves with duplex ultrasound while simultaneously measuring calf volume (stress gauge plethysmography) and venous pressure in the lower extremity veins of 51 normal and/or low risk patients and 36 high-risk patients with superficial venous insufficiency. The high-risk group showed diminished vein wall elasticity ($p < 0.001$) and increased arterial inflow ($p < 0.005$). It is plausible that a lifetime of physical stress and changes in venous elastic properties could cause veins to dilate so that valve cusps fail to come properly into apposition. Anatomically, these valves appear redundant and distorted leading to poor coaptation of the leaflets. Valve incompetence leads to venous reflux which may be present within the superficial, deep or perforating venous systems alone or in any combination.[13] This can lead to CVI with the usual stigmata that was once thought only to be secondary to a previous history of deep venous thrombosis (DVT).

The association between age and prevalence of venous insufficiency may be further elucidated by an evidence-based study currently being carried out in Europe by Schultz-Ehrenburg et al.[24] Presence of varicose veins in school-age children is the focus of the study. Duplex ultrasonography and photoplethysmography supplement clinical examination. In a preliminary report, presence of long or short saphenous vein incompetence was found to be four times as common in the 14–16 year age group compared to the 10–12 year age group.[24] Ongoing follow-up of this important patient cohort may shed light on some of the causal relationships associated with varicose veins.[25,26]

Genetic Predisposition

Although it is commonly thought that family history is one of the strongest influences for the development of CVI, in fact, factual Level 1 (large, prospective studies with definite conclusions) or Level 2 (smaller studies with less certain results) evidence of the contributory role of this risk factor is limited because of methodological difficulties of published data.[8] Nevertheless, Cornu-Thenard et al.[27] demonstrated the influence of genetic predisposition by comparing the clinical examination of the parents of 67 patients with varicose veins to the parents of 67 patients without varicose veins. They found that mothers and fathers of patients with varicose veins were more likely to also have varicose veins. Furthermore, these parents were more likely to have had a history of treatment for the varicose veins. Belcaro et al.[28] objectively studied saphenofemoral incompetence using Doppler ultrasound in parents and offspring with varicose veins and found a positive familial association. In the Basle study, varicose veins were also found to be more common in patients with a positive family history.[17]

Other studies support a familial association in the development of CVI. However, these studies are open to bias because family history was verbally obtained from the patient. Family members with a positive history of CVI were not examined clinically.[29,30] On the other hand, Weindorf and colleagues[25,26] found no proof of a familial association. However, based upon current evidence it would be safe to say that an individual with a genetic predisposition would be more likely to develop varicosities with age or when exposed to risks that seem to have a causal relationship to CVI such as phlebitis, leg trauma, pregnancy or obesity.

Sex

Evidence from numerous epidemiological studies demonstrate a female predominance in the prevalence of varicose veins.[31] In fact, the female-to-male incidence of varicosities apparently increases with advancing age. This may, in part, be related to hormonal influences in addition to the fact that women are more likely than their male counterparts to notice and self-report varicose veins.[31] Nevertheless, notable exceptions have been published. Nobl[32] found a male predominance in his evaluation of 47,140 patients and Nicholson[33] demonstrated a male preponderance in the incidence of varicose veins in his analysis of 112 hospital patients. However, both of these studies were biased towards men and published long before there was a better understanding of venous disease. Therefore, these conclusions may not be entirely accurate as the overall weight of evidence-based study clearly supports a female predominance in the development of varicose veins.

In contradistinction, more severe forms of chronic venous insufficiency such as leg ulceration tend to be more common in men. This was demonstrated by Scott et al.[22] in their dual case–control study of patients with varicose veins. The authors compared patients with CVI displaying venous ulcers to a general population control group. They found the majority of patients within the venous ulcer group to be male. However, there remained a strong female predominance in the varicose vein group. These results are consistent with numerous other studies.[3,9,34–36] In our current practice environment, patients presenting for treatment of varicose veins are usually younger, female, have a history of phlebitis and often have a family history of varicose veins.

Hormones and Pregnancy

Estrogens cause smooth muscle proliferation and increase connective tissue content within vein walls. These changes are often circumferential and can lead to decrease in or loss of vein wall elasticity resulting in valvular incompetence.[24,37] However, they can be segmental which may account for the noncontiguous array in which varicosities often appear. Structural alterations in venous endothelium may occur secondary to estrogen use including increased capillary permeability, vasodilation with edema formation and neovascularization.[24,37]

Natural estrogens taken by mouth increase coagulation factor I concentration and decrease antithrombin III levels. This effectively increases DVT risk. Similarly, pregnancy and the postpartum state are associated with a fivefold increased risk of venous thrombosis.

Progesterone is a potent smooth muscle relaxer and has been shown to inhibit smooth muscle contraction.[8] This, in turn, hinders venous contraction and results in valve incompetence. Ultimately, there is development of venous reflux. In addition, there is increased venous and arterial compliance, leading to stasis and vasodilation. Even so, progesterones are thought to have little effect on the development of DVT. Overall, there has been a precipitous decrease in hormone-related vascular problems with the advent of low-dose oral contraceptive agents except in patients with a significant vascular past medical history.[38,39]

Vin and colleagues[38] studied a population of females (21–40 years old) who took oral contraceptive agents (OCA) of various types. In their review of 2,295 medical records, analysis of variance showed a difference in venous symptomatology as a function of the consumed type of OCA. A minimum-dose estroprogesterone was associated with less venous symptomatology compared to normal dose OCA. This phenomenon of symptoms related to hormonal concentration is readily apparent during the menstrual cycle where venous distensibility follows the rise of progesterone rather than estrogen. Though there is slight distensibility of veins when estrogen levels peak at about cycle day 12–14, venous distensibility is at its greatest when progesterone reaches its highest level during the last half of the cycle.[8] Clinically, this is coincident with the development of maximal pain in telangiectasias or varicose veins days before menses.

Some controversy exists regarding the effect of pregnancy on the development of CVI even though an estimated 8–20% of females develop varicose veins during pregnancy.[40] Evidence-based studies, conducted in English-speaking countries as well as Israel, have demonstrated that prevalence of varicosities increases with multiparity.[41] However, it has also been found that women in countries with a low incidence of varicose veins have, on average, more pregnancies than women in countries with a higher incidence of CVI.[8] Number of pregnancies has also not explained differences in varicose vein preva-

lence in at least one study conducted in the South Pacific.[8] Multiparous women are likely overall to be older than women with fewer pregnancies, and as noted previously, age is an important factor in the development of venous insufficiency. Other factors, such as genetic predisposition could be at play in this scenario. Therefore, for reasons other than parity alone, multivariate analysis may show no difference in incidence of CVI in some groups of women.[42] These apparent inconsistencies with some studies clearly showing a prevalence of varicose veins with number of pregnancies and others showing no increased incidence with multiparity highlight the lack of a unifying theory for the development of CVI.

Nevertheless, any tendency toward varicosities is exacerbated by pregnancy.[15,31] In addition, pregnancy may trigger or aggravate lower extremity venous insufficiency. The clinical observation that varicosities appear in the first trimester of pregnancy strongly implicates progesterone from the corpus luteum (and not pressure of the gravid uterus on iliac veins and vena cava) as the inciting element. In general, it has been found that there is a large increase in venous distensibility during pregnancy with a return to normal at about 8–12 weeks after parturition.[8] This tendency toward venous distension is amplified in women who already have varicosities. The rapid onset and aggressiveness of signs and symptoms of CVI with pregnancy and the rapid regression with childbirth favors this association even though some studies have not demonstrated an evidence-based link.[43]

Deep Venous Thrombosis

Evidence-based data demonstrate that there is a positive association between DVT and the development of chronic venous ulcers.[31] However, the strength of this association is a subject of considerable debate. Meissner et al.[44] demonstrated valve incompetence in vein segments which had had intraluminal thrombus previously seen by duplex ultrasound examination. As expected, recanalization and thrombus propagation occurred early after the initial thrombotic event. However, rethrombosis and thrombus extension to previously uninvolved vein segments occurred later. This dynamic process may be associated with an insidious clinical presentation of CVI which lags decades following the original deep venous thrombotic event. The primary mechanism may involve reflux, obstruction, or a combination of reflux and obstruction. For example, post-thrombotic collaterals may form and become a source of massive reflux in addition to axial reflux caused by incompetent valves. Abnormalities are also noted at the level of the calf muscle pump including reduced venous capacitance and compliance which leads to worsening reflux and obstruction.[24] Despite the above, some patients have little to no symptoms following an episode of DVT. As a corollary, only 37% of patients in one series with venous ulcers had a previous history of DVT.[31] Therefore, not all forms of CVI are positively linked to a previous episode of DVT. This observation has lead to new treatment possibilities for the patient previously thought to be "postphlebitic" and without hope.[45-47]

Lifestyle

Lifestyle factors, such as standing occupation, have been implicated in the development of CVI. For example, duplex ultasound imaging demonstrated venous reflux to be more frequently seen among symptom-free vascular surgeons compared to nonmedical individuals in a study from St. Mary's Hospital Medical School.[48] The superficial, deep and perforating venous systems were evaluated in 28 vascular surgeons (56 limbs) and 25 normal volunteers (50 limbs). Although there was no measurement of calf pump function and retrograde flow greater than 1.0 s was considered positive for reflux instead of 0.5 s, the authors found that vascular surgeons had a significantly ($p < 0.04$) greater degree of all types of reflux compared to age- and sex-matched controls.[49-51] The study by Stvrtinová and Kolesár also found a positive correlation between a lifestyle of prolonged standing and the incidence of varicose veins.[11] An interesting study from New Guinea demonstrated that men who sat on low stools or logs with their feet dangling were more likely to be diagnosed with varicose veins than women who sat cross-legged on the ground.[31] The

implication here is that prolonged chair sitting may result in venous stasis and increased lower extremity venous pressure.

Race/Geography

The 1961 US National Health Survey revealed that 24% of whites complained of varicose veins compared with 10.4% of the African-Americans surveyed.[52] This information was survey-based and nonobjective. However, an association between Westernized, developed Caucasian countries and an increased incidence of varicose veins has been consistently noted. A study by Mekky and colleagues assessed 500 female cotton wool workers in England and Egypt and demonstrated a 32% prevalence of varicose veins in the English women compared to 5.8% incidence in the Egyptians.[53] Another survey found that migrant men born in North Africa had a lower incidence of varicosities than their immigrant counterparts who were born in Europe, America and Israel.[31] The studies discussed above have been used to link race and geography with incidence of CVI. Yet, lifestyle and/or genetic predisposition may also play important roles in this association. Evidence-based data on this topic is lacking, as subjective survey data comprises much of the current knowledge.

Obesity

The balance of evidence suggests that a large body mass is related to CVI. Current data suggest that this association is more convincing in women than in men.[8] The Basel study demonstrated varicose veins to be more common in overweight women.[17] Telangiectasias and reticular varicosities were more common than truncal varices in obese men (> 20% ideal weight).[17] A recent study on risk factors for CVI by Scott and colleagues from Boston University Medical Center found obesity to be a statistically significant independent risk factor for CVI.[22] Obesity may lead to a perturbation of lower extremity venous outflow, especially in gynecoid obesity. This can cause chronic venous insufficiency with an increased risk for thromboembolism and lymphatic insufficiency or capillary permeability disorders. Despite the seemingly reasonable relationship between obesity and CVI, other studies fail to support the contention that obesity, even in women, is a primary risk factor.[8,31]

Diet, Tight Clothes and Toilet Posture

Other lifestyle factors such as low-fiber diet, tight undergarments and toilet posture have been suggested to cause distal venous hypertension, perhaps leading to venous wall stretching and elongation of venous valves. However, such associations have been difficult to explain statistically. No doubt that a Western diet of refined foods and reduced fiber content leads to a higher incidence of constipation. This, in turn, results in increased intra-abdominal pressure and straining during defecation. Cleave has suggested that that increased intra-abdominal pressure causes iliac vein compression.[54] Over years, this effective outflow obstruction results in distal venous hypertension, venous insufficiency and varicose veins.[54] Burkitt has suggested that venous dilation and valvular incompetence develop when constipation (from a low-fiber diet), related to a rise in intra-abdominal pressure, is transmitted to the veins of the lower extremities.[55] Raised toilet seats and tight undergarments have also been implicated in causing distal venous hypertension. Yet, evidence for these is tenuous and such factors certainly have less than a direct causal relationship to the development of CVI.

Conclusions

Despite some general agreement, controversy and lack of evidence-based study surrounds the definition of risk factors for CVI. Some links can only be suggested as likely causes of CVI, while others clearly have not been factually established. Among the mostly agreed upon are age, sex, genetic predisposition, hormonal influences (including pregnancy and the menstrual cycle), history of deep venous thrombosis, and lifestyle. Others that are less agreed upon include race, geography, body mass, dietary habits, tight clothing, toilet posture, cigarette smoking and lack of exercise.

References

1. White GH. Chronic venous insufficiency. In: Veith F, Hobson RW, Williams RA, Wilson SE (eds) Vascular surgery, 2nd edn. McGraw-Hill, New York, 1993: 865–88
2. Porter JM, Rutherford RB, Clagett GP et al. Reporting standards in venous disease. J Vasc Surg 1988; 8:172–81
3. Callam MJ, Harper DR, Dale JJ, Ruckley CV. Chronic ulcer of the leg: clinical history. Br Med J 1987; 294:1389–91
4. Coon WW, Willis PV, Keller JB. Venous thromboembolism and other venous diseases in the Tecumseh community health study. Circulation 1973; 48:838–46
5. Capeheart JK. Chronic venous insufficiency: a focus on prevention of venous ulceration. J Wound Ostomy Continence Nurs 1996; 23(4):227–34
6. Callam MJ, Harper DR, Dale JJ, Ruckley CV. Chronic leg ulceration: socioeconomic aspects. Scott Med J 1988; 33:358–60
7. Callam MJ. Epidemiology of varicose veins. Br J Surg 1994; 81(2):167–73
8. Bergan JJ, Ballard JL. Controversies surrounding the diagnosis and treatment of varicose veins. Chapter 14A. In: Schein M, Wise L (eds) Crucial controversies in surgery 1998. Karger Landes Systems, Basel, 1997: 235–47
9. Carpentier P, Priollet P. Epidemiology of chronic venous insufficiency. Presse-Med 1994; 23(5):197–201
10. Capitao LM, Menezes JD, Gonveia-Oliveira A. A multivariate analysis of the factors associated with the severity of chronic venous insufficiency. Acta Med Port 1993; 6:501–06
11. Stvrtinová V, Kolesár J. Prevalence of varicose veins of the lower limbs in the women working at a department store. Int Angiol 1991; 10:2–5
12. Rudofsky G. Epidemiology and pathophysiology of primary varicose veins. Langenbecks Arc Chir 1988; Suppl 2:139–44
13. Abramson JH, Hopp C, Epstein LM. The epidemiology of varicose veins. A survey in Western Jerusalem. J Epidemiol Community Health 1981; 35:213–17
14. Widmer LK, Kamber V, da Silva A, Madar G. Overview: varicosis. Langenbecks Arch Chir 1978; 347:203–7
15. McEnroe CS, O'Donnell TF, Mackey WC. Correlation of clinical findings with venous hemodynamics in 386 patients with chronic venous insufficiency. Am J Surg 1988; 156:148–52
16. Hanrahan LM, Aronki CT, Rodriguez AA, Kechejian GJ, LaMorte WW, Menzoian JO. Distribution of valvular incompetence in patients with venous stasis ulceration. J Vasc Surg 1991; 13:805–12
17. Becker F. Mechanisms, epidemiology and clinical evaluation of venous insufficiency of the lower limbs. Rev Prat 1994; 44(96):726–31
18. Ibrahim S, MacPherson DR, Goldhaber SZ. Chronic venous insufficiency: ulcerations and management. Am Heart J 1994; 132(4):856–60
19. Krijnen RW, deBoer EM, Ader JH, Bruynzeel DP. Venous insufficiency in male workers with a standing profession. Part I: epidemiology. Dermatology 1997; 194(2):111–20
20. Nelzen O, Bergquist D, Fransson I, Lindhagen A. Prevalence and etiology of leg ulcers in a defined population of industrial workers. Phlebology 1996; 11:50–4
21. Depalma RG, Talieh YJ. Discussion of: Nelzen O, Bergquist D, Fransson I, Lindhagen A. Prevalence and etiology of leg ulcers in a defined population of industrial workers. Phlebology 1996; 11:50–54. Venous Digest 1997; 4(9):4–5
22. Scott TE, LaMorte WM, Gorin DR, Menzoian JO. Risk factors for chronic venous insufficiency: a dual case–control study. J Vasc Surg 1995; 22:622–8
23. Clarke GH, Vasdekis SN, Hobbs JT, Nicolaides AN. Venous wall function in the pathogenesis of varicose veins. Surgery 1992; 111:402–8
24. Schultz-Ehrenburg U, Weindorf N, Von Uslar D, Hirche H. Prospective epidemiological investigations on early and pre-clinical stages of varicosis. In: Davy A, Stemmer R (eds) Phlebology. John Libbey Eurotext, Paris, 1989: 163–5

25. Weindorf N, Shultz-Ehrenburg N. Development of varicosis in children and adolescents. Phlebologie 1990; 43(4):573–7
26. Weindorf N, Shultz-Ehrenburg N. Early and preclinical stages of varicose veins. Bochum Study I–III. Phlebologie 1992; 45(4):497–500
27. Cornu-Thenard A, Moivin P, Baud JM, deVincenzi I, Carpentier PH. Importance of the familial factor in varicose disease: clinical study of 134 families. J Dermatol Surg Oncol 1994; 20:318–26
28. Belcaro GV. Saphenofemoral incompetence in young asymptomatic subjects with a family history of varices of the lower limbs. In: Negus D, Jantet G (eds) Phlebology 1985. John Libbey Eurotext, Paris, 1986: 30–2
29. Hirai M. Prevalence and risk factors of varicose veins in Japanese women. Angiology 1990; 3:228–32
30. Matousek V, Prevorsky J. A contribution to the problem of the inheritance of primary varicose veins. Hum Hered 1974; 24:225–35
31. Lawrence PF, Gazak CE. Epidemiology of chronic venous insufficiency. Chapter 3. In: Gloviczki P, Bergan JJ (eds) Atlas of endoscopic perforator vein surgery. Springer-Verlag, London, 1998: 31–44
32. Nobl G. Der varicose symptomen complex (phlebectasie, stauungsdermatose, ulcus crusis) Seine Grundlagen und Behandlung, Berlin, Wein, Urban and Schwarzenberg, 1910
33. Nicholson BB. Varicose veins: etiology and treatment. Arch Surg 1927; 15:351–72
34. Madar G, Widmer LK. Varicose veins and chronic venous insufficiency – minor disorder or disease? A critical review of the literature. Z Lymphol 1990; 14(1):36–46
35. Borschberg E. The prevalence of varicose veins in the lower extremities. Karger, Basel, 1967
36. Petruzzellis V, Florio T, Quaranta D, Trocolli T, Serra MA. Epidemiologic observations on the subject of phlebopathy of the legs and its dermatologic complications. Minerva Med 1990; 81(9):611–16
37. Clarke GH, Smith SR, Vasdekis SN et al. Role of venous elasticity in the development of varicose veins. Br J Surg 1989; 76:577–80
38. Vin F, Allaert FA, Levardon M. Influence of estrogens and progesterone on the venous system of the lower limbs in women. J. Derm Surg Oncol 1992; 18:888–92
39. Cohen J. Venous insufficiency and oral contraception. Rev Fr Gynecol Obstet 1991; 86 (2.2):187–9
40. Nabatoff RA. Varicose veins of pregnancy. JAMA 1960; 174:1712–14
41. Dindelli M, Parazzini F, Basellini A et al. Risk factors for varicose disease before and during pregnancy. Angiology 1993; 361–7
42. Maffei FH. Varicose veins and chronic venous insufficiency in Brazil: prevalence among 1755 inhabitants of a country town. Int J Epidemiol 1986; 15:210–17
43. Porte H, Erny R. Venous insufficiency of the lower limbs in pregnancy. Rev Fr Gynecol Obstet 1991; 86 (2.2):181–3
44. Meissner MH, Caps MT, Bergelin RO, Manzo RA, Strandness DE. Propagation rethrombosis and new thrombus formation after acute deep venous thrombosis. J Vasc Surg 1995; 22:558–67
45. Bergan JJ, Ballard JL, Sparks SR, Murray JS. Subfascial perforator vein surgery (SEPS): the open technique. Phlebologie (Fr.) 1996; 49:467–73
46. Gloviczki P, Bergan JJ, Menawat SS et al. Safety, feasibility and early efficacy of subfascial endoscopic perforator surgery (SEPS): a preliminary report from the North American Registry. J Vasc Surg 1997; 25:94–105.
47. Sparks SR, Ballard JL, Bergan JJ, Killeen JD. Early benefits of subfascial endoscopic perforator surgery (SEPS) in healing venous ulcers. Ann Vasc Surg 1997; 11:367–73
48. Labropoulos N, Delis KT, Nicolaides AN. Venous reflux in symptom-free vascular surgeons. J Vasc Surg 1995; 22:150–4
49. Bays RA, Healy DA, Atnip RG et al. Validation of air plethysmography, photoplethysmography, and duplex ultrasonography in the evaluation of severe venous stasis. J Vasc Surg 1994; 20:721–7
50. Masuda EM, Kistner RL, Eklof B. Prospective study of duplex scanning for venous reflux: comparison of Valsalva and pneumatic cuff techniques in the reverse Trendelenburg and standing position. J Vasc Surg 1994; 20:711–19
51. Polak JF. Chronic venous thrombosis and venous insufficiency. In: Polak JF (ed.) Peripheral vascular sonography. A practical guide. William & Wilkins, Baltimore, 1992: 223–45
52. Department of Health, Education and Welfare. Health statistics from the US National Health Survey. Chronic conditions causing limitation of activities. United States July 1959–June 1961. Series B, No. 36. Washington DC, 1962
53. Mekky S, Schilling RSF, Walford J. Varicose veins in woven cotton workers. An epidemiological study in England and Egypt. Br Med J 1969; 2:591–5
54. Cleave TL. Varicose veins – nature's error or man's? Lancet 1959; ii:172–5
55. Burkitt DP. Varicose veins, deep vein thrombosis, and hemorrhoids: epidemiology and suggested aetiology. Br Med J 1972; 2:556–61

Pathogenesis of Chronic Venous Insufficiency

3

Jeffrey L. Ballard, John J. Bergan and Steven Sparks

Until pharmacologic methods are available to block the fundamental processes which lead to venous ulceration, a surgical approach will continue to be necessary. Chronic venous insufficiency (CVI) occurs when the fundamental mechanisms of venous blood transport are deranged. Abnormalities can occur in either the superficial venous system, the deep venous system, the perforating veins, or combinations of these. Furthermore, it is important to recognize that venous ulceration may be caused by simple varicose veins and this occurs in some 20 to 50% of venous leg ulcers. Conversely, the venous abnormality may be in the deep venous system with reflux occurring only there and not in superficial veins. In a percentage as small as 4 or 5%, the valve dysfunction may occur in the perforating veins alone.

The chief reason for misconception about the etiology of venous insufficiency has been caused by the methods of evaluation of the venous system. Clinical examination is flawed, as is evaluation of the deep venous system by phlebography. It is now known that duplex ultrasound can miss as many as 20% of perforating veins with bidirectional flow. Despite these imperfections, it is necessary to understand the pathogenesis of chronic venous insufficiency in order to prescribe proper surgical care.

Outmoded Concepts

Forty years ago, chronic venous leg ulcers were defined as a break in the epidermis which persists for a month or longer and occurs as a result of venous hypertension and calf muscle pump dysfunction.[1] From the vantage point of the late 1990s, the link to venous hypertension remains solid. However, increasing questions are asked about what constitutes calf muscle pump dysfunction. That term arises from experience in assessing ambulatory venous pressure with a cannula placed in the dorsal foot vein. Experience taught that patients with "severe calf muscle impairment" could not reduce foot vein pressure below the resting level and the presence of substantial venous reflux refilled the veins of the calf after exercise. As experience was gained, it was clear that some patients could tolerate what was called severe muscle pump impairment without forming venous ulcers or even suffering from lipodermatosclerosis but others suffered from gross, non healing ulcers with only moderate calf muscle pump impairment. It was obvious that other factors were important in the pathogenesis of ulceration.

Venous Stasis

Among the theories describing additional elements was the concept of stasis. This gave rise to the term venous stasis ulceration. This concept suggested that stagnant blood accumulates within tortuous, non-functioning, dilated channels close to the skin and implies that consequent tissue anoxia causes cell death. Before 1930, Alfred Blalock showed that oxygen content of blood in varicose veins was higher not lower than oxygen content of normal veins[2] and, more recently, it has been shown that with a supine patient, hemoglobin saturation in varicose vein blood is greater than in the veins of normal limbs.[3] As there is an increased interest in what happens when the patient stands, it has also been shown that there is no difference between normal subjects and patients with varicose veins in the standing position. The raised blood oxygen tension in varicose veins has suggested to some that arteriovenous fistulae were present. Recent studies have shown a faster circulation time in limbs with varicosities and stigmata of chronic venous insufficiency.[4,5] It has been suggested that the presence of the arteriovenous fistula might deprive the skin of oxygen[6,7] but microsphere research has failed to demonstrate any increase in arteriovenous shunting in patients with chronic venous insufficiency.[8]

The Fibrin Cuff

Pursuing the subject of cutaneous deoxygenation further, Browse and Burnand proposed that oxygen diffusion was restricted by a pericapillary fibrin cuff.[9] That theory has so dominated modern thinking that it permeates all textbooks describing venous pathophysiology. However, the theory has fallen from influence in light of increasing evidence that leukocyte adhesion and activation is a more satisfactory explanation for the skin changes which occur.

The Postphlebitic Leg

Just as the term venous stasis is unsatisfactory, so is the term postphlebitic. This term originated in the 1950s[10] when one large study showed that the post-thrombotic state was present in nearly 80% of limbs with CVI. The term postphlebitic is still in use on both sides of the Atlantic.[11-14] but modern experience teaches that only a minority of the limbs seen with venous ulcers are truly post-thrombotic.

Venous Hypertension

The link of hyperpigmentation, lipodermatosclerosis and venous ulcer to venous hypertension has not been broken. Venous pressure studies show that at rest in the erect position, the superficial and deep venous systems have approximately the same hydrostatic pressure. At rest, this is defined as the weight of a column of blood between the point of measurement and the right atrium. During calf muscle contraction, a transient pressure rise occurs in the deep veins. This propels blood cephalad. Functioning perforating vein–valves close during muscle contraction preventing transmission of high compartmental pressure to the superficial venous system. After calf muscle contraction and during relaxation, deep venous pressure falls abruptly to a very low level (Fig. 3.1). This allows valves in the perforating veins to open and blood rushes into the deep veins from the superficial veins. This causes the superficial venous pressure to drop, and a drop of 30% is to be expected. Calf muscle pump dys-

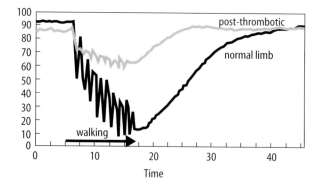

Fig. 3.1. These curves plot venous pressure in a normal and post-thrombotic limb. During calf compression, venous pressure falls to a low level in the normal limb, less so in the postthrombotic limb. Return of venous pressure to baseline because of venous reflux occurs rapidly in the postthrombotic limb. Return to baseline pressure occurs more slowly in the normal limb and is dependent upon arterial inflow. (From: Coleridge-Smith PD. Chapter 3. In: Goldman MP, Weiss RA, Bergan JJ (eds). Varicose veins and telangiectasias: diagnosis and treatment, 2nd edn. Quality Medical Publishers, St Louis, 1998.)

function occurs when either the ejection is incomplete or the residual volume is maintained at a high level after calf contraction. It has been said that "studies… clearly show that calf pump failure leads to venous ulceration."[15]

While one would expect that there is a direct linear relationship between ambulatory venous pressure and severity of venous dysfunction, in fact this is not true.[16] Using venous pressure alone, it is impossible to clearly separate limbs with dermatitis or eczema from those with hyperpigmentation from those with lipodermatosclerosis from those with venous ulceration. In fact, most studies would separate limbs with lipodermatosclerosis and healed and open ulceration from those with edema and/or varicose veins. Thus, ambulatory venous pressure studies have taught a great deal but at best these give a global assessment of the entire limb and do not give specific information about individual venous segments. In a study on the subject, van Bemmelen has said, "The correlation of a high ambulatory venous pressure with ulceration is evident but the contribution of the superficial and deep systems to an increased ambulatory venous pressure is unclear."[17] An attempt to extend the measurement of ambulatory venous pressure to a continuous pressure reading has added very little to our knowledge of venous ulceration.[18]

Water-Hammer Effect: Perforating Veins

Today's emphasis on detecting and dealing with perforating veins is supported by the observations of Raju and Fredericks.[19] They find that severe changes of chronic venous insufficiency are linked to a velocity of reflux, (water-hammer effect) and that this is important exactly where perforating veins transmit compartmental pressure to the skin. Raju's studies confirmed that 20–25% of patients with venous ulcer have normal ambulatory venous pressure measurements. However, a special test called the Valsalva-induced venous pressure showed a relationship between the water-hammer effect of high pressure being transmitted to the skin and venous ulceration. Thus, ambulatory venous pressure and Valsalva-induced venous pressure do give an index which provides excellent cor-

relation with venous ulceration. In the past, Negus has referred to this water-hammer effect as venous blowout.[20]

Leukocyte Trapping

The hypothesis that white blood cell trapping resulted in neutrophil activation and this caused damage to the tissues was published in the late 1980s by the Middlesex Hospital group.[21] Further investigations have suggested strongly that white blood cell activation is truly an important part of the process (Fig. 3.2). This results in release of proteolytic enzymes, superoxide radicals, and chemotactic substances.[22]

Our own investigations have been in genesis of valvular insufficiency and venous wall weakening.[23] These observations have implicated the monocyte. Monocytes might very well become activated in the periphery causing the skin damage of chronic venous insufficiency by release of cytokines such as interleukin-1 (IL-1) and tumor necrosis factor-α

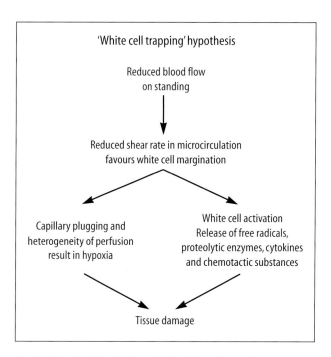

Fig. 3.2. The white blood cell trapping hypothesis of tissue damage explains the causes of lipodermatosclerosis and venous ulceration. White blood cells are not only trapped but are literally driven into the endothelium of elongated, tortuous veins which are subjected to venous hypertension and high-pressure perforating vein outflow. (From: Coleridge-Smith PD. Chapter 3. In: Goldman MP, Weiss RA, Bergan JJ (eds) Varicose veins and telangiectasias: diagnosis and treatment, 2nd edn. 1998.)

(TNF-α). These might activate endothelial cells to allow passage of large protein molecules. This, in combination with decreased fibrinolysis, leads to vascular occlusion.[24] Decreased fibrinolysis has been observed in patients with venous disease[25] and is due to production of fibrinolytic inhibitor, the plasminogen-activator inhibitor-1 (PAI-1).

The above observations confirm the obvious. That is, that lipodermatosclerosis is a chronic inflammatory process that is linked to venous hypertension by the mechanisms explained earlier. That is, reflux in superficial and/or deep veins and outflow through failed perforating veins drives leukocytes into enlarged and elongated precapillary venules. Immunohistological methods have shown that capillaries in the region of venous hypertension contain macrophages and T lymphocytes. Further, it has been shown that patients with venous disorders have greater neutrophil activation than controls. Experimental venous hypertension produces neutrophil degranulation and it is possible that clinical venous hypertension can produce this also. This, in turn, may cause endothelial injury and significant inflammatory response which results in the plaque formation of lipodermatosclerosis. It is hypothesized that massive activation of large numbers of macrophages in lipodermatosclerotic skin results in severe destruction of tissues by free radical attack. Other triggering events such as minor trauma may also contribute. While the explanation is partly speculative at the present time, it is still a useful explanation when designing strategies of treatment for the individual patient.[26,27]

Increased Endothelial Area

It is a common observation that microvascular changes in chronic venous insufficiency are characterized by skin capillaries which are dilated, elongated, and tortuous.[28] Their appearance with intravinyl staining and direct observation is very much like glomerular capillaries. These elongated, dilated, tortuous vessels can be seen in the epidermis as telangiectasias and in the subdermal tissues as reticular varicosities. These can almost always be traced with contrast media to perforating veins.

This shows that dilated and elongated vessels in the epidermis and subdermal areas are related to failed check valves in tiny perforating veins. Elongation and dilation is the product of muscular compartmental pressure transmitted to unsupported vessels in the skin and subcutaneous tissues.

The histologic changes of lipodermatosclerotic skin have been observed by the Middlesex group.[29] They confirm that the increased surface area of endothelium is exposed to circulating blood and that white-cell–endothelium interactions might very well occur to stimulate lipodermatosclerosis.

While calf muscle pump failure has been linked to changes of severe chronic venous insufficiency, there is very little evidence that it is muscular activity itself which fails. Instead, there is a great deal of support for the relationship between ulceration and increasing values of reflux and decreased values of venous ejection. A poor ejection fraction is directly related to venous ulceration and a good ejection fraction reduces the incidence of ulceration in limbs with marked reflux.[30]

Distribution of Incompetence

There has been difficulty in discovering the presence of perforating veins and determining their direction of blood flow. This has hampered investigations. However, it is now generally acknowledged that perforating veins are important. Isolated deep reflux is present in 2% of limbs with uncomplicated varicose veins, 7% of limbs with lipodermatosclerosis and 8% of limbs with healed ulceration. In contrast, superficial reflux alone is found in 55% of limbs with uncomplicated varicose veins, 39% of limbs with lipodermatosclerosis and 38% in limbs with healed or present ulceration. Outward flow in medial calf perforating veins is seen in 57% of complicated varicose veins, 67% of limbs with lipodermatosclerosis and 66% of limbs with healed ulceration. Such outward flow in perforating veins occurs more frequently in limbs with complications. Isolated outward flow in perforating veins without any other abnormality is found in 10% of limbs with varicose veins, 10% of limbs with lipodermatosclerosis and 2% of limbs with ulceration.[31] These figures may be confusing, but in fact it is clear that correction of superficial reflux and perforator outward flow could have a profoundly beneficial effect.

While direct relationship of perforating veins to ulceration is hypothesized but not proven, it is well known that large calf perforating veins permitting outward flow are commonly associated with the severe changes of chronic venous insufficiency.[32]

Use of the directional Doppler has confirmed the fact that blood flow in medial calf perforating veins may be both inward and outward.[32] Fifteen percent of normal limbs show outward flow in perforating veins but clinical correlation with perforating vein outflow teaches that in limbs with severe chronic venous insufficiency, a significant number of perforating veins demonstrate outward flow. This is true whether or not there is accompanying superficial venous incompetence.[33] Use of manual compression or cuff compression suffices to demonstrate such outward flow. In examination of limbs with chronic venous insufficiency, one should use one or the other or both maneuvers above and below any suspected perforating vein. During the relaxation phase after proximal compression, many perforating veins demonstrate flow from deep to superficial as well as superficial to deep.

Unifying Concept: Venous Hypertension/Leukocyte Activation

When the concept of white blood cell adhesion and activation is taken into consideration, it is not surprising that normal limbs might have perforating veins with outward flow and not have signs of severe chronic venous insufficiency. It is, after all, the limbs that do suffer from white cell trapping that will show the skin changes. Large dilated perforating veins would be associated with the cutaneous changes of chronic venous insufficiency if leukocyte sequestration and activation were present.

Assuming that superficial reflux and deep reflux produce distal venous hypertension and perforating vein incompetence transmits both static and dynamic exercise pressure to the skin, it is not surprising that in some limbs, lipodermatosclerosis and ulceration occur and in others, skin changes are absent or trivial. The differentiating factor between these extremes could be white blood cell trapping and activation (Fig. 3.3). Limbs with normal skin would have an absence or decrease in trapping and activation while those with the most profound

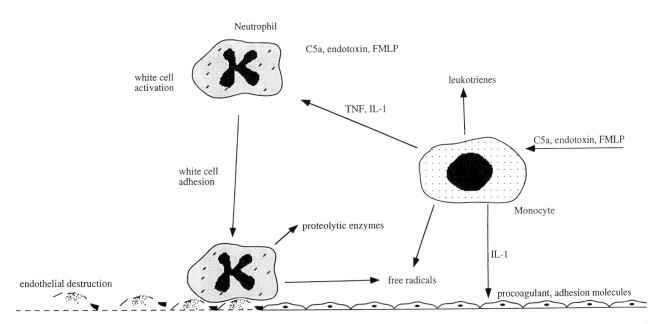

Fig. 3.3. Neutrophils and monocytes in response to a variety of stimuli adhere to endothelium when a variety of reactions occur. Among these is a release of proteolytic enzymes and free radicals.

changes would have maximal tissue destruction by toxic factors liberated by activated leukocytes.

Using this concept, one can learn from reports in the literature.[34] In one study, a total of 300 limbs in 153 patients were examined by duplex ultrasound. The focus of the study was the presence of venous reflux in superficial veins, deep veins, and medial perforating veins both above and below the knee. Ninety-eight limbs had skin changes of chronic venous insufficiency. In only 2% of these was there no evidence of venous reflux. In fact, knowing the error rate in detecting perforating veins, these may have had undetected perforator dysfunction. In this group of limbs with severe chronic venous insufficiency, 39% had deep venous reflux and 57% had superficial venous incompetence. In fact, 2% had isolated medial perforating vein reflux without other abnormality. Of the 25 limbs with open ulceration, 13 had superficial reflux and 12 had deep venous reflux. In the 202 limbs, including 20 normals, there were no skin changes. Of these, 22.3% had no venous reflux, 8.4% had deep vein incompetence, and 65.3% had superficial incompetence with 4% having isolated medial calf perforat-

ing vein incompetence. Clearly, keeping in mind the phenomenon of leukocyte trapping and activation, the differentiating factor in these limbs could have been that phenomenon; those limbs with intact skin having no leukocyte trapping and activation and those with advanced skin changes having that as the cause of the skin changes. It is clear that a very large number of patients with advanced skin changes could profit by removal of the superficial reflux. If this were done, 52% of the limbs with ulceration and 57% of those with skin changes would be improved. Furthermore, treatable superficial reflux combined with perforating vein incompetence was present in 77% of ulcerated limbs (Fig. 3.4). The inescapable conclusion in this observation is that ablation of superficial reflux and interruption of perforating veins can be of benefit in those limbs with the most advanced skin changes.

There is corroborating evidence for this.[35] In her study, McMullin et al. demonstrated that two-thirds of the patients presenting with symptoms of severe chronic venous insufficiency had only superficial venous incompetence detected by duplex ultrasound.[36] This confirms once again that attention to

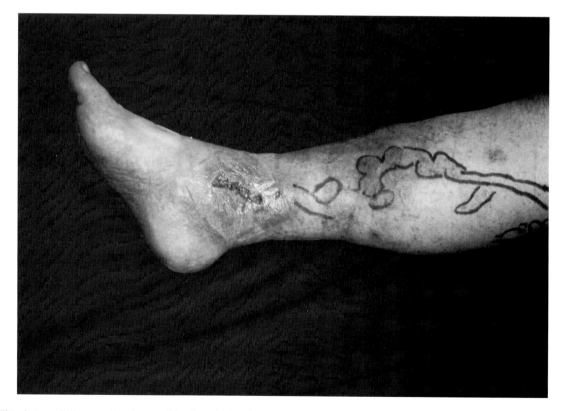

Fig. 3.4. This photograph illustrates the stigmata of the class 6 limb with severe chronic venous insufficiency. Note the elongated, dilated, incompetent superficial veins and their relationship by way of reflux to the unhealed ankle ulceration.

superficial incompetence will benefit many limbs with chronic venous insufficiency.

The potential for curing chronic venous insufficiency ranges from 16.8% in the study at Boston University[37] to 53% in the study at the Middlesex Hospital.[38] In the Boston study, if one adds perforator reflux to the limbs with superficial reflux, the potential for cure is present in 45.2% of limbs. Finally, several workers have confirmed the possibility of correcting deep venous reflux by superficial venous surgery.[39-43]

Conclusion

The pathophysiology of chronic venous insufficiency suggests that venous hypertension is linked to severe changes of chronic venous insufficiency. Furthermore, these changes can be favorably modified by ablation of superficial venous reflux. If that is done in combination with interruption of perforating veins, then the water-hammer effect of downward flow and outward flow through perforating veins will be halted, leukocyte trapping and activation decreased and skin changes reversed. It may very well be that the favorable observations by surgical intervention of ulcer healing, correction of lipodermatosclerosis and fading of hyperpigmentation are related to correction of the causes of these changes by surgical intervention.

References

1. Douglas WS, Simpson NB. Guidelines for the management of chronic venous leg ulceration. Report of a multidisciplinary workshop. Br J Dermatol 1995; 132:446–52
2. Blalock A. Oxygen content of blood in patients with varicose veins. Arch Surg 1929; 19:898–905
3. Blumhoff RL, Johnson G. Saphenous vein Pp02 in patients with varicose veins. J Surg Res 1977; 23:35–6
4. Shami SK, Chittenden SJ, Scurr JH, Coleridge Smith PD. Skin blood flow in chronic venous insufficiency. Phlebology 1993; 8:72–6
5. Shami SK, Cheatle TR, Chittenden SJ, Scurr JH, Coleridge Smith PD. Hyperaemic response in the skin microcirculation of patients with chronic venous insufficiency. Br J Surg 1993; 80:433–5
6. Pratt GH. Arterial varices: a syndrome. Am J Surg 1949; 77:456–60
7. Brewer AC. Arteriovenous shunts. Br Med J 1950; ii:270
8. Lindmayr W, Lofferer O, Mostbeck A, Partsch H. Arteriovenous shunts in primary varicosis: a critical essay. Vasc Surg 1972; 6:9–14
9. Browse NL, Burnand KG. The cause of venous ulceration. Lancet 1982; ii:243–5
10. Anning JT. Leg ulcers: their cause and treatment. Churchill Livingstone, London, 1954
11. Debure C. La maladie postphlebitique des membres inferieurs: quoi de neuf en 1993? Actualites D'Angiologie 1993; 18;147–50
12. Owens JC. Management of postphlebitic syndrome. Vasc Diagn Ther 1981; 3:34–40
13. Mudge M, Leinster SJ, Hughes LE. A prospective 10 year study of the post-thrombotic syndrome in a surgical population. Ann Roy Coll Surg Engl 1988; 70:249–52
14. Ludbrook J. Post-thrombotic venous obstruction in the lower limb. Editorial. Arch Surg 1973; 106:11–12
15. Gourdin FW, Smith Jr, J. Etiology of venous ulceration. South Med J 1993; 86:1142–6
16. Payne SPK, London NJM, Newland CJ et al. Ambulatory venous pressure: correlation with skin condition and role in identifying surgically correctable disease. Eur J Vasc Endovasc Surg 1996; 11:195–200
17. van Bemmelen PS. Invasive methods – radiology and venous pressure. In: van Bemmelen P (ed.) Quantitative measurement of venous incompetence. R.G. Landes Co, Austin, 1992: 29
18. Taheri SA, Pendergast D, Lazar E et al. Continuous ambulatory venous pressure for diagnosis of venous insufficiency. Am J Surg 1985; 150:203–6
19. Raju S, Fredericks R. Hemodynamic basis of stasis ulceration: a hypothesis. J Vasc Surg 1991; 13:491–5
20. Negus D. Perforating vein interruption in the postphlebitic syndrome. In: Bergan JJ, Yao JST (eds) Surgery of the veins. Grune & Stratton, Orlando, 1985: 196
21. Coleridge Smith PD, Thomas P, Scurr JH, Dormandy JA. Causes of venous ulceration: a new hypothesis. Br Med J 1988; 296:1726–7
22. Adams DO, Hamilton TA. The cell biology of macrophage activation. Ann Rev Immunol 1984; 2:283–318
23. Ono T, Bergan JJ, Schmid-Schönbein GW, Takase S. Monocyte infiltration into venous valves. J Vasc Surg 1998; 27:158–66
24. Pober JS. Cytokine-mediated activation of vascular endothelium. Am J Pathol 1988; 133:426–33
25. Schleef RR, Bevilaqua MP, Sawdey M, Gimbrone MA, Loskutoff DJ. Cytokine activation of vascular endothelium: Effects on tissue-type plasminogen activator and type 1 plasminogen activator inhibitor. J Biol Soc 1988; 163:5797–803
26. Coleridge Smith PD. Conclusions and future directions. In: Coleridge-Smith PD (ed.) Microcirculation in venous disease. R.G. Landes Co., Austin, 1994: 192–4
27. Coleridge Smith PD. Etiology and pathophysiology of chronic venous insufficiency. http://www.ucl.ac.uk/~rehk999/pdcs.htm
28. Wilkinson LS, Bunker C, Edwards JCW, Scurr JH, Coleridge Smith DP. Leukocytes: Their role in the etiopathogenesis of skin damage in venous disease. J Vasc Surg 1993; 17:669–75
29. Coleridge Smith PD. Venous ulcer. Br J Surg 1994; 81:1404–5
30. Leu AJ, Leu H-J, Franzeck UK, Bollinger A. Microvascular changes in chronic venous insufficiency: a review. Cardiovasc Surg 1995; 3:237–45
31. Bradbury AW, Murie JA, Ruckley CV. Role of the leucocyte in the pathogenesis of vascular disease. Br J Surg 1993; 80:1503–12.
32. Christopoulos D, Nicolaides AN, Cook A, Irvine A, Galloway JMD, Wilkinson A. Pathogenesis of venous ulceration in relation to the calf muscle pump function. Surgery 1989; 106:829–35
33. Myers KA, Ziegenbein W, Zeng GE, Matthews PG. Duplex ultrasonography scanning for chronic venous disease: patterns of venous reflux. J Vasc Surg 1995; 21:605–12
34. Shami SK, Sarin S, Cheatle TR, Scurr JH, Coleridge Smith PD. Venous ulcers and the superficial venous system. J Vasc Surg 1993; 17:487–90
35. Sarin S, Scurr JH, Coleridge Smith PD. Medial calf perforators in venous disease: the significance of outward flow. J Vasc Surg 1992; 16:40–6
36. McMullin GM, Scott HJ, Coleridge Smith PD, Scurr JH. A comparison of photoplethysmography, Doppler, and duplex in the assessment of venous insufficiency. Phlebology 1989; 4:75–82
37. Darke SG, Penfold C. Venous ulceration and saphenous ligation. Eur J Vasc Surg 1992; 6:4–9

38. Hanrahan LM, Araki CT, Rodriguez AA et al. Distribution of valvular incompetence in patients with venous stasis ulceration. J Vasc Surg 1991; 13:805–12

39. Shami SK, Sarin S, Cheatle TR, Scurr JH, Coleridge Smith PD. Venous ulcers and the superficial venous system. J Vasc Surg 1993; 17:487–90

40. Walsh JC, Bergan, Beeman S, Comer TP. Femoral venous reflux abolished by greater saphenous vein stripping. Ann Vasc Surg 1994; 8:566–70

41. Goren G. Letter to the Editor – Regarding venous ulcers and the superficial venous system. J Vasc Surg 1996; 18:716–19

42. Sales CM, Bilof ML, Petrillo KA, Luka NL. Correction of lower extremity deep venous incompetence by ablation of superficial venous reflux. Ann Vasc Surg 1996; 10:186–90

43. Padberg Jr FT, Pappas PJ, Araki CT, Back TL, Hobson II RW. Hemodynamic and clinical improvement after superficial vein ablation in primary combined venous insufficiency with ulceration. J Vasc Surg 1996; 24:711–18

Venous Anatomy of the Lower Limb   4

Géza Mózes, Peter Gloviczki, Anna Kádár and Máté Dzsinich

"The (leg) veins may be divided into three sets, the saphenous, the deep and the intercommunicating (veins)…perforating the intervening aponeurosis…"[1]

John Gay, The Lettsomian Lectures, 1868

❖

Our knowledge of the anatomy of lower extremity veins is based on description of three main groups of veins more than a century ago by John Gay.[1] Since Gay's original communication, important data have accumulated on venous components of the cutaneous microcirculation, the functional anatomy of venous muscle pump, distribution and function of venous valves and the location and possible role of perforating veins. These observations have allowed a functional approach to understand the complex and intriguing anatomy of the venous system of the lower extremity.

The venous system of the lower limb is composed of parallel networks. These include the *superficial venous system*, with venules and venous plexuses of the cutaneous microcirculation and axial superficial veins and their tributaries; the *deep venous system*, with axial main veins and venous sinuses of the calf, and the interconnecting *perforating veins* (Fig. 4.1). Perforating veins penetrate the fascia and connect the superficial with the deep venous system. Communicating veins connect veins within the same network.

Superficial Venous System

Cutaneous Microcirculation

Microcirculation of the skin plays an important role in the thermoregulation of the human body. Cutaneous blood supply, therefore, exceeds ten times that of the nutritional requirements of the skin.[2] Cutaneous branches of major arteries reach the skin either directly or through perforating branches from the skeletal muscles.[3] In the skin the arteries form two horizontal dermal plexuses: subpapillary and reticular.[4] Capillary loops in the dermal papillae, that rise from the subpapillary arterial plexus, drain through venules into the subpapillary venous plexus situated 1–1.5 mm below the surface of the skin.[5] The subpapillary venous plexus drains into a deeper, reticular venous plexus at the dermal–subcutaneous junction (Fig. 4.1). Small, vertically oriented valved veins connect the reticular venous plexus to the superficial epifascial veins.

Axial Superficial Veins and their Tributaries

Superficial epifascial veins course outside the fascia in subcutaneous tissue (Fig. 4.1). These superficial

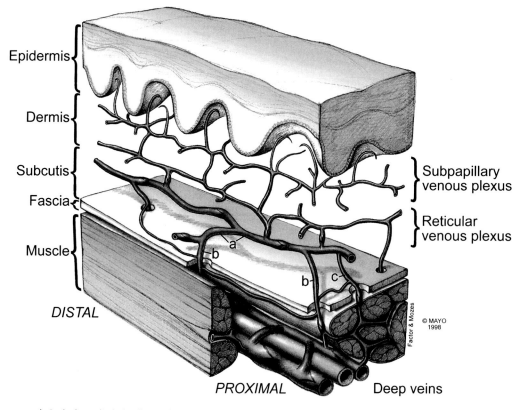

Epidermis

Dermis

Subcutis

Fascia

Muscle

DISTAL

Subpapillary
venous plexus

Reticular
venous plexus

a

b

b   c

Factor & Mozes

© MAYO
1998

PROXIMAL   Deep veins

Fig. 4.1. Venous networks in the lower limb. Capillaries of dermal papillae are drained by the subpapillary venous plexus which joins the reticular venous plexus. Superficial veins **a** drain dermal veins and empty into deep axial veins through direct perforating veins **b**. Muscular venous sinuses may fill from superficial veins through indirect perforating veins **c** and are drained into the deep axial veins.

veins, which include greater and lesser saphenous veins and their tributaries, collect blood from the skin and the subcutaneous tissues.[6] They empty into deep veins through the saphenofemoral and saphenopopliteal junctions as well as through direct or indirect perforators (Fig. 4.1). Direct perforators join the main axial deep veins, while indirect perforating veins ensure connection between superficial veins and venous sinuses of the leg muscles.

Few veins of the human body have more variability in their topographic anatomy than the superficial lower extremity veins. The venous drainage of the foot developed to meet specific requirements of ambulation. The dorsal and plantar superficial venous networks communicate extensively with each other and with the corresponding deep pedal plexuses. Superficial veins of the sole form an anastomosing network, which is particularly rich in small communicating tributaries at the heel and over the metatarsophalangeal joints.[7] Superficial plantar veins and the underlying deep plantar venous plexus are rhythmically compressed at each footstep. During ambulation, therefore,

mechanical forces propel blood from the foot into the more proximal veins and prime the calf muscle pump.[8] On the dorsum of the foot, digital veins form dorsal metatarsal veins. These empty into the dorsal venous arch at about the level of the proximal end of the metatarsals (Fig. 4.2). The dorsal venous arch receives blood from several other veins from the dorsum of the foot and from the medial and lateral plantar surfaces. The medial end of this venous arch continues in the greater saphenous vein and the lateral end in the lesser saphenous vein (Fig. 4.2).

The *greater saphenous vein*, similar to other superficial veins, courses mostly in the subcutaneous fat; however, in the leg and in the lower third of the thigh it often has a fibrous sheath that in the calf is attached to the outer surface of the crural fascia. The greater saphenous vein begins anterior to the medial malleolus, crosses the tibia and ascends medial to the knee (Fig. 4.3). At the knee it courses 8–10 cm dorsal to the medial edge of the patella.[6] In the leg it collects blood from two main tributaries: a less constant anterior venous tributary and the posterior

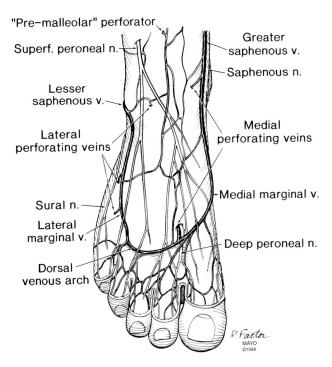

Fig. 4.2. Anatomy of the superficial and perforating veins of the foot.

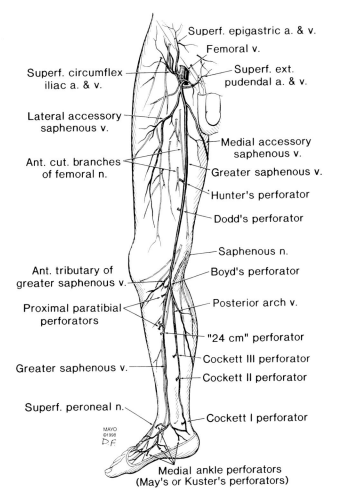

Fig. 4.3. Anatomy of medial superficial and perforating veins of the leg.

arch vein. The anterior tributary ascends from the dorsum of the foot and joins the greater saphenous vein at the knee.[9] The *posterior arch vein*, or Leonardo's vein (presumably first depicted on Leonardo da Vinci's drawings),[10] is a relatively constant tributary. It begins around the medial ankle, ascends on the posteromedial aspect of the leg and joins the greater saphenous vein distal to the knee (Fig. 4.3). Major medial perforating veins connect the posterior arch vein with the posterior tibial veins. In the thigh, the greater saphenous vein ascends anteriorly, enters the fossa ovalis below the inguinal ligament and empties into the femoral vein at about two finger breadths (4 cm) distal to the inguinal ligament, inferior and lateral to the pubic tubercle.[11] Just before the greater saphenous vein ends, it receives one or two large tributaries from the thigh, the lateral and medial accessory saphenous veins. The medial accessory saphenous vein, if present (~8–20%), drains mainly the posterior surface of the thigh.[7] The lateral accessory saphenous vein is almost always present; it originates from the suprapatellar region and receives tributaries from both the lateral and the anterior surfaces of the thigh. Additional, small saphenous tributaries include the superficial circumflex iliac, the superficial epigastric and the superficial external puden-

dal veins (Fig. 4.3).[12] The number of anatomic variations of these tributaries is significant (Fig. 4.4).[7] A duplicated greater saphenous system may be found in up to one fourth of the limbs.[13,14]

The *lesser saphenous vein* begins on the lateral side of the foot as a continuation of the dorsal venous arch and ascends on the posterolateral aspect of the leg along the lateral border of the Achilles' tendon.[15] It runs in the subcutaneous fat until the mid or upper third of the leg, where it pierces the deep fascia and courses either in a fascial duplication or under the fascia, between the two heads of the gastrocnemius muscle. The lesser saphenous vein joins the popliteal vein in two thirds of limbs in the proximal popliteal fossa (Fig. 4.5).[7] Less frequently, the lesser saphenous veins ends high and empties directly into the femoral vein.[7] Uncommonly, the lesser saphenous vein ends below the knee and empties into the posterior tibial veins

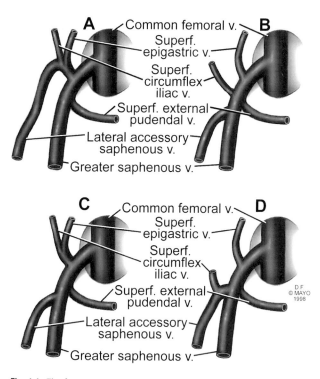

Fig. 4.4. The four most common anatomical variations of tributaries of the saphenofemoral junction (A, 33%, B, 15%, C, 15%, D, 13%), according to Daseler.

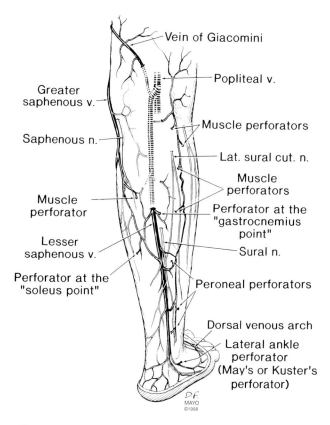

Fig. 4.5. Anatomy of posterior superficial and perforating veins of the leg.

or it may have several common anastomotic tributaries with the greater saphenous vein. In about 15% of limbs, a vein in the posterior thigh called the vein of Giacomini, connects the lesser with the greater saphenous vein.[7,16] There can be several other, smaller connections between the two saphenous veins.

Bicuspid valves in the superficial veins assure unidirectional blood flow toward the heart. There are some more constant valve sites which are usually at the termination of major venous trunks. These valves have strong, white cusps and a bulging sinus of the venous wall at their origin. Other valves are more delicate structures with almost transparent cusps.[9]

The number of valves in the greater saphenous vein is at least six, although in some studies it has ranged from 14 to 25.[7] In most limbs there is a valve in the greater saphenous vein within 3 cm of the saphenofemoral junction.[17] Below the knee, the frequency of valves is greater than above the knee.[9]

In the lesser saphenous vein, valves are more closely spaced. In more than half of limbs this vein has 7–11 valves.[15] Similar to the greater saphenous vein, the lesser saphenous vein has a valve close to its confluence with the deep vein.[7] Valves in communicating tributaries between the two saphenous systems are always oriented to direct blood from the lesser to the greater saphenous vein.[15]

In the leg, the greater saphenous vein is accompanied by the *saphenous nerve*.[18] These two structures are closely adherent in the mid and distal thirds of the leg (Fig. 4.3).[19] In the thigh, the greater saphenous vein is accompanied by small cutaneous nerve branches of various origin.[19] The lesser saphenous vein is accompanied by the sural nerve in the lower part of the leg and ankle (Fig. 4.5). They are closest to each other in the retromalleolar space at the lateral aspect of the ankle.[16,19]

Deep veins

Deep axial veins in the lower extremity accompany major arteries and their branches. They are frequently doubled, and pairs of veins are connected by multiple anastomoses (Fig. 4.1).

In the foot, plantar digital veins unite into four plantar metatarsal veins, which empty into the *deep plantar venous arch*. The plantar venous arch continues into *medial* and *lateral plantar veins*, which flow into the posterior tibial veins behind the medial ankle (Fig. 4.6). The plantar venous arch and medial and lateral plantar veins are part of the *deep plantar venous plexus*. This plexus is composed of veins coursing diagonally from a lateral position in the forefoot to a medial position at the ankle.[8] On the dorsum of the foot, the main deep veins are the *dorsalis pedis veins*, which form the paired anterior tibial veins.[20]

In the calf, paired *posterior tibial veins* run under the fascia of the deep posterior compartment (the deep lamina of the posterior fascia) between the edges of the flexor digitorum longus and tibialis posterior muscles (Fig. 4.7). These veins course under the soleal arcade, close to the tibia and unite with the paired peroneal veins. They continue in the popliteal

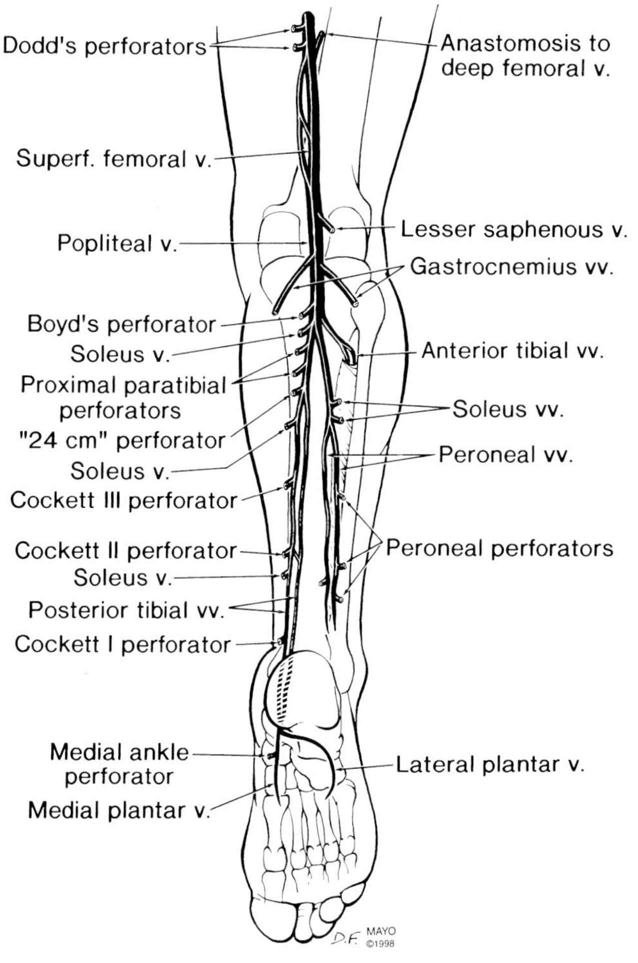

Fig. 4.6. Anatomy of the deep veins of the lower extremity.

vein, following union with the paired anterior tibial veins.[20] The posterior tibial veins drain muscles in the deep and superficial posterior compartments and collect blood through the perforating veins from the posterior arch and greater saphenous veins (Fig. 4.6). The *anterior tibial veins* are the continuation of the dorsalis pedis veins and ascend between muscles in the anterior compartment of the calf. They drain blood from muscles of the anterior compartment and receive perforators from the anterior aspect of the leg. In the distal leg, they also communicate with the peroneal veins.[9,21] Paired *peroneal veins* originate in the distal third of the leg and ascend deep to the flexor hallucis longus. In the distal half of the leg they receive blood through lateral, peroneal perforators (Fig. 4.6). Large venous sinuses from the soleus muscle also empty into the peroneal veins.[6,9]

The *popliteal* and *femoral veins* rarely (~16%) form a single large channel, rather they are usually duplicated in segments of various length or even form a plexus around the corresponding arteries similar to the deep veins of the leg (Fig. 4.6).[9] Main tributaries of the popliteal vein are the gastrocnemius veins and the lesser saphenous vein. In the adductor canal, the popliteal vein becomes the *superficial femoral vein* which runs first lateral, then medial to the femoral artery. It drains muscles from the medial side of the thigh and receives blood from the greater saphenous vein through the Dodd and Hunterian perforators. The superficial femoral vein unites with the *profunda femoris (deep femoral) veins* at the groin.[9] The profunda femoris vein drains muscles of the lateral aspect of the thigh and may receive perforators from the lateral accessory saphenous vein. In the adductor canal or more distal there is a frequent (~84%) communication between the profunda femoris and the superficial femoral or popliteal veins. This is an important collateral pathway in limbs with thrombosis of the femoral vein (Fig. 4.6). It is important to remember that the segment of the femoral vein between the adductor canal and the confluence with the profunda femoris vein is called "superficial" femoral vein, although this segment is part of the deep venous system.

The *common femoral vein* is formed following the union of the superficial and deep femoral veins. It runs medial to the respective artery and continues at the inguinal ligament in the *external iliac vein*.[7,20] The greater saphenous vein empties into the common femoral vein at the saphenofemoral junction (Fig. 4.4).

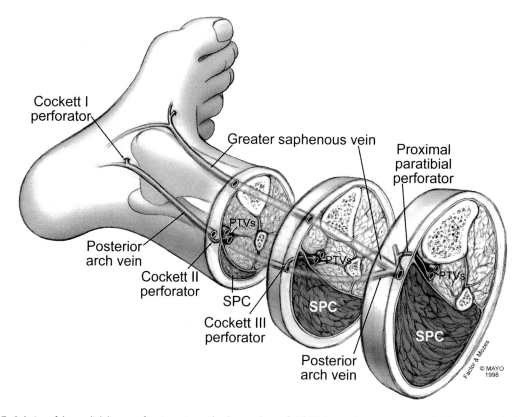

Fig. 4.7. Relation of the medial direct perforating veins to the deep and superficial (SPC) posterior compartments (PTVs, posterior tibial veins).

The frequency of *valves* in deep veins decreases from distal to proximal.[6] Deep veins of the foot, posterior tibial, anterior tibial and peroneal veins all have many valves. The popliteal vein has one or two valves, and there are three or more valves in the superficial femoral vein.[9] The most proximal valve is found constantly just distal to the sapheno-femoral junction.[6,22] There may be one valve in the common femoral vein, but in one-third of the cases, the external iliac and common femoral veins proximal to the saphenofemoral junction are valve-less. This exposes the greater saphenous vein to increased transmitted intra-abdominal venous pressures. There are no valves in the common iliac veins or in the inferior vena cava.[9]

Venous Sinuses of Calf Muscles

Venous sinuses are thin walled, large veins in the calf muscles, which have a capacity to hold great volumes of venous blood. They are embedded in skeletal muscles which contract rhythmically during ambulation, therefore, they serve as chambers of the "peripheral heart", the calf muscle pump.[9] The soleus muscle is particularly rich in venous sinuses, containing as many as 18 of them.[6] Venous sinuses are less developed in the gastrocnemius muscle. These sinuses are valveless, but the small intramuscular veins that connect them to axial veins contain numerous valves.[6,9]

Venous sinuses receive blood from superficial veins through indirect perforators and from small muscular veins (Fig. 4.1). Venous sinuses of the soleus muscle are drained into the posterior tibial and peroneal veins by the *soleus veins* (Fig. 4.6). These veins are large, short and tortuous and can accommodate considerable range of muscular movements.[9] In the lower third of the leg, they frequently join direct perforating veins before entering the deep veins.[9] Bilateral *gastrocnemius veins* draining the two heads of the gastrocnemius muscle usually empty into the popliteal vein, distal to the saphenopopliteal junction. In patients with valvular incompetence these veins can enlarge considerably.[23]

Perforating Veins

Perforating veins take their origin from the superficial epifascial veins. At one point of their course, they perforate the fascia underlying the subcutaneus fat and join either the deep (axial) veins or venous sinuses of calf muscles.[24] The term "*communicating vein*" is reserved for venous tributaries, which connect veins within the same system i.e., veins of the superficial system or those of the deep.[25-26] Small communicating branches on both sides of the fascia may also connect perforating veins (Fig. 4.1). As early as 1867, Le Dentu distinguished direct and indirect perforating veins. *Direct* perforating veins connect superficial to deep axial veins, while *indirect* perforators connect superficial veins to veins and venous sinuses of leg muscles.[27] Direct perforating veins show a relatively constant anatomic distribution, while the more frequent indirect ones are irregularly distributed.[7] Differentiation between these two types of perforators may seem somewhat arbitrary as direct perforating veins often have small side tributaries communicating with muscle veins as well (Fig. 4.1). In the thigh and leg, perforating veins may be accompanied by cutaneous arteries. It is only in the foot where veins pass through fascia by themselves.[28] Otherwise, small nerves or arteries may accompany perforators as they pass through fascia. In the thigh and leg, perforating veins usually have one to three *valves*, which are all located in the subfascial part of the perforator.[29] Bicuspid valves are oriented to direct blood from superficial to deep veins. Small (< 1 mm) perforating veins, however, rarely have valves.[23] In addition to valves, the oblique lie of perforating veins between fascia and muscles and the course of these veins in intermuscular septa are helpful in maintaining superficial to deed unidirectional blood flow. In the foot, perforating veins are either valveless or valves are oriented to allow outward flow.[23]

The number of perforating veins identified in different anatomic studies has been variable and largely dependent on the applied method of detection. Corrosion cast models demonstrate as many as 150 perforating veins in the lower limb, although, most of these are very small perforators accompanying cutaneous arteries and have no clinical significance. Dissection and radiologic studies have revealed four groups of clinically significant perforating veins: those of the foot, medial calf, lateral calf, and thigh (Table 4.1).[9,24,30-34]

In the foot, eight to 10 perforators connect the deep to the superficial veins.[35] A large perforator at the first interosseous space between the metatarsals joins the dorsal venous arch with the dorsalis pedis veins (Fig. 4.2).[36] Medial and lateral ankle perforators (Kuster's or May's perforators)[25] collect blood from deep veins and distribute it to the greater and lesser saphenous veins, respectively (Fig. 4.3).

Medial calf perforators are clinically the most significant ones. In our anatomic study of cadaver legs an average of seven to eight direct, and five to six indirect, perforators were found in this region.[30]

Table 4.1. Studies on the location of direct medial perforating veins in the leg

1st Author	Number of legs		Location of medial perforating veins*		
(Year)	Anatomic dissections	Surgical findings	Cockett II	Cockett III	Proximal paratibial PVs
Linton (1938)	10	50	Distal third of the leg	Middle third of the leg	Proximal third of the leg
Sherman (1948)	92	901	13.5 cm	18.5 cm	24 cm, 30 cm, 35 cm, 40 cm
Cockett (1953)	21	201	13–14 cm	16–17 cm	At the knee
O'Donnell (1977)	–	39	Half of the incompetent PVs is between 10–15 cm† (15–20 cm*)		Few incompetent PVs
Fischer (1992)	–	194	Random distribution of incompetent PVs		
Mózes (1996)	40	–	7–9 cm† (12–14 cm*)	10–12 cm† (15–17 cm*)	18–22 cm†, 23–27 cm†, 28–32 cm† (23–27 cm*), (28–32 cm*), (33–37 cm*)

*Distances measured from the sole.
†Distances measured from the lower tip of the medial malleolus.

Indirect muscle perforators were randomly distributed, mostly located in the proximal half of the calf. Direct perforating veins are clustered in three groups in the distal half of the medial side of the leg (Table 4.1). The lowest, the retromalleolar group (*Cockett I*) is situated just behind the medial ankle (Fig. 4.3).[32,37,38] *Cockett II* and *III perforators* are located usually at 7–9 and 10–12 cm proximal to the tip of the medial malleolus and within 2 to 4 cm of the medial edge of the tibia (Fig. 4.3).[30] These perforating veins connect the posterior arch vein or other tributaries of the greater saphenous vein with the posterior tibial veins (Fig. 4.6). In the proximal part of the medial leg, direct perforating veins are paratibially located usually within 1 cm of the tibia. Paratibial direct perforators located 18–22 cm proximal to the medial malleolus were originally described as "*24 cm perforators*" because of their usual distance from the sole.[25] Two other groups of paratibial perforators are located at 23–27 and 28–32 cm from the medial malleolus (Fig. 4.3).[30] Less than half of these perforators make immediate connections between the greater saphenous and posterior tibial veins. The majority drain tributaries of the greater saphenous vein (Fig. 4.6). *Boyd's perforators,* located distal to the knee, usually directly connect the greater saphenous vein to the deep veins (Figs 4.3 and 4.6).[36,39]

Most medial calf perforators run across the superficial posterior compartment (Table 4.2 and Fig. 4.7).[29,40,41] However, a significant number run in the intermuscular septum or under the fascia of the deep posterior compartment (Fig. 4.8A–C).[42]

Lateral calf perforators include *peroneal perforators,* that connect the lesser saphenous system with the peroneal veins (*Bassi's perforator* located at 5–7 cm and the "*12 cm perforator*" at 12–14 cm from the lateral ankle) (Fig. 4.5).[7,25] More proximal indirect muscle perforators are referred as *gastrocnemius* and *soleus points* (Fig. 4.5).[25]

On the *anterior* side of the calf, direct perforators connect the anterior tributary of the greater saphe-nous vein to the anterior tibial veins.[33] Anterior perforators are situated in an irregular linear distribution between 2 and 5 cm lateral from the edge of the tibia.[21,43] The premalleolar and the midcrural perforators are constant (Fig. 4.2).[9,21]

In the thigh, clinically important direct perforating veins include *Dodd's perforators* and *Hunterian perforators*.[9,25,34] Both connect the saphenous with the popliteal or femoral veins (Figs 4.3 and 4.6). Additional perforators may connect accessory saphenous veins or the vein of Giacomini to the profunda femoris vein.[23] There are several indirect perforators in the thigh connecting the saphenous system to deeper muscular veins.

Histology

The venous wall contains three layers: the intima, the media and the adventitia.[44,45] *Intima* is fairly uniform. It is made up of a single layer of endothelial cells and subendothelium, which is composed of few connective tissue fibers and extracellular matrix. The internal elastic lamina is a layer of thick elastic fibers located at the base of the intima. It is absent in smaller veins and frequently incomplete even in medium-sized ones. Bicuspid venous valves are infoldings of the intima covered bilaterally by endothelium (Fig. 4.9A, B). Normally, there is only scant connective tissue skeleton between the two layers of endothelial cells (Fig. 4.10A, B). At the origin of valve cusps, veins are distended, forming small sinusoids. These undoubtedly form as a result of focally reversed blood flow.

The *media* is a distinct layer even in small veins draining venous capillaries. Its thickness and ratio of smooth muscle cells and connective tissue vary considerably depending on vein size and function. Large superficial veins, like the saphenous vein, have thick, muscular media, with contractile ability

Table 4.2. Percentage of direct perforating veins (PVs) accessible from the superficial posterior compartment

Direct medial perforating vein	Percentage of perforators accessible from the superficial posterior compartment (%)
Cockett I	~0
Cockett II	32
Cockett III	84
Proximal partibial PVs including "24 cm" PV	25

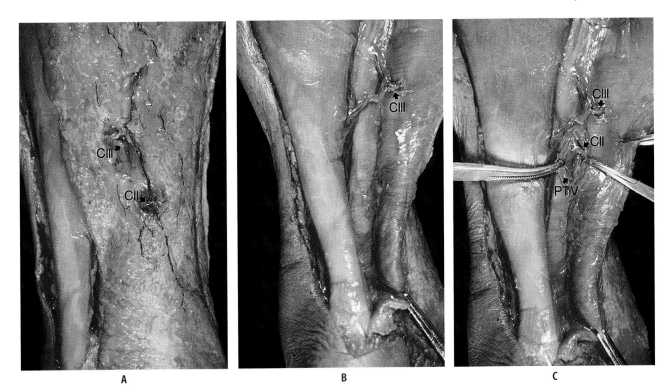

Fig. 4.8. Corrosion cast model of the posteromedial aspect of a left leg. **A** Note Cockett II (CII) and Cockett III (CIII) perforating veins branching from the posterior arch vein. The greater saphenous vein ascends on the right side of the leg. On the left side the Achilles' tendon is exposed. **B** The fascia and the subcutaneous fat have been been rolled up to expose the superficial posterior compartment. Note that the only visible perforating vein is a Cockett III perforator. **C** Following incision of the intermuscular septum between the superficial and deep posterior compartments Cockett II perforating veins are uncovered. (PTV, posterior tibial vein)

that helps to resist the development of varicosities.[46] Tributaries of the saphenous veins have thinner, weaker walls. Therefore, they become tortuous and varicose sooner and more frequent than their respective main axial vein. The media of the deep veins contain as much smooth muscle as saphenous

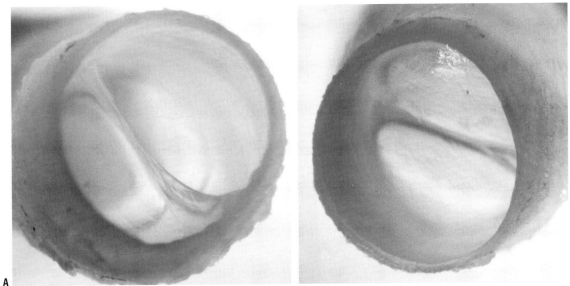

Fig. 4.9. Proximal **A** and distal **B** aspect of a valve in the greater saphenous vein. (Stereo microscopy, magnification: ×14).

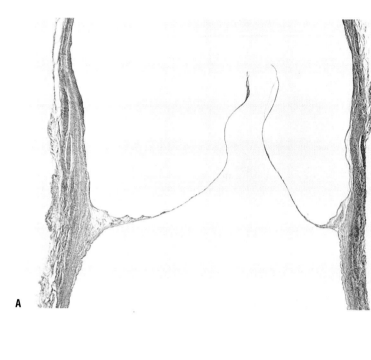

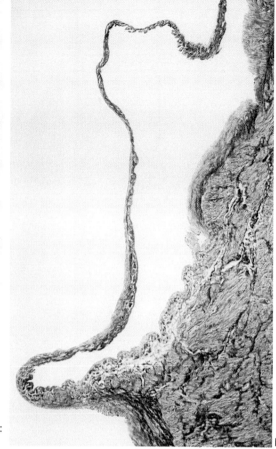

Fig. 4.10. Histology of valves in the greater saphenous vein. (**A**, orcein, magnification: ×2.5; **B**, AZAN magnification: ×10).

veins do; however, their collagen content is more abundant. Deep veins are supported from outside by surrounding skeletal muscle and a strong fibrous sheath as well. Therefore, their wall is considerably rigid.[47]

The *adventitia* of veins is poorly demarcated from surrounding tissues. It is made up of loose connective tissue, lymphatics, vascular channels (vasa vasorum) and adrenergic nerve fibers.

References

1. Gay J. On varicose disease of the lower extremities. John Churchill and Sons, London, 1868
2. Bannister LH. Integumental system: skin and breasts. In Gray's anatomy, 38th edn. Churchill Livingstone, New York, 1995: 375–424
3. Zbrodowski A, Gumener R, Gajisin S, Montandon D, Bednarkiewicz M. Blood supply of subcutaneous tissue in the leg and its clinical application. Clin Anat 1995; 8:202–7
4. Braverman IM. Ultrastructure and organization of the cutaneous microvasculature in normal and pathologic states. J Invest Dermatol 1989; 93:2S–9S
5. Braverman IM. The cutaneous microcirculation: ultrastructure and microanatomical organization. Microcirculation 1997; 4:329–40
6. Moneta GL, Nehler MR. The lower extremity venous sysrem: anatomy and physiology of normal venous function and chronic venous insufficiency. In: Gloviczki P, Yao JST (eds) Handbook of venous disorders. Guidelines of the American Venous Forum. Chapman & Hall Medical, London, 1996: 3–26
7. Hollinshead WH (ed). Anatomy for surgeons: the back and limbs, Volume 3. Harper & Row Publishers, New York, 1969: 617–31, 754–8, 803–7
8. White JW, Katz ML, Cisek P, Kreithen J. Venous outflow of the leg: anatomy and physiologic mechanism of the plantar venous plexus. J Vasc Surg 1996; 24: 819–24
9. Dodd H, Cockett FB. Surgical anatomy of the veins of the lower limb. In: Dodd H, Cockett FB (eds) The pathology and surgery of the veins of the lower limb. E & S Livingstone, London, 1956: 28–64
10. Negus D. The blood vessels of lower limb: applied anatomy. In: Negus D (ed) Leg ulcers: a practical approach to management, 2nd edn. Butterworth-Heinemann, London, 1995: 14–29
11. Gardner E, Gray DJ, O'Rahilly R. Anatomy – a regional study of human structure, 5th edn, Vessels and lymphatic drainage of the lower limb. WB Saunders, Philadelphia, 1986: 190–6
12. Daseler EH, Anson BJ, Reimann AF, Beaton LE. The saphenous venous tributaries and related structures in relation to the technique of high ligation: based chiefly upon a study of 550 anatomical dissection. Surg Gynecol Obstet 1946, 82:53–63

13. Kaiser A, Duff C, Scherrer C, Enzler M, Hauser M, Brunner U. Proximo-distal course of the diameter of the greater saphenous vein and the distribution of the number of side branched as an inherent difficulty in infra-inguinal arterial *in-situ* bypass (in German). Helv Chir Acta 1993; 59:893–6

14. Thomson H. The surgical anatomy of the superficial and perforating veins of the lower limb. Ann R Coll Surg Engl 1979; 61:198–205

15. Kosinski C. Observations on the superficial venous system of the lower extremity. J Anat 1926; 60:131–42

16. Bergan JJ. Surgical management of primary and recurrent varicose veins. In: Gloviczki P, Yao JST (eds) Handbook of venous disorders. Guidelines of the American Venous Forum. Chapman & Hall Medical, London, 1996: 394–415

17. Pang AS. Location of valves and competence of the great saphenous vein above the knee. Ann Acad Med Singapore 1991; 20:248–50

18. Garnjobst W. Injuries to the saphenous nerve following operation for varicose veins. Surg Gynecol Obstet 1964; 119: 359–61

19. Murakami G, Negishi N, Tanaka K, Hoshi H, Sezai Y. Anatomical relationship between saphenous vein and cutaneous nerves. Okajimas Folia Anat Jpn 1994; 71:21–33

20. Williams PL, Warwick R, Dyson M, Bannister LH (eds). Gray's anatomy. Churchill Livingstone, New York, 1989: 812–14

21. Green NA, Griffiths JD, Lavy GAD. Venous drainage of anterior tibio-fibular compartment of leg, with reference to varicose veins. Br Med J 1958; 1:1209–10

22. Basmajian JV. Distribution of valves in femoral, external iliac and common iliac veins and their relationship to varicose veins. Surg Gynecol Obstet 1952; 95:537–42.

23. Tibbs DJ. Varicose veins and related disorders. Butterworth-Heinemann, Oxford, 1992: 204–32

24. Linton RR. The communicating veins of the lower leg and the operative technique for their ligation. Ann Surg 1938;107:582–93

25. May R. Nomenclature of the surgically most important connncecting veins. In: May R, Partsch H, Staubesand J (eds) Perforating veins. Urban & Schwarzenberg, Baltimore, 1981: 13–18

26. May R, Nissl R. Phlebography of the lower limb (in German), 2nd edn. Thieme, Stuttgart, 1973

27. Le Dentu A. Anatomic research and physiologic considerations of the venous circulation of the foot and leg (in French). Thése Agrégat, Paris, 1867

28. Schäfer K. The course, structure and passage through the fascia of the perforating veins. In: May R, Partsch H, Staubesand J (eds) Perforating veins. Urban & Schwarzenberg, Baltimore, 1981: 37–45

29. Pirner F. On the valves of the perforating veins. In: May R, Partsch H, Staubesand J (eds) Perforating veins. Urban & Schwarzenberg, Baltimore, 1981: 46–8

30. Mozes G, Gloviczki P, Menawat SS, Fisher DR, Carmichael SW, Kadar A. Surgical anatomy for endoscopic subfascial division of perforating veins. J Vasc Surg; 24:800–8

31. O'Donnell TF, Burnand KG, Clemenson G, Thomas ML, Browse NL. Doppler examination vs clinical and phlebographic detection of the location of incompetent perforating veins. Arch Surg 1977; 112:31–5

32. Fischer R, Fullemann HJ, Alder W. About a phlebological dogma of the localization of the Cockett perforators (in French). Phlébologie 1992; 45:207–12

33. Sherman RS. Varicose veins: Further findings based on anatomic and surgical dissections. Ann Surg 1949; 130:218–32

34. Sherman RS. Varicose veins: anatomic findings and an operative procedure based upon them. Ann Surg 1944; 120:772–84

35. Kuster G, Lofgren EP, Hollinshead WH. Anatomy of the veins of the foot. Surg Gynecol Obstet 1968; 127: 817–23

36. Stolic E. Terminology, division and systematic anatomy of the communicating veins of the lower limb. In: May R, Partsch H, Staubesand J (eds) Perforating veins. Urban & Schwarzenberg, Baltimore, 1981: 19–34

37. Cockett FB, Jones DEE. The ankle blow-out syndrome: a new approach to the varicose ulcer problem. Lancet 1953; 1:17–23

38. Cockett FB. The pathology and treatment of venous ulcers of the leg. Br J Surg 1956; 44:260–78

39. Boyd AM. Discussion on primary treatment of varicose veins. Proc Royal Soc Med 1948; XLI:633–9

40. Gloviczki P, Cambria RA, Rhee RY, Canton LG, McKusick MA. Surgical techniques and preliminary results of endoscopic subfascial division of perforating veins. J Vasc Surg 1996; 23: 517–23

41. Gloviczki P, Canton LG, Cambria RA, Rhee RY. Subfascial endoscopic perforator vein surgery with gas insufflation. In: Gloviczki P, Bergan JJ (eds) Atlas of endoscopic perforator vein surgery. Springer-Verlag, London, 1998: 125–38

42. Mozes G, Gloviczki P, Kadar A, Carmichael SW. Surgical anatomy of perforating veins. In: Gloviczki P, Bergan JJ (eds) Atlas of endoscopic perforator vein surgery. Springer-Verlag, London, 1998: 17–28

43. Fischer R. Insufficient perforating vein on the antero-medial surface of the tibia (in German). VASA 1985; 14:168–9

44. Patrick JG. Blood vessels. In: Strenberg SS (ed.) Histology for pathologist. Raven Press, New York, 1992: 195–213

45. Parum DV. Histochemistry and immunochemistry of vascular disease. In: Stehbens WE and Lie JT (eds) Vascular pathology. Chapman & Hall, London, 1995: 313–27

46. Thomson H. The surgical anatomy of varicose veins. Phlebologie 1982; 35:11–8

47. Rickenbacher J. The microscopic structure of the walls of the perforating veins. In: May R, Partsch H, Staubesand J (eds) Perforating veins. Urban & Schwarzenberg, Baltimore, 1981: 60–3

Editors' Commentary

The first section of this volume lays the groundwork for clinical investigation of limbs with chronic venous insufficiency (CVI) and the prescription for specific therapy for patients who are so afflicted. CVI represents the end stage of a complex mix of risk factors, which are best determined by epidemiology, anatomic abnormalities, venous hypertension and molecular events.

In discussing the epidemiology of chronic venous insufficiency, Dr Lawrence and colleagues summarize what is known worldwide about the prevalence of venous disorders. It is clear that each epidemiological study uncovers more patients with venous insufficiency than would be expected by surveying medical practices. This report, and the one that follows describing risk factors for venous insufficiency, both emphasize the importance of genetics, female sex, pregnancy and a standing occupation. Of interest to vascular surgeons is the fact that their legs show more venous reflux on duplex examination than those of general surgeons. Presumably, this relates to longer time spent at the operating table. More importantly, the incidence of severe chronic venous insufficiency is documented to be approximately 4% in a general population and even greater in the population of individuals over 80 years.

Epidemiological studies, such as reported in the first chapter, uncover the fact that patients with apparently normal legs without previous deep venous thrombosis also experience severe chronic venous insufficiency. Thus, the term postphlebitic ulcer is incorrect in many cases. Risk factors are more thoroughly discussed in the second chapter which emphasizes that age, genetics, female sex and pregnancy predispose individuals to venous insufficiency in general and a fraction of those to severe chronic venous insufficiency in particular. In discussing parity as a risk factor, it is emphasized that it is progesterone from the corpus luteum and not pressure of the gravid uterus on iliac veins that appear to be an inciting element for varicosities that begin during pregnancy. Among the less well understood risk factors are the controversial elements of lifestyle, tight clothing and toilet posture. However, it is clear that obesity remains an important risk factor for the development of CVI. However, the reason for obesity being linked to venous insufficiency is entirely unknown.

Some of the observations on epidemiology and risk factors are brought together in the discussion of pathogenesis of chronic venous insufficiency. Here the link between chronic venous insufficiency and apparent uncomplicated varicose veins is explained. It is emphasized that total venous hypertension as expressed by gravitational pressure as well as compartmental pressure transmitted through failed check valves are additive in the most dependent portions of the medial leg. There, the apparent disparity between limbs that have only varicose veins and limbs that have varicose veins and severe changes of chronic venous insufficiency is explained by the inflammatory reaction related to leukocyte trapping. The elements of venous hypertension, activation of leukocytes, expression of adhesion molecules and the elongation and dilation of venules thus producing an excessive endothelial surface are linked in a unified concept of pathogenesis of severe chronic venous insufficiency. Clearly, all of the factors mentioned before, including genetics, standing occupation, female sex and parity can be linked to venous hypertension. However, the trigger mechanism in activation of leukocytes remains unknown.

Not all physicians interested in venous pathophysiology embrace the leukocyte trapping theory of chronic venous insufficiency. However, it is most plausible and does explain the observed phenomena of venous insufficiency, in which hemodynamically identical limbs have a widely different clinical appearance.

In preparation for discussions of therapy, the explication of lower extremity venous anatomy by Mózes is particularly helpful. Here, not only are the traditional pathways of venous return but also the anatomy of perforating veins and their relationship to the superficial posterior compartment and the deep posterior compartment, are described in detail. Experience with surgery in this area has verified the observations of Dr Mózes and colleagues that important perforating veins originate in the deep posterior muscular compartment and traverse the intermuscular septum between the superficial posterior compartment and the deep posterior compartment. Simple exploration of the superficial posterior compartment and sectioning of veins, which traverse this area, would be ineffective in producing total perforator ablation. Thus, the blind procedures advocated by some must be discredited.

Section B _____
PRIMARY VENOUS INSUFFICIENCY

Practical Application of the CEAP Classification

5

Elna M. Masuda, Robert L. Kistner, Bo Eklof and Danian Yang

Introduction

When Rene Leriche described the "obliteration of the terminal abdominal aorta" in 1923, his approach included an organized discussion of the clinical state, etiology, location of the problem and the involved pathophysiology.[1] Such an organized approach to arterial disease has become well established in the modern era of vascular surgery since the 1940s. It is surprising that a similar organized approach to the venous system has lagged so far behind its arterial counterpart. Like the treatment of arterial disease, progress in the management of venous disease requires clear identification of four basic elements that describe the venous limb. Ultimately, by knowing the clinical symptom or sign, the etiology of the venous problem, the site involved and the physiologic abnormality, one can formulate a logical treatment plan for the patient.

The "CEAP" classification for chronic venous disease was developed in 1994 by an international *ad hoc* committee of the American Venous Forum to address this need. The product of the meeting was a consensus document that classified venous disease into four categories: clinical state (C), etiology (E), anatomy (A), and pathophysiology (P). Since its inception, the classification has been endorsed in the United States by the American Venous Forum, the Joint Council of the Society for Vascular Surgery (SVS) and North American-

International Society for Cardiovascular Surgery (ISCVS) and was published in 1995.[2] It also became an integral part of the updated Reporting Standards in Venous Disease[3] and has been accepted as a standard by many societies in Europe, Asia and South America.

Purpose of CEAP

The purpose of the classification of chronic venous disease is to provide a standard for a thorough diagnosis in chronic venous disease, and a means for improving the precision of communication in the field of venous disease in a way that can benefit both clinicians and researchers. Clearly, its usefulness can be seen as a tool for research. The CEAP classfication is now a standardized method for reporting data considered for publication, as recommended by the SVS and ISCVS in their *Reporting Standards in Venous Disease: An update.*[3] When applied in academia, the CEAP classification provides a template for institutions to use in reporting variables found to be clinically important in the management of chronic venous insufficiency (CVI).

Less obvious, however, is how CEAP can be used by the clinician to manage the venous patient on a day-to-day basis. The focus of this chapter is to show how the CEAP classification can become a useful tool in clinical practice and how to overcome some of its perceived disadvantages. By first identifying symptoms and signs of venous disease (*C*linical class), the CEAP classification can be used to develop an orderly work-up and treatment plan. Once objective testing is completed, the last three categories of the CEAP classification (*E*tiology, *A*natomy, *P*hysiology) can be extracted from test results. Then, data can be formulated into meaningful conclusions that lead to the best treatment option.

Table 5.I. Clinical class (C)

Class 0:	No visible or palpable signs of venous disease
Class 1:	Telangiectases or reticular veins
Class 2:	Varicose veins
Class 3:	Edema
Class 4:	Skin changes ascribed to venous disease (e.g. pigmentation, Venous eczema, lipodermatosclerosis.)
Class 5:	Skin changes as defined above with healed ulceration
Class 6:	Skin changes as defined above with active ulceration

Decision Making Based on the CEAP Classification

In the setting where therapy is limited to external compression alone for the treatment of all patients with venous disease, regardless of the severity of symptoms or location of disease, the CEAP classification has little value. This approach to treatment would not benefit from deciphering details of the venous abnormality through the CEAP classification, as management would not be affected.

However, for the clinician who chooses from a number of therapeutic options available for treatment of venous disease (such as ligation and stripping, sclerotherapy, laparoscopic perforator interruption, deep vein–valve reconstruction, or endovascular therapy with balloon angioplasty/stenting), fundamental knowledge of the venous abnormality is necessary to make the correct choice of therapy. These treatment options can be organized based on information acquired by the CEAP classification.

The Work-up of Chronic Venous Disease

Applying the Clinical Class "C"

Defining clinical class or presenting symptom is the first step toward arrival at a plan for treatment for the patient with CVI. Clinical presentation may fall into one or more classes as shown in Table 5.1. A simple method to organize the diagnostic evaluation of a patient with venous disease is to utilize one of three levels of testing. Level I is the office examination and assessment of the venous system with a hand-held continuous wave Doppler. Level II consists of noninvasive vascular lab testing including color flow duplex scanning and/or plethysmography. Level III indicates invasive examination by venography either ascending or descending or both, and/or venous pressure measurements. The level of work-up can be assigned to the appropriate clinical class(es) as shown in Table 5.2.

As the clinical severity increases, the work-up of the patient becomes more detailed. With a low level of severity, such as a patient presenting with simple telangiectasias or asymptomatic varicose veins (class 1–2a), the work-up should be kept to a simple evaluation by Level I testing. Examination by more extensive testing such as duplex scanning or plethysmography is seldom necessary, and the CEAP classification may be truncated to a simple "C" description, without need for the identification of the "EAP" categories. However, if a patient presents with painful varicose veins, hyperpigmentation and long saphenous vein reflux by continuous wave Doppler examination, and surgical ligation and stripping is being considered, work-up should include color-flow duplex scanning and/or plethysmography. Rationale for the noninvasive examination is to obtain information which the bedside examination cannot provide. For instance, duplex scanning may detect axial reflux, perforator disease, deep venous obstruction or reflux that may ultimately lead to the better choice of sclerotherapy, surgery or endovascular treatment.

Table 5.2. Suggested work-up for chronic venous insufficiency, based on the maximal severity of symptoms Clinical Class (C) of CEAP. Note: in patients with more than one class, use the class with the highest level of work-up

Clinical class	Level I Clinical exam Continuous wave Doppler	Level II Non-invasive test Duplex scanning Plethysmography	Level III Invasive test Venography Vein pressures
Asymptomatic (C0-2)	X		
Symptomatic			
0 No signs	X	X*	
1 Telangiectasia or reticular veins	X	X*	
2 Varicose veins	X	X*	
3 Edema	X	X	X*
4 Skin Changes	X	X	X*
5 Ulcer healed	X	X	X*
6 Ulcer active	X	X	X*

X*: Proceed with this level of diagnostic testing if treatment requires a higher level of testing.

Diagnostic Testing

Duplex ultrasound has been shown to be an accurate and reliable tool in determining the anatomic site of venous disease.[4] It can also be used to estimate whether etiology is primary versus secondary in most instances. This is especially true if post-thrombotic changes are found such as mural thickening, intraluminal filling defects and venous obstruction with collaterals. The various types of plethysmography (air, photo and strain gauge) can be used to determine the global pathophysiology of disease, whether dealing with reflux or obstruction or both.

Venography provides clear delineation of the etiology, anatomy and pathophysiology of the limb. When used as an *ascending* study, the contrast is injected into a dorsal foot vein with tourniquet at the ankle. This allows contrast to flow into the deep system. Incompetent perforators can be found and isolated using this method. Secondary causes for venous disease such as post-thrombotic changes or venous obstruction can also be identified. *Descending* venography involves injecting contrast into the iliac or common femoral vein with the patient in a 60° semi-erect position. With Valsalva, the contrast descends down the leg toward the foot in cases of reflux. This method is ideal for identifying the presence or absence of valves, for distinguishing primary disease (intact, floppy or nonfunctional valves) from secondary disease (destroyed valves with loss of morphology from prior deep vein thrombosis (DVT)), and to test for reflux and obstruction.

Because of its invasive nature, however, venography should be reserved for those cases where deep venous valve reconstruction or endovascular treatment with balloon angioplasty and stenting is being considered. The details provided by venography are substantial, but because of the small, but recognized, risks involved such as allergic reaction to contrast and rare venous thrombosis, it should be used only if treatment depends on it.

Treatment based on "*Etiology, Anatomy, Physiology*"

Etiology (E)

Treatment of venous insufficiency may be altered based on whether the patient has one of three underlying causes of chronic venous disease: congenital, primary or secondary as shown in Table 5.3.

Table 5.3. Etiologic classification

Congenital (E$_c$)
Primary (E$_p$) – with undetermined cause
Secondary (E$_s$) – with known cause
Post-thrombotic
Post-traumatic
Other

With congenital maldevelopment, there may be venous aplasia or total absence of a vein, hypoplasia, reduplication or persistence of vestigial vessels.[5] The importance of identifying the rare case of congenital malformation is that despite the unsightliness of these abnormalities, direct surgical intervention may make it worse, especially if details of the abnormality are not properly investigated. One of the most common abnormalities is the Klippel–Trenaunay syndrome (KTS) which is defined by the presence of cutaneous nevus, varicose veins, and bone or soft tissue hypertrophy involving one or both limbs. For most patients with KTS, management with elastic stockings will suffice. For others, however, stripping or excision of superficial veins may reduce symptoms. In these cases, knowledge of the deep venous system is absolutely necessary as removal of the superficial veins should not be done if aplasia of the deep veins is present.

The most common type of venous disease is known to be primary (E_p) with undetermined cause, and the great majority fall under the category of saphenous or superficial venous reflux disease.[6] Secondary causes (E_s) are also common and are most frequently caused by prior venous thrombosis. The importance of distinguishing primary from secondary disease is that with primary disease, ligation and stripping with or without perforator interruption can be curative, even with patients presenting with longstanding skin changes and ulceration. Prognosis is very good with surgery for primary disease, especially in those with isolated greater saphenous vein reflux and no involvement of the deep system.[7] Those with secondary disease usually have other involved venous segments and do not usually present with isolated greater saphenous reflux. Results of ligation and stripping alone in this setting has not been as successful as when this treatment is applied to patients with primary disease.

In 1976, Burnand and others[8] showed that when patients with ulceration were treated with perforator ligation for venographically proven incompetence, those with ulcers associated with secondary or post-thrombotic changes (E_s) in the deep system fared poorly when compared to those with no post-thrombotic changes or presumably primary (E_p) disease. There was a tenfold greater chance of ulcer recurrence when perforator disease was associated with the post-thrombotic syndrome. In a more contemporary report, deep venous valve reconstruction was applied to patients with severe symptoms of chronic venous insufficiency. Better clinical results were achieved with surgery for primary valvular disease than secondary or post-thrombotic disease at a mean follow-up of 10 years.[9] With primary valvular disease, good to excellent clinical results are achieved in 73%, whereas only 43% of those with post-thrombotic syndrome gain the same benefit. Although one cannot exclude the possibility that this discrepancy may reflect a difference in type of procedure used for primary (valve repair) versus secondary reflux (valve transposition), it appears that the physiologic effects of deep venous thrombosis (E_s) on the venous system is notably worse than the primary etiology (E_p). With post-thrombotic syndrome, there may be reduction of venous compliance and production of physiologic obstruction as a direct result of thrombosis, which is not present with primary venous disease.

Anatomy (A)

Knowledge of venous anatomy is critical for the clinician to make a decision regarding best treatment. By dividing up anatomic segments into superficial, deep and perforator groups (Table 5.4), a logical approach to treatment can be made. In

Table 5.4. Anatomic classification

Segment No.	
	Superficial veins (A_s)
1	Telangiectases/reticular veins
2	Greater (long) saphenous (GSV)
3	Above knee
4	Below knee
5	Lesser (short) saphenous (LSV)
6	Nonsaphenous
	Deep veins (A_D)
7	Inferior vena cava iliac
8	Common
9	Internal
10	External
11	Pelvic – Gonadal, broad ligament, other femoral
12	Common
13	Deep
14	Superficial
15	Popliteal
	Crural – Anterior tibial, posterior tibial, peroneal (all paired)
16	Muscular – gastrocnemial, soleal, other
	Perforating Veins (A_p)
17	Thigh
18	Calf

Table 5.5. Treatment alternatives for chronic venous insufficiency based on Etiology, Anatomy and Physiology.

	Anatomy (physiology)			
	Perforator (reflux)	Superficial (reflux)	Deep (reflux)	Deep (obstruction)
Etiology				
Congenital	S, Sc, L&S	S, VR	S	S, Sc, Interrupt
Primary	S, Sc, L&S	S, VR (valvuloplasty)	Not applicable	S, Sc, Interrupt
Secondary	S, Sc, L&S	S, VR (valve transposition, transplant)	S, E, B	S, Sc, Interrupt

S, stockings; Sc, Slerotherapy; L&S, Ligation and stripping; E, Endovascular techniques, balloon angioplasty, stenting; B, Surgical bypass; VR, Valve reconstruction.
Interrupt*= with open or laparoscopic technique

Note: Categories for superficial and perforator obstruction were omitted due to lack of therapeutic significance.

Table 5.5, treatment options are shown based on *Etiology*, *Anatomy* and *Physiology*. If a patient has swelling, pain and venous claudication, the finding of venous obstruction in the iliac vein (A7) could lead to endovascular manipulation with balloon angioplasty and/or stenting, and subsequent relief of venous hypertension.[10] In contrast, if the patient presents with venous ulceration and is found to have primarily perforator incompetence (A_p), then the preferred treatment may be laparoscopic or standard open perforator vein interruption. Finally, if all three anatomic levels (superficial, perforator and deep: A_{spd}) are affected with reflux, it may be best to manage the problem with external compression stockings. Alternatively, all three anatomic levels could be addressed with ligation and stripping, perforator interruption, venous valve reconstruction, or a combination of these methods.

Pathophysiology (P)

Whereas the arterial system primarily consists of obstructive disease (with the exception of aneurysms), the venous system has obstruction and reflux, or a combination of both (Table 5.6). It is well accepted that the most common physiologic state associated with clinical symptoms is reflux.[11] If reflux is found, treatment may consist of stock-ings and/or ablative procedures such as ligation and stripping of the superficial veins or perforator interruption (Table 5.5). If deep veins are incompetent, reconstructive procedures on the deep venous system such as valve repair, transposition or valve transplantation may be indicated. The final option may be elastic support stockings, especially in those who are elderly and less active.

If physiologic obstruction is discovered, treatment may be limited to stockings or may include restorative procedures such as reopening areas of obstruction with balloon angioplasty and/or stenting, or surgical cross-pubic or saphenopopliteal bypass.[12,13]

Anatomic, Clinical and Disability Scores

The scoring system was designed to estimate functional capacity of the venous patient (disability score), capture severity of symptoms (clinical score), and incorporate importance of extent of disease (anatomic score). The anatomic score is the sum of anatomic segments each counted as one point in Table 5.4. The disability and clinical scores are shown in Tables 5.7 and 5.8, respectively. They

Table 5.6. Pathophysiologic classification

Reflux (P_r)
Obstruction (P_o)
Reflux and obstruction (P_{ro})

Table 5.7. Disability score

0	Asymptomatic
1	Symptomatic, can function without support device
2	Can work 8-hour day *only* with support device
3	Unable to work with support device

Table 5.8. Clinical score

Pain	(0 = none; 1 = moderate, not requiring analgesics; 2 = severe, requiring analgesics)
Edema	(0 = none; 1 = mild/moderate; 2 = severe)
Venous claudication	(0 = none; 1 = mild/moderate; 2 = severe)
Pigmentation	(0 = none; localized; 2 = extensive)
Lipodermatosclerosis	(0 = none; localized; 2 = extensive)
Ulcer – size (largest ulcer)	(0 = none; 1 = <2 cm diameter; 2 = >2 cm diameter)
Ulcer – duration	(0 = none; 1 = <3 months; 2 = >3 months)
Ulcer – recurrence	(0 = none; 1 = once; 2 = more than once)
Ulcer – number	(0 = none; 1 = single; 2 = multiple)

are important, but from a practical standpoint are probably more useful to the academician than to the clinician for every day application. For research, scoring can be used to describe a group of patients before and after treatment as illustrated in Fig. 5.1, where the cumulative score can be used to measure benefit (or lack of benefit) of intervention.

Limitations of CEAP

There are at least three features of CEAP classification that at first glance may be perceived as disadvantages. The first and most obvious is its complexity. The CEAP classification was not deliberately made to be complex, but was designed to reduce the confusion that existed between different centers and individuals reporting their clinical experience. The complexity of the classification reflects the detail that is inherent in the description of the venous limb. One way to apply CEAP in a simplistic form when referring to groups of patients, is to describe the four major categories without using all of the numbered segments. By using the general four categories with delineation of subgroups, data from different institutions can be compared. For example, it is easy to see that the group of patients with varicose veins from Maywood, Illinois (Fig. 5.2) are similar to the group of patients found in a general population of venous patients seen in Honolulu, Hawaii shown in Fig. 5.3.

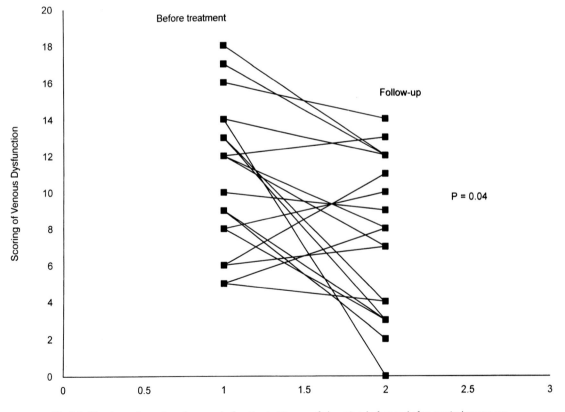

Fig. 5.1. The change in scoring of venous dysfunction in 19 cases of ulceration, before and after surgical treatment.

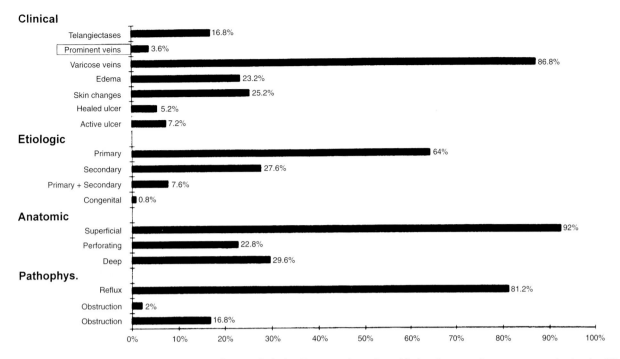

Fig. 5.2. Clinical, etiologic, anatomic and physiologic data from 250 limbs in 182 consecutive patiens with chronic venous disease encountered at London, UK and Maywood, IL, USA. (Adapted from: Labropoulos, N. CEAP in clinical practice. Vasc Surg 1997; 31:224–5).

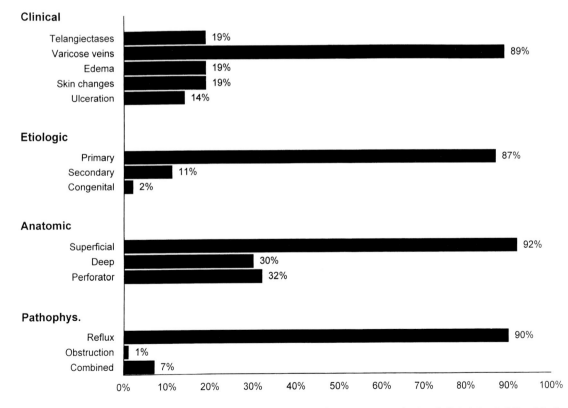

Fig. 5.3. CEAP data from 166 limbs in consecutive patients with chronic venous disease encountered in Straub Clinic & Hospital, Honolulu, Hawaii.

In contrast, the group of patients with general venous symptoms from Maywood and Honolulu in Figs 5.2 and 5.3, are very different from the second group of patients from Honolulu presenting with venous ulceration (Fig. 5.4). By using the CEAP format for comparison, one can see that the venous ulceration group differs from the other two in that they have more severe symptoms, more secondary disease, more involvement of the deep and perforator systems, and a greater number have obstructive disease which may explain the increased severity of symptoms.

When applying CEAP to the patient encountered in practice, details of the numbered segments are particularly useful in tracking the clinical course of the patient over time. For example, if a patient with varicose veins has pain, ulceration, deep venous and greater saphenous vein reflux, the code would be: C2,6$_s$, E$_p$, A2,13,18 P$_r$. Following surgical removal of the varicose veins, greater saphenous vein, interruption of calf perforators and subsequent resolution of the ulcer, the new CEAP classification would be: C$_a$, E$_p$, A13, P$_r$.

The second limitation of CEAP is that not all patients with venous disease can be classified into all four categories because classification is based upon objective testing, and not all receive testing. As not all patients undergo vascular lab testing with duplex, plethysmography or venography, the "EAP" data may be lacking. Hence, the usefulness of the CEAP classfication gains more applicability the more complex the case of venous disease. Patients with asymptomatic varicose veins or telangiectasias may never require color flow duplex, and CEAP will only be limited to the clinical class (C), whereas the complex patient with recurrent ulcerations, lipodermatosclerosis and previous deep venous thrombosis may be an excellent candidate to describe in a CEAP format, in which all details can be captured by a single code.

The third limitation of CEAP has to do with the limited accuracy or reliability of the various tests for venous disease currently available. There is a lack of standardization of the tests used for chronic venous disease. For example, depending on the institution, the technique of duplex scanning for chronic venous disease may vary: supine versus standing, Valsalva versus cuff deflation versus manual compression. Furthermore, accuracy between institutions may be variable and the type of study done to determine the

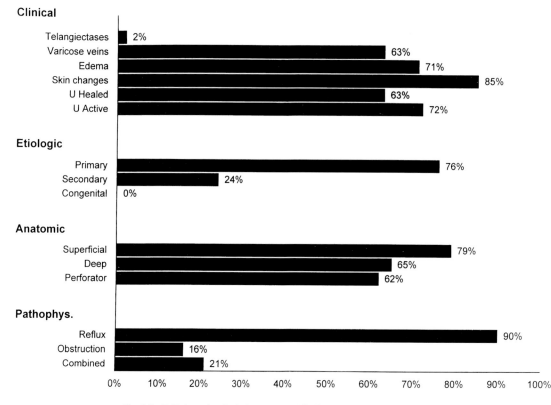

Fig. 5.4. CEAP data of 82 limbs in patients with ulceration, in Honolulu, Hawaii.

etiology, anatomy, and physiology may differ. Some centers may use plethysmography, whereas others prefer color flow duplex scanning or venography. This lack of standardization is what will hopefully be sorted out and organized into a more uniform level of reporting in the future. CEAP may be the means by which "rules for reporting" will be standardized so that appropriate testing will ensue. The type and method of testing will need to evolve as the field of venous disease grows.

In summary, the classification can be modified for simplicity especially when it is applied to large groups. For simple, straightforward venous cases with minimal symptoms, the entire CEAP description will not be applicable. A shorter version using only categories where data is available may be reasonable.

Conclusions

The CEAP classification was designed to improve the quality of work-up, diagnosis, treatment and further the advancement of our understanding of chronic venous insufficiency. Although it has some limitations, its many strengths should be reason for adoption in clinical practice and academia. During this modern era of vascular surgery and medicine, and with our growing knowledge of the venous system, a systematic method of acquiring and presenting data on venous disease is needed. By using this method of categorizing the many facets of venous disease into a universal code, interpretation of data between institutions will be facilitated, and

clinicians will benefit by having an organized approach to the diagnosis and treatment of the venous patient.

References

1. Leriche R. Des obliterations arterielles hautes (obliteration de la terminaison de l'aorte) comme causes des insuffisances circulatoires des membres inferieurs. Bull Mem Soc Chir (Paris) 1923; 49:1404
2. Beebe HG, Bergan JJ, Bergqvist D et al. Classification and grading of chronic venous disease in the lower limbs, a consensus statement. Vasc Surg 1996; 30:5–11
3. Porter JM, Moneta GL, An International Consensus Committee on Chronic Venous Disease. Reporting standards in venous disease: an update. J Vasc Surg 1995; 21:635–45
4. Masuda EM, Kistner RL. Prospective comparison of duplex scanning and descending venography in the assessment of venous insufficiency. Am J Surg 1992; 164:254–9
5. Browse NL, Burnand KG, Thomas ML. Congenital venous abnormalities. In: Browse NL, Burnand KG and Thomas ML (eds) Diseases of the veins, pathology_diagnosis and treatment. Edward Arnold, London, 1988: 603–25
6. Kistner RL, Eklof B, Masuda EM. Diagnosis of chronic venous disease of the lower extremities: the "CEAP" classification. Mayo Clin Proc 1996; 71:338–45
7. Sarin S, Scurr JH, Coleridge Smith PD. Assessment of stripping the long saphenous vein in the treatment of primary varicose veins. Br J Surg 1992; 79;889–93
8. Burnand K, Thomas ML, O'Donnell T, Browse NL. Relation between postphlebitic changes in the deep veins and results of surgical treatment of venous ulcers. Lancet 1976; 936–38
9. Masuda EM, Kistner RL. Long-term results of venous valve reconstruction: a four- to twenty-one year follow-up. J Vasc Surg 1994; 19:391–403
10. Semba CP, Dake MD. Catheter-directed thrombolysis for iliofemoral venous thrombosis. Semin Vasc Surg. 1996; 9:26–33
11. Killewich LA, Martin R, Cramer M et al. Pathophysiology of venous claudication. J Vasc Surg 1984; 1:507–11
12. Palma EC, Esperon R. Vein transplants and grafts in the surgical treatment of the postphlebitic syndrome. J Cardiovasc Surg 1960; 1:94
13. Warren R, Thayer TR. Transplantation of the saphenous vein for postphlebitic stasis. Surgery 1954; 35:867

Compression Sclerotherapy for Large Veins and Perforators

6

Joseph G. Sladen and J.D.S. Reid

Introduction

Large varicose veins and incompetent perforators have been injected effectively since the early 1950s when Sigg[1] added compression to sclerotherapy. Henry and Fegan reported success in the treatment of venous ulcers in 1971.[2] The procedure described in this chapter is an "empty vein" technique used by the above mentioned practitioners.

Surgery has been the traditional approach to treatment of complicated venous insufficiency in North America.[3,4,5] Subfascial endoscopic perforator ligation (SEPS) and direct valve repair and replacement are more recent additions to this armamentarium. Saphenofemoral, thigh and short (lesser) saphenous reflux should be controlled surgically. Most surgeons now agree on the importance of perforator control in the management of tissue changes secondary to venous insufficiency (clinical, etiologic, anatomic, physiologic (CEAP) clinical class 3–6).[6] In 1974 Hobbs[7] demonstrated that compression sclerotherapy treated perforators effectively and that at six years results were better than subfascial ligation. We have used compression sclerotherapy to the exclusion of surgery for 20 years in the treatment of complicated venous disease below the knee.[8] In addition, we have had a very satisfactory experience in controlling perforators with this technique.[9]

Clinical Examination and Investigation

Careful clinical examination is important in the management of complicated venous disease. The patient is examined after standing for 10 minutes. The aim is to identify specific anatomical sites of reflux (Table 6.1).

Perforators and Control Points

Clinical demonstration of perforators (in fact, the venous lake fed by the high pressure perforator) and control points is mandatory if one is to practice effective compression sclerotherapy without a duplex scanner. The calf is examined, with the patient

Table 6.1.

Area	Clinical examination	Investigation
Thigh	– sapheno femoral reflux	Doppler
	– thigh varices and perforators	Duplex
	– short (lesser) saphenous	Duplex
Calf & Foot	– perforators	Duplex
	– control points	
	– manifestations of venous insufficiency *	Duplex, A.P.G.

*CEAP, Clinical 3–6: edema, skin changes, healed or active ulcer.

standing, searching for perforator tenderness over anatomical perforator sites. The edema is "milked" away by pressing with a thumb over tender areas. A venous lake must be seen or at least palpated to be injected (Fig. 6.1). Control points can be identified by digitally stripping the blood out of the vein, working upwards. Sudden reappearance of the blood from above marks a control point. These areas will be sclerosed at the time of compression sclerotherapy. Findings should be recorded on a venous form (Fig. 6.2).

Duplex examination of the leg identifies 80% of incompetent perforators[10,11] and demonstrates a few areas thought to be perforators on physical examination, which in fact are control points. From a practical standpoint, this is not critical before compression sclerotherapy because all perforators, tender areas and control points should be sclerosed. Duplex examination does shorten the learning curve if the physician is not confident in venous examination.

Saphenofemoral and Thigh Reflux

Although not the primary focus of this chapter, effective treatment of saphenofemoral reflux as well as reflux in thigh perforators and short saphenous vein is mandatory in the treatment of complicated venous insufficiency. Burnand et al.[12] have shown that an incompetent long saphenous vein may contribute more than 50% of the increase in ambulatory venous pressure at the ankle seen in venous disease, even in the presence of incompetent perforators. Superficial reflux alone may be the cause of venous ulceration[13] and more frequently, alone accounts for lesser degrees of venous insufficiency. Surgery is the treatment of choice for saphenofemoral and thigh reflux. The most definitive approach is ligation and thigh stripping,[14,15] with careful attention to groin tributaries.[16] The option of saving the saphenous vein in the thigh but treating saphenous varices locally at the time of flush ligation under local anesthesia has been our choice as these patients are not concerned about a few residual veins.

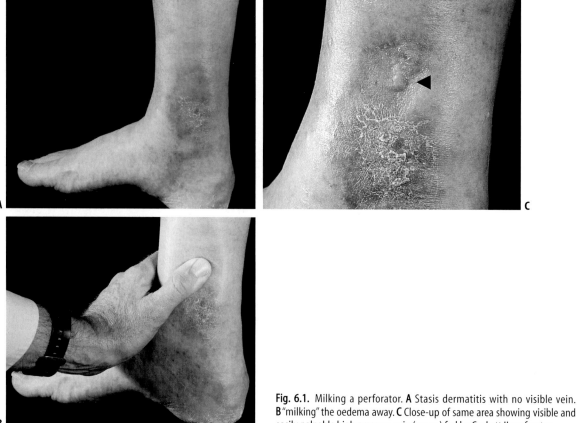

Fig. 6.1. Milking a perforator. **A** Stasis dermatitis with no visible vein. **B** "milking" the oedema away. **C** Close-up of same area showing visible and easily palpable high pressure vein (arrow) fed by Cockett II perforator.

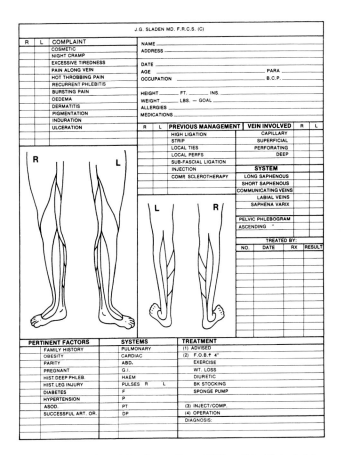

Fig. 6.2. Venous form (after Fegan, Henry, Milliken; Vein Clinic, Dublin, Ireland).

Preparation of Patient

The patient must understand the basic principles of venous disease for satisfactory management. Concepts of venous drainage, valves and the calf muscle pump are discussed. We stress control of disease, not cure. As an integral part of treatment, all patients are fitted with a below-knee compression stocking (30–40 mmHg). If there is a history of phlebitis, we use the stocking as a "therapeutic trial" to be sure there is adequate venous outflow in the leg to allow treatment of perforators.

If diffuse tenderness, induration or ulceration is present on the medial lower calf, a "sponge pump" is added rather than increasing the pressure of the stocking (Fig. 6.3). This is because very few patients initially tolerate stockings with a pressure gradient of 40–50 mmHg or greater. A sponge pump is made from soft, 1.25 cm latex foam rubber, measuring approximately 8 × 20 cm. The sponge is rounded

and beveled so that the edges do not indent the tissue. It can be modified to apply more pressure behind the medial malleolus. The sponge pump is placed over the medial perforator area on top of the compression stocking and wrapped with about one-half of a 10 cm tensor bandage. The bandage is applied tightly with crisscrossing wraps on the lower part of the sponge pump. As the bandage is applied upward, the pressure is reduced by spreading the wraps and easing the pressure.

Characteristically, venous ulcers are not painful and only slightly tender. If the ulcer is painful, there is either a significant infective component or it is a combined ulcer, associated with occlusive disease or severe venous hypertension. After the ulcerated area is cultured and cleansed, it is covered with sterile cotton gauze. The gauze is backed with a portion of abdominal padding to absorb moisture and held in place with a nylon stocking. A compression stocking is applied over the nylon and then wrapped with a sponge pump for additional pressure. This dressing is changed morning and evening. The patient is instructed to walk 2 miles daily and to resume normal activities as much as possible. It usually takes one or two follow-up visits to be certain the patient is using the sponge pump effectively. When the ulcer is clean and relatively dry, Telfa is substituted for gauze and the need for the abdominal pad is soon eliminated. An alternative method of applying pressure is by use of the "four layer wrap"[17] and hydrophilic (Allevyn, Smith + Nephew Medical Limited, Hull, UK) dressing. Compliance is high with both methods as tenderness and induration subside quickly. Patients are carefully taught that pressure heals. They are fully mobile and can easily monitor the progress of healing. This education is helpful later as the patient becomes involved in the treatment and can reapply pressure dressings after treatment is completed if the involved area deteriorates. Perforators proximal to the ulcer can be injected to accelerate healing of the ulcer.

Compression Sclerotherapy

We first described our technique in 1983[8] and the details more recently.[18] Essentially it is an empty vein technique tailored after Sigg, Fegan and Hobbs. After learning to inject efficiently, which comes fairly quickly with practice, by far the most important component is bandaging of the leg.[19] An organized

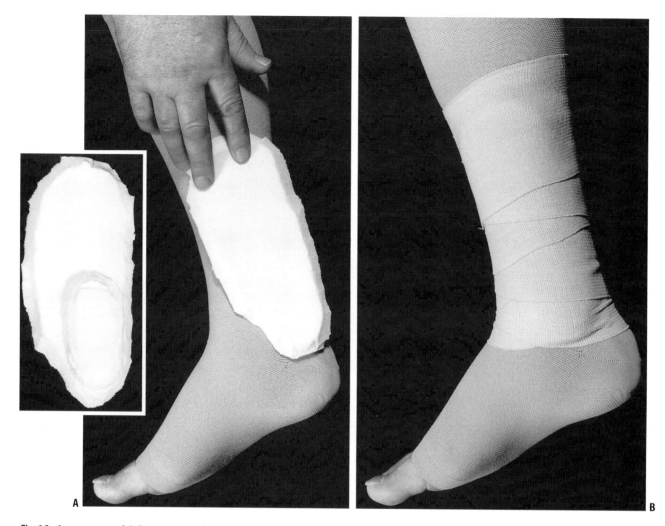

Fig. 6.3. Sponge pump. **A** Soft 1.25-cm latex foam rubber sculpted to fit the area (inset) – applied over 30–40 mmHg stocking. Additional foam may be used to apply more pressure behind medial maleolus. **B** Ten-centimeter elasticized bandage applied tightly over lower part of sponge, easing pressure above.

injection tray is mandatory to accomplish the procedure expediently. The suggested syringe and needle size provide good tactile feedback while the physician is injecting.

Injection Tray

- Prefilled 3 ml syringes with 0.5 ml solution and 25 G needles:
- 1% Sodium tetradecyl sulfate (STS)* for small superficial veins.

- 3% STS for perforators and control points, coded with tape.
- Pre-cut 1.25 cm tape, 8 cm. lengths.
- Cotton fluffs.
- Crepe bandages.
- Sponge.
- Adhesive elastic bandage (Elastoplast).
- Scissors.
- Porous plastic tape (Micropore).
- Old nylon stocking.

A layer of carpeting under each end of the examination table allows the table to slide easily over a smooth floor. There should be a footstool for the patient and a sitting stool for the physician.

It is important that the patient understands the basic principles of venous disease and learns to

---

*Editor's note: Wyeth-Ayerst Laboratories (Philadelphia), the manufacturer of STS, does not advise allowing STS to remain in contact with the rubber stopper of a syringe for longer than a few hours because of degradation of the rubber (personal communication, 1992).

master the use of pressure gradient stockings. Therefore, compression sclerotherapy is not performed at the initial office visit.

Technical Steps in Compression Sclerotherapy

1. Have patient stand for 10 minutes.
2. Make multiple oblique punctures, note flash of blood in syringe.
3. Elevate the patient's leg.
4. Inject the sclerosant and trap with cotton fluffs.
5. Hold the cotton fluffs in place with a crepe bandage applying moderate pressure.
6. Apply latex sponge to the course of the vein.
7. Wrap with crepe bandage in random criss-crossing fashion.
8. Apply Elastoplast to stabilize the bandage.
9. Cover the bandage with an old nylon stocking.
10. Add compression through the use of a below-knee compression stocking 30–40 mmHg).

When all sites have been punctured, the patient lies supine on the examination table with the leg elevated and foot resting on the physician's shoulder to empty the veins. The sclerosant is then injected slowly; it is trapped by digital pressure applied over cotton fluffs placed approximately 5 cm proximal to the injection site. Assistance from a nurse is necessary at this stage. We usually avoid the saphenous vein and never inject the saphenofemoral or saphenopopliteal areas.

If the sclerosant extravasates, it burns severely, like a bee sting. The patient is warned of this and the injection is stopped if there is any suggestion of extravasation. Infiltration of 1% lidocaine solution controls the pain and may reduce the incidence of injection ulceration. Injection sites and areas of suspected extravasation are recorded for future reference.

Large veins on the foot, perforators at the ankle (Cockett I) and medial aspect of the foot and residual perforators after SEPS, can be treated effectively with compression sclerotherapy. A few modifications are helpful. Bandages that incorporate the ankle may cause blisters and sometimes ulceration over the Achilles' tendon because of pressure and friction. It is always necessary to protect this area when treating veins of the foot. Friction on the Achilles' tendon can be reduced by covering the area with Telfa or Tegaderm. Smaller cotton fluffs are used on the foot supplemented with a piece of

1.25 cm foam, custom fitted and beveled to cover injection sites. This method reduces dressing bulk so that a shoe can be worn and allow comfortable walking. Perforators and varices of the foot and ankle are more easily managed separately, after treatment of the calf.

The option of real-time duplex to help locate and guide injection has been proposed by a number of authors. In a time of cut backs and cost control, a controlled trial would be necessary to justify its use. With good preparation and control of edema, localizing the injection site has not been a problem in our experience.

Management After Compression Sclerotherapy

Advice

The patient is advised to walk 2 miles a day, and to return to the clinic if the foot swells to the point that a shoe is unmanageable. The stocking is worn when the leg is dependent and every second night if tolerated. Bandages are removed at 3 weeks. Compression bandaging for more than 3 weeks after compression sclerotherapy does not improve results,[20] but use of a stocking for at least another 3 weeks is always recommended. The patient is told that scar tissue, which heals these veins, is like "slow glue" and takes 6 weeks to set.

Sessions

The patient returns a few days after removing the bandage. If there are residual veins they are injected at this time. Local areas of phlebitis are aspirated. These veins are usually low pressure so unless a perforator is reinjected, 10 days of compression bandaging is usually adequate. We try to minimize the number of sessions. Approximately 75% of the patients are treated in one session, 20% in two sessions and 5% in three sessions. An average of six or seven sites are injected at the first session. Thereafter, two or three sites are injected with subsequent office visits.

Compression Stocking

Most patients who present with lipodermatosclerosis, induration and ulceration require a Class II (30–40 mmHg) compression stocking indefinitely to control residual deep venous insufficiency. This was true after surgical fasciotomy and remains unchanged today, regardless of how perforators are managed. When treatment is complete the patient is advised to "listen to the leg." If the leg feels better with the stocking it usually reflects residual reflux or deep venous insufficiency. In this case, continued use of a compression stocking is strongly encouraged.

Complications

The patient should be warned about superficial phlebitis (usually localized), pigmentation and injection ulcers. Aspiration of thrombus at follow-up immediately reduces pain and reduces pigmentation. Pigmentation improves during the first year, but residual staining may be permanent. It compares favorably with the appearance of a large vein prior to treatment. Saphenous neuritis is rare. Itchiness following injection is a warning of developing sensitivity. Anaphylactic reaction is extremely rare (1 in 10,000).

Reducing the concentration of sclerosant from 3 to 1% decreases the incidence of injection ulcer also decreases success in controlling perforators or large high-pressure varicosities in our experience. Injection ulcers may be more than 2 cm in diameter and tend to occur in the lower half of the calf. Large ones may take 3 or 4 months to heal, as subcutaneous fat and the capillary bed are necrosed as well as the skin. Fortunately, they are not painful and are easily managed by covering the ulcer with Telfa or a plastic Band-Aid under the compression stocking.

Results of Pressure and Compression Sclerotherapy

Healing time and recurrence rate of venous ulcers are time-honored clinical methods of assessing treatment of venous insufficiency as these end-points are definitive. Total CEAP scores are a refinement which allows the clinician to classify severity of venous insufficiency before and after treatment. Air plethysmography and duplex examination for reflux in superficial, deep and perforator veins are useful noninvasive methods of assessment.[13,21–25] Ulcer clinics, which dressed ulcers week after week with healing potions or Unna's paste boots, without reduction of ulcer size, are no longer acceptable from a social or economic standpoint. In 1969, Stemmer[26] showed that a pressure of 40 mmHg at the ankle increased healing rate of venous ulcers. A myriad of clinical trials mounted by Christine Moffat[17,27] with four layer bandaging have established that about 67% of venous ulcers will heal in 12 weeks and at least 75% in 24 weeks. Size and duration of the ulcer were the primary determinants of healing time. Mayberry and Moneta[28] report healing of venous ulcers in 97% of patients who were compliant with the use of a Grade II (30–40 mmHg) compression stocking. Our experience confirms this as it usually takes 1–2 months to heal ulcers approximately 1 cm. in minimum diameter. Larger ulcers heal at a rate of approximately 1 cm. per month; i.e. 5–6 months for a 6 cm ulcer. If we eliminate ulcers associated with ischemia, hypertension, arthritis and arteritis – it is extremely rare to fail to heal a true venous ulcer with pressure.

Mayberry and Moneta[28] reported a recurrence rate of 16% at a mean time of 30 months, or approximately 30% at 5 years by life table analysis, in patients who were compliant with the use of Grade II compression stockings after initial ulcer healing. Fegan, the father of compression sclerotherapy in the English literature, reported an ulcer cure rate of 82% at 4–5 years in 73 patients after compression sclerotherapy[2]. These ulcers had an original mean diameter of 11.3 cm. In 1987, we reviewed 67 patients treated with compression sclerotherapy who presented with venous ulceration. Our patients with complicated venous disease, including those with healed ulcers, are followed at 2 year intervals where we continue sclerosing veins and perforators as necessary. Recurrent perforators are not uncommon (20% at 4 years), but they were easily retreated with compression sclerotherapy. Ulcer recurrence was rare after compression sclerotherapy. Incidence was about 5% through the same interval. Like assisted patency in vascular surgery this may be more a reflection of the persistence of the follow-up rather than the mode of treatment. These figures for compression sclerotherapy compare very favorably with open fasciotomy in the 1980s[29,32] and set a standard for SEPS.

Comment

Large varicose veins and perforators in the calf are easily managed with compression sclerotherapy. Saphenofemoral and thigh reflux should be controlled surgically. We see no place for sclerotherapy of the saphenofemoral junction, whether ultrasound guided or not, as tributaries are not sclerosed with this technique and the surgical option is so easily tolerated. Our only experience with deep vein phlebitis after compression sclerotherapy followed injection of a lesser saphenous recurrence in the popliteal fossa. Dermatitis, dermatosclerosis, induration and ulceration have been known to resolve with pressure for decades.[8,26,28] We should not forget this lesson. Moneta and Porter[33] question whether additional treatment of perforators or valves is necessary at all. In our opinion, treatment of perforators makes it easier for the patient to protect superficial tissue and skin from reflux from the deep system, which behaves like an internal water hammer with calf systole. With the introduction of SEPS, a new surgical option for perforator ligation which is relatively non invasive, there is renewed interest in treatment of perforators. A randomized trial between open fasciotomy (modified Linton's) and SEPS by Pierik[34] demonstrates an advantage for SEPS, on the basis of decreased postoperative infection rate. This may encourage surgeons with little experience in the management of the spectrum of venous disease to enter the field. However, it is well to remember that SEPS is simply another method of treating perforators – an important but relatively small part of managing chronic venous insufficiency. Direct valve surgery or interposition of a competent valve containing segment, is exciting in concept and associated with some good mid-term results when the deep system is incompetent. In the cooler climate of Vancouver we see little need for this more aggressive approach as patients are quite satisfied to wear a 30–40 mmHg compression stocking over the long haul. Our aim is to control venous disease to the point that the leg is comfortable and the skin is safe from ulceration. When necessary, which includes practically all patients with healed ulcers, a compression stocking easily controls residual swelling or symptoms. Compression sclerotherapy is an ideal way to accomplish this end and is easily repeated.

To our knowledge, there has been no trial between SEPS and compression sclerotherapy. One might expect more complete and long lasting control of perforators by SEPS. However, it is clear that a number of important perforators are not accessible with the operation and some are missed.[35] Current techniques must be supplemented by either direct surgery or compression sclerotherapy. Venous disease recurs and veins reform. The most common type of recurrence after carefully performed high ligation is neovascularization – true new vein formation.[15,36] Perforators reform along fasciotomy incisions in areas where they were obviously ligated and divided. Therefore, we control but do not cure. Compression sclerotherapy is appropriate as a primary treatment in cooler climates and certainly very useful in other situations: the single perforator, supplementary to SEPS, recurrent perforators and in treating the elderly patient. In this age of cost containment, it may be that ever-diminishing medical resources are best directed to conditions which treat life- or limb-threatening conditions. In our setting, compression sclerotherapy is certainly less costly to the system. The real question is: what is the best bargain for the patient? The answer may be quite different in Vancouver, Portland and Dublin, Ireland than it is in San Diego, Jackson, MS and Hawaii.

Summary

Symptomatic venous insufficiency is effectively managed through surgical control of saphenofemoral and thigh reflux combined with compression sclerotherapy for perforating veins and major control points. Treatment can be repeated easily when necessary. Patients with edema, dermatosclerosis or ulceration (clinical class 3–6) are ideal candidates for compression sclerotherapy if perforators are present. This method is particularly applicable to patients who are elderly, obese or at high risk for other reasons. An air mattress foot pump is a useful "exerciser" if the patient's walking distance is limited. Compression sclerotherapy with its attendant bandaging, is well accepted by patients in the temperate regions of North America and is an extremely useful tool in the management of symptomatic venous disease both primarily and secondarily after open surgical ligation of perforators or SEPS.

References

1. Sigg K. The treatment of varicosities and accompanying complications. Angiology 1952; 3:355–79
2. Henry MEF, Fegan WG, Pegum JM. Five year survey of the treatment of varicose ulcers. Br Med J 1971; 2:493–4
3. Homans J. The operative treatment of varicose veins and ulcers. Surg Gynecol Obstet 1916; 22:143–158
4. Linton RR. The post-thrombotic ulceration of the lower extremity: its etiology and surgical treatment. Surgery 1953; 138:415
5. Larson RH, Lofgren DF, Meyers TT et al. Long term results after vein surgery: Study of 1,000 cases after 10 years. Mayo Clin Proc 1974; 49:114–17
6. Porter JM, Moneta GL and International Consensus Committee. Reporting standards in venous disease: an update. J Vasc Surg 1995; 21;4:635–45
7. Hobbs JI. Surgery and sclerotherapy in the treatment of varicose veins. A random trial. Arch Surg 1974; 109:793–6
8. Sladen JG. Compression sclerotherapy: preparation, technique, complications and results. Am J Surg 1983; 146:228–32
9. Sladen JG. Complicated deep venous insufficiency: conservative management, Canadian J Surg 1986; 29(1):17–18
10. Hanrahan LM, Araki CT, Fisher JB, Rodriguez AA et al. Evaluation of the perforating veins of the lower extremity using high resolution duplex imaging. J Cardiovasc Surg (Torino) 1991; 32(1):87–97
11. Pierik EGJM, Toonder IM van Urk H, Wittens CHA. Validation of duplex ultrasonography in detecting competent and incompetent perforating veins in patients with venous ulceration of the lower leg. J Vasc Surg 1997; 26:49–52
12. Burnand JC, O'Donnell TF, Thomas ML, Browse NL. The relative importance of incompetent communicating veins in the production of varicose veins and venous ulcers. Surgery 1977; 82:9–14
13. Labropoulos N, Leon M, Geroulakos G, Volteas N, Chan P, Nicolaides AN. Venous hemodynamic abnormalities in patients with leg ulceration. Am J Surg 1995; 169:572–4
14. McMullin GM, Coleridge-Smith PD, Scurr JH: Objective assessment of ligation without stripping the long saphenous vein, Br J Surg 1991; 78:1139–42
15. Neglen P. Treatment of varicosities of saphenous origin: comparison of ligation, sclerotherapy and selected stripping. In: Bergan JJ, Goldman MP (eds) Varicose veins and telangiectasias: diagnosis & management. Quality Medical Publishing Inc., St Louis, 1993: Chapter 9
16. Hobbs JT. Operations for varicose veins. In: De Weese JA, (ed.) Rob and Smith's Operative Surgery, Vascular Surgery, 4th edn. St. Louis, Mosby, 1985, and London, Butterworths, 1985: 278
17. Moffatt CJ, Dickson D. The Charing Cross high compression four layer bandaging system. J Wound Care 1993; 2(2):91–4
18. Sladen JG, Reid JDS. Compression sclerotherapy for large veins and perforator veins. In: Bergan JJ, Goldman MP (eds) Varicose veins and telangiectasias. Quality Medical Publishing Inc., St Louis, 1993: Chapter 12
19. Gunderson J. Bandaging of the lower leg. Phlebology 1992; 7:50–3
20. Reddy P, Wickers J, Terry T, Lamont P, Moller J, Dormandy JA. What is the correct period of bandaging following sclerotherapy? Phlebology 1986; 27
21. Weingarten MS, Czeredarczuk BA, Scovell S, Branas CC, Mignogna GM, Wolferth CC. A correlation of air plethysmography and color flow assisted duplex scanning in the quantification of chronic venous insufficiency. J Vasc Surg 1996; 24:750–4
22. Padberg FT, Pappas PJ, Araki CT, Back TL, Hobson RW. Hemodynamic and clinical improvement after superficial vein ablation in primary combined venous insufficiency with ulceration. J Vasc Surg 1996; 24:711–8
23. Beckwith, RC, Richardson GD, Sheldon M, Clarke GH. A correlation between blood flow volume and ultrasonic Doppler wave forms in the study of valve efficiency. Phlebology 1993; 8:12–16
24. Hanrahan LM, Araki CT, Rodriguez AA et al. Distribution of valvular incompetence in patients with venous stasis ulceration. J Vasc Surg 1991; 13(6):805–11
25. Welch HJ, Young CM, Semegran AB, Iafrati MD, Mackey WC, O'Donnell TF. Duplex assessment of venous reflux and chronic venous insufficiency: the significance of deep venous reflux. J Vasc Surg 1996; 24:755–62
26. Stemmer, R. Ambulatory elastocompressive treatment of the lower extremities particularly with elastic stockings. Der Kassenarzt 1969; 9:1–8
27. Moffatt CJ, O'Hare L. Venous leg ulceration: treatment by high compression bandaging. Ostomy Wound Manag 1995; 41(4): 16–8, 20, 22–25
28. Mayberry JC, Moneta GL, Taylor LM, Porter JM. Fifteen year results of ambulatory compression therapy for chronic venous ulcers. Surg 1991; 109:575–81
29. Hyde GL, Litton TC, Hull DA. Long term results of subfascial vein ligation for venous stasis disease. Surg Gynecol Obstet 1981; 153:683
30. Negus D, Friedgood A. The effective management of venous ulceration. Br J Surg 1983; 70:623
31. Johnson WC, O'Hara ET, Corey C et al. Venous stasis ulceration: effectiveness of subfascial ligation. Arch Surg 1985; 120:797
32. Cikrit DF, Nichols WK, Silver D. Surgical management of refractory venous stasis ulceration. J Vasc Surg 1988; 7:473
33. Moneta GL, Porter JM. Varicose veins and venous ulceration: rationale for conservative treatment. In: Bergan JJ, Goldman MP (eds) Varicose veins & telangiectasias. Quality Medical Publishing Inc., St Louis, 1993: Chapter 17
34. Pierik EGJM, van Urk, H, Hop WCJ, Wittens CHA. Endoscopic versus open subfascial division of incompetent perforating veins in the treatment of venous leg ulceration: A randomized trial. J Vasc Surg 1997; 26:1049–54
35. Gloviczki P, Cambria RA, Rhee RY, Canton LG, McKusick MA. Surgical technique and preliminary results of endoscopic subfascial division of perforating veins. J Vasc Surg 1996; 23:517–23
36. Darke SG. Recurrent varicose veins. In: Goldman MP, Bergan JJ (eds) Ambulatory treatment of venous disease. Mosby, St Louis, 1996: Chapter 19

Principles and Technique of Ambulatory Phlebectomy

7

Robert A. Weiss and Albert-Adrien Ramelet

Introduction

Phlebectomy, first described by Cornelius Celsus (25 BC–45 AD), was performed until the Middle Ages. Not until the 1500s did phlebectomy resume with phlebectomy hooks illustrated in the *Textbook of Surgery* by WH Ryff, published in 1545.[1] Lost again, this technique was rediscovered in 1956 by Dr Robert Muller, a Swiss dermatologist in private practice in Neuchâtel (Switzerland). Dr Muller developed his method,[2,3] modestly calling it Celsus' phlebectomy, and eagerly taught this technique to over 300 physicians who visited his office.[4,5,6]

This cosmetically elegant, safe, effective and low-cost technique allows the physician to remove incompetent saphenous veins (except sapheno-femoral and in most cases saphenopopliteal junctions), major tributaries, perforators or reticular veins, including veins connected with telangiectasias. Specially designed phlebectomy hooks enable venous extraction through minimal skin incisions (1–3 mm) or needle puncture, assuring complete eradication in most cases. Visual evidence of the vein being extracted typically confirms its eradication.

In contrast to traditional venous ligation, the small size of the skin incision or puncture usually results in little or no scar. Performed under local anesthesia, ambulatory phlebectomy leads to greatly reduced surgical risks compared to traditional surgery for truncal (axial), reticular varicose veins and incompetent perforators. In contrast, for these larger veins, sclerotherapy involves risks including intra-arterial injection, iatrogenic phlebitis, deep vein thrombosis and pulmonary embolism, skin necrosis and residual hyperpigmentation. Unlike sclerotherapy, ambulatory phlebectomy prohibits venous recanalization with recurrence. A comparison of advantages and disadvantages of both techniques is listed in Table 7.1.

Indications

This technique provides excellent and definitive results for treating truncal and reticular varicose veins, as long as junctional reflux has been treated and eliminated. When proximal reflux is ignored, only short-term improvement may be realized. Occasionally this is deliberately performed to address an acute problem. Examples include avulsion of a single painful varicose vein in a young mother post-partum who is unwilling or unable to consider more extensive surgery, eradication of a single symptomatic varicose segment or a feeding vein causing a leg ulcer in an elderly individual.[4–8]

All types of primary or secondary varicose veins (truncal, reticular, telangiectatic, perforators) may be removed by Muller's phlebectomy. Most of the

Table 7.1. Comparative indications of phlebectomy and sclerotherapy

	Phlebectomy		Sclerotherapy	
Pudendal veins		+++		+++
Greater saphenous (without SFJ insufficiency)		+++		+
Saphenous accessory	+++		+	
Perforators (Dodd, etc.)		+++		++
Reticular varicosities	+++		+++	
Subdermic lateral venous system		+++		++
Prepatellar		+++		+
Popliteal perforator		+++		+
Popliteal fold veins		+++		++
Lesser saphenous		+++		++
Saphenous accessory	+++		++	
Perforators (Boyd, Cockett)	+++		+	
Foot perforators		+++		+
Dorsal venous network of the foot	+++		–	
Feeding veins of telangiectasias		++		+++
Telangiectatic webs	+		+++	
Postsurgical residual varicosities		++		+++
Postsurgical recidivism		+++		++
Superficial thrombophlebitis	+++		–	

SFJ, saphenofemoral junction.
+, poor indication; ++, good indication; +++, excellent indication; –, not indicated.

procedures are ambulatory, but the technique may also be used in conjunction with other surgical procedures such as flush ligations and stripping of incompetent proximal saphenous veins in ambulatory or bedridden patients.

Regions particularly appropriate for ambulatory phlebectomy include accessory saphenous veins of the thigh, groin pudendal veins, reticular varices (popliteal fold, lateral thigh and leg), veins of the ankles and the dorsal venous network of the foot. Superficial phlebitis may also be effectively and easily treated by Muller's phlebectomy. Following the incision, the clot is expressed and the vein wall may be removed by the hook, assuring definitive treatment and immediate relief of pain.

Preoperative Evaluation of the Patient

A detailed general and phlebological examination is mandatory before any varicose vein treatment. Minimal evaluation includes medical history including general health assessment. Contraindications to local anesthesia or the surgical procedure itself must be elicited. Clinical observation and duplex ultrasound mapping of varicosities with determination of origin of reflux is performed. Correction of insufficient perforator reflux, reflux of the saphenofemoral or saphenopopliteal junctions, must either precede or accompany any attempt to avulse superficial varicose veins. In addition, evaluation of the integrity of the deep venous system and calf muscle pump must also be performed. Hematologic or other laboratory investigations are not normally required, unless indicated by previous disorders revealed by patient history.

Technique

This ambulatory procedure is usually performed in an office surgical facility or the hospital outpatient operating room. An operating table permitting Trendelenburg positioning and availability of good lighting is required. Direct intraoperative support is seldom necessary, but the presence of a nurse or an assistant in the procedure room is helpful to aid with the unexpected. Resuscitation equipment should be readily available.

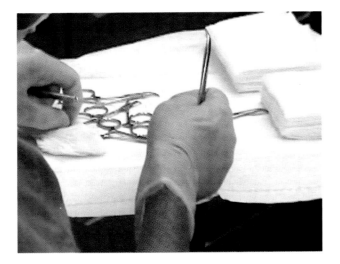

Fig. 7.1. Ambulatory phlebectomy surgical tray.

Very few surgical instruments are required to perform Muller's phlebectomy (Fig. 7.1) and these include: number 11 scalpel or 18 gauge needle to perform the incisions/punctures, mosquito forceps to grasp and avulse the veins and several sets of phlebectomy hooks with different tip designs. The ideal hook to begin the procedure should have a sharp harpoon to engage the adventitia of the vein, allowing its extraction through a minimal incision and a comfortable grip to prevent fatigue. Blunt hooks (boot hook type) are to be avoided as these require a larger incision and more aggressive venous dissection, possibly causing excessive tissue damage.

Two hook sizes are the minimal requirement for most types of phlebectomies. A large hook with a thicker stem is indicated in extraction of larger truncal varicosities and perforators. A thinner hook is necessary to remove reticular venous networks. Several types of hooks have been developed. The Ramelet hook (Fig. 7.2A) is used to initially engage the adventitia from above and the Oesch hook, with a short barb, can be used to grasp the vein from the side (Fig. 7.2B). The traditional "Muller" hook is designed with a large curve to allow grasping the vein from below (Fig. 7.2C).

The Muller hook, available in four sizes, was the first device to be developed. The Oesch hook, available in three sizes, is characterized by a massive grip, although one cannot roll it between the

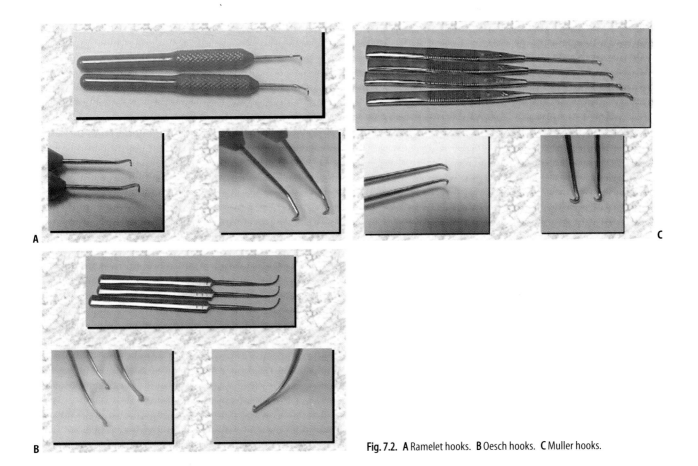

Fig. 7.2. A Ramelet hooks. **B** Oesch hooks. **C** Muller hooks.

fingers. The "barb" or spike end can be used for lateral "harpooning" of the vein. The Oesch hook, like the Muller hook, is very effective for removing larger veins, but less efficacious for reticular veins. The Oesch hook is best to grasp a vein from the side between a finger and the skin.

The Ramelet hook is relatively inexpensive and is produced in two sizes that are easily distinguishable by different handle colors.[9] A smaller, fine hook is designed to remove reticular or medium-sized varicose veins. Another has a thicker stem, which is useful for large truncal and perforating veins. The hook angulation facilitates vein dissection and anchoring. Individual adjustments of hook angulation permit customization to individual surgeon preference. The grip is easy to grasp allowing finger placement near the tip for leverage and precise touch. Because the stem is short, precise movement is permitted. It is well adapted to the operator's hand and does not slip, minimizing the risk of tearing surgical gloves. The cylindrical shape of the grip permits a gentle rolling of the hook between the fingers, diminishing the amount of rotation of the wrist. This handle shape minimizes wrist and hand stress during the procedure as well as during removal of long venous segments.

Varady's phlebextractor combines two devices on one stem. The vein is first dissected with the spatula end, then grasped with the hook end of the phlebextractor. The device must be frequently reversed in the operator's hand. Because the hook end is blunt, "harpooning" is not possible. In our opinion, the spatula-dissector portion has no advantage over using the hook itself as a dissector.

Patient Preparation and Anesthesia

Premedication is rarely required and it should be avoided as it may hinder postoperative walking. Immediate ambulation is the best means of prevention of potential vascular complications. To begin, varicose veins are carefully drawn on the standing patient with $KMnO_4$ or an indelible marking pen. The patient is then placed supine for further marking. Cutaneous transillumination may be helpful as

veins shift relative to the skin surface when the patient changes from the standing to supine position.[10] Local anesthesia, using the tumescent technique, is injected after standard cleansing skin preparation.

Several modalities of local anesthesia have been developed for this procedure. Perivenous infiltration with lidocaine (0.25–1%) or lidocaine-epinephrine is used primarily. Occasionally regional nerve blocks may be utilized. The lidocaine--epinephrine solution can be buffered to a near neutral pH with 8.4% sodium bicarbonate (add 10% bicarbonate to the anesthetic: 5 ml in 50 ml). This diminishes pain from an otherwise acidic solution. This preparation may be stored up to 2 weeks when properly refrigerated.[11]

The maximal recommended amount of lidocaine is 200 mg (i.e. 20 ml lidocaine 1%) and 500 mg for lidocaine–epinephrine (i.e. 50 ml lidocaine 1% epinephrine) for an adult of 70 kg. Larger amounts, however, may be well tolerated using tumescent anesthesia and placement into the subcutaneous area of the leg.[12,13] Use of tumescent anesthesia, in which lidocaine is highly diluted in saline or in Ringer's solution (1/10) offers several major advantages:[14,15] these include decreased pain with injection, low toxicity, advanced dissection of the vein, perioperative compression effect for hemostasis, postoperative rinsing effect and long-lasting anesthetic properties.

Technique

Cutaneous incisions or punctures performed with a #11 scalpel blade or 18 gauge needle (Fig. 7.3) should be vertical along the thigh and lower leg and follow the skin lines in flexural areas such as the knees or ankles. The distance between the incisions varies from 2 to 15 cm, according to the size of the vein, presence of perforators, previous episodes of phlebitis or previous sclerotherapy.

The varicose vein is gently dissected by undermining with the stem of the phlebectomy hook, mainly along its course, slightly perpendicularly to its axis (Fig. 7.4). When freed of its fibroadipose attachments, the liberated vein can then be grasped by the hook and easily removed with the help of a

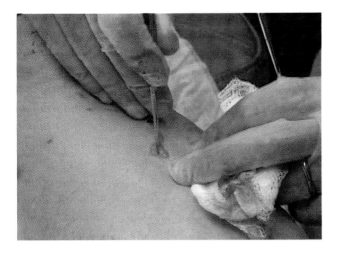

Fig. 7.3. Minimal cutaneous incision with the edge of a #11 blade.

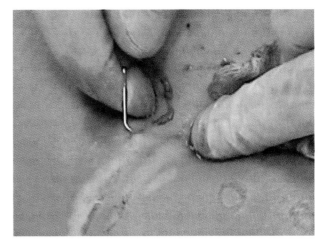

Fig. 7.4. Introduction of Ramelet's phlebectomy hook through the incision.

mosquito forceps held in the nondominant hand. The nondominant hand also grips a sterile gauze and assures hemostasis by local compression of the already removed venous network. The whole varicose vein is then extracted progressively from one incision to the other (Figs 7.5 and 7.6). Associated perforators are carefully dissected and eliminated by gentle traction or torsion.

Some areas may be more surgically difficult than others and require more persistence. These include popliteal fold, dorsum of the foot, prepatellar or pretibial areas, and recurrent varicose veins after phlebitis or sclerotherapy. Hemostasis is achieved with intra- and postoperative local compression. Venous ligation is not necessary. No skin sutures or

Steri-Strips are required if the operator respects the basic principle of a minimal incision (1–3 mm) and good postoperative compression. Usually both legs, even with extensive varicosities, may be operated upon in a single session (60–90 min). Areas in which hemostasis is more difficult to achieve (popliteal fossa, thighs, groin, major perforators) are surgically removed first, allowing intravascular clotting while the patient remains supine. Gentle local compression for several minutes by an assistant may be required.

Sclerotherapy of telangiectasias can be performed immediately before or after avulsion of connecting points to reticular veins.[16,17] Larger telangiectasias may also be destroyed by gentle

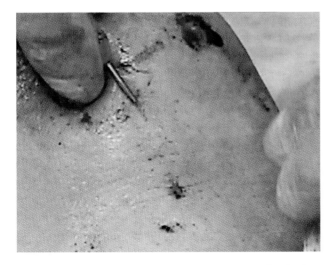

Fig. 7.5. Gentle dissection by undermining with the stem of the hook.

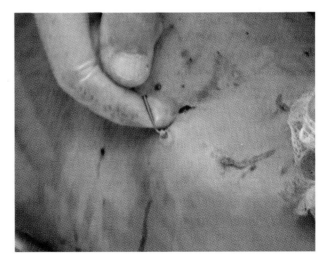

Fig. 7.6. The varicose vein is removed and exposed. Hook is seen harpooning the adventitia.

subcutaneous curettage (scratching technique) with the harpoon of the hook. Debris of these venules that have been shredded by the hook can be removed through tiny incisions.

Once all targeted veins are avulsed, the leg is thoroughly cleansed with hydrogen peroxide. Persistent bleeding of one incision is easily controlled by additional local compression. Application of antiseptic powder is ineffective and must be avoided as it has been reported to induce silicotic granuloma, even years later.[18]

Postoperative Medication and Prophylactic Anticoagulation

Postoperative pain seldom occurs. Nonprescription acetaminophen or ibuprofen is usually adequate for the possible slight discomfort during the initial postoperative evening. Prophylactic anticoagulation is not indicated, as the patient moves during the operation and is immediately ambulatory after phlebectomy with a compression bandage.

Postoperative Care and Bandaging

The compression dressing is an essential and critical step to conclude the procedure. The bandage should be applied by the surgeon or a well-trained assistant. The incisions may covered with a protective film but punctures may require no covering. Overlapping sterile gauzes or absorbent pads firmly attached by adhesive tape or nonflexible strips are then placed over the operative sites. The initial compression wrap to hold the absorbant gauze in place consists of a short-stretch material to achieve a low resting pressure but a high working pressure.

A second dressing is typically placed over the first with the second consisting of a high elasticity (long-stretch) bandage or gradient compression stocking. This achieves compression along operating zones minimizing postoperative hemorrhage

and pain. This second dressing covers the entire extremity uniformly to prevent isolated edema, constriction or pinching between gauze pads.

The patient is required to walk regularly over the first few days postoperatively. The patient is also allowed to work but driving an automobile should be avoided in the ensuing few hours postoperatively since the motor nerves may be not be functioning properly due to local anesthesia effects. This is of greatest concern for local anesthesia delivered in the popliteal fold.

Dressings are changed after 24 or 48 h and the wounds cleansed with antiseptic and sprayed with a protective film. No further dressings are needed at this point if the incisions size is minimal, but compression therapy (elastic bandages or compression stockings) is mandatory for 7–21 more days, depending on the size of the removed veins, degree of treated reflux and amount of hematoma. Short showers are allowed 4 days postoperatively or sooner if the compression is protected by a waterproof covering.

Sclerotherapy of any residual varicosities may be undertaken at 3 weeks postoperation or later. Some telangiectasias may progressively and spontaneously disappear following varicose vein removal by ambulatory phlebectomy, so that if sclerotherapy is performed too soon, it may be unnecessary. Sun exposure should be avoided until the fine erythematous marks have faded or they may become hyperpigmented.

Results

Surgical puncture sites usually clear within several months, but may persist much longer in younger patients with tighter skin. These patients should be warned about this possibility. Hematomas rapidly disappear and pigmentation usually fades in a few weeks. Meticulous application of the postoperative compressive dressing diminishes incidence of bleeding, pain, hematoma and residual pigmentation. The rare complications are discussed below. Figs 7.7 and 7.8 demonstrate some pre- and postoperative results. Good results are also achieved when treating varicophlebitis and superficial phlebitis.

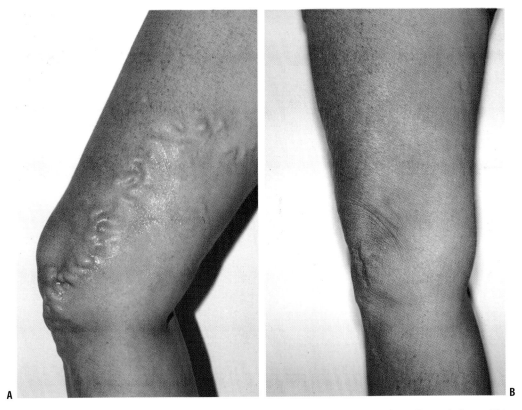

Fig. 7.7. **A** Truncal varicose vein (greater saphenous accessory). **B** Excellent cosmetic result, 5 weeks after Muller's ambulatory phlebectomy.

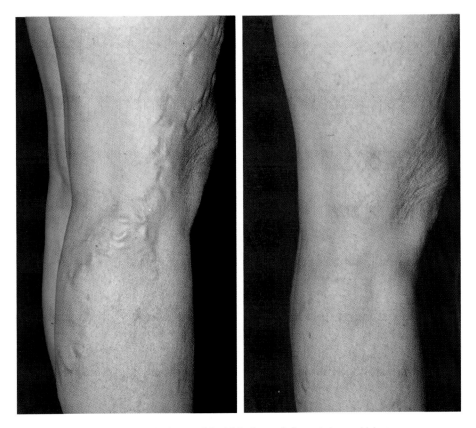

Fig. 7.8. Anterolateral tributary of the GSV before and after ambulatory phlebectomy.

Ambulatory Phlebectomy of Body Areas Other than the Lower Extremities

This procedure may also be utilized for removing cosmetically unacceptable dilated periorbital, temporal or frontal venous networks, and venous dilatation of the abdomen, arms or dorsum of the hands. However, removal of functional veins for purely aesthetic reasons is presently debatable.

Complications and their Treatment

Most complications are benign and resolve spontaneously, although patients must understand the common risks. Relatively few publications have been devoted to the complication rate after ambulatory phlebectomy,[8,19,20] although a recent article summarizes them with fair completeness.[21]

Poor results may be the consequence of inappropriate patient selection, inaccurate initial diagnosis or suboptimal intraoperative or postoperative procedures. A patient with rapid postoperative recurrence of varicose veins or new matting indicates insufficient correction of venous reflux. Complications such as edema, hemorrhage, hematomas or blisters can be attributed to inadequate postoperative compression. Other complications such as scars and matting may result from excessive tissue trauma.

No matter how much experience the operator has, some complications are relatively unavoidable.[4,21] Complications may be classified as cutaneous, vascular, neurological or general, as illustrated in Table 7.2.

Table 7.2. Postoperative complications

Frequent
Cutaneous
Skin blisters (from friction of compressive Dressing)
Transient pigmentation
Rare
Infections
Contact dermatitis
Tattooing with marking pen
Keloids
Silicon (foreign body) granuloma
Vascular
Hematomas
Telangiectatic matting
Rare
Postoperative hemorrhage
Superficial phlebitis
Edema (frequent after phlebectomy of dorsum of the foot)
Lymphatic pseudocyst
Neurological – all rare
Postoperative pain
Concomitant anaesthesia of deeper nerves
Carpotarsal syndrome after improper compression of the dorsum of the foot
Transitory or long-term sensory defect (primarily foot dorsum)
Neuroma

Cutaneous Complications

Transitory hyperpigmentation usually fades in few months without any treatment. Hyperpigmentation incidence is much lower for ambulatory phlebectomy than for sclerotherapy. Vesicles secondary to skin shearing from adhesive tape may induce postbullous depigmentation or transitory hyperpigmentation. Contact dermatitis secondary to antiseptic solutions or adhesives is rare, and this generally heals quickly with topical steroid application.

Infection is highly unusual (4 out of 7,000 procedures (0.06%) in our experience) and controlled by local application of a topical antibiotic without concomitant systemic antibiotics. Keloids almost never occur, even in predisposed patients, because of the minimal size of the incisions or punctures. Hypertrophic scars may rarely be seen on the dorsum of the foot and respond to typical treatment by intralesional triamcinolone injection, cryotherapy or intense pulsed light.

Tattooing with marking pen ink is unusual. We have observed it only on two occasions with no treatment required as the tattoos were barely visible. Silicotic granulomas occur several years after the postoperative application of antiseptic powder. The only treatment is excision of every foreign body granuloma.[18] In one case, an association of silicotic granuloma and necrobiosis lipoidica at each incision site was noted.[22]

Vascular Complications

Hematomas are frequent and depend on skin fragility (Fig. 7.9). Immediate postoperative hemorrhage may occur. We routinely re-evaluate the postoperative dressing after 10–30 min of walking in or near the office, in case tightening or readjustment is necessary. This is particularly important for patients who may have a long journey home. Postoperative compression plays an important preventative role, but individual variations in coagulation can oppose the action of compression. Some patients rarely complain of persistent (months) subcutaneous nodules, corresponding to deep hematomas in the "tunnel" of the removed vein.

Superficial phlebitis of incompletely removed varicose veins or along neighboring veins may occur. This is best treated conservatively with compression and nonsteroidal anti-inflammatory agents but rarely may require incision and phlebectomy of the inflamed vein. Deep vein thrombosis has not yet been reported after ambulatory phlebectomy.

Lymphatic pseudocyst may complicate phlebectomy of the ankle, pretibial or popliteal areas. When a soft subcutaneous nodule develops within a few days postoperatively, this lymph collection may be punctured and drained. The best treatment is compression along with gentle circular massage and, in resistant cases, lymphatic drainage.

Neotelangiectasias ("telangiectatic matting") are the most annoying complication of phlebectomy, but also an unwanted and frequent complication of sclerotherapy and traditional surgical methods. The etiology is multiple and poorly understood. In some cases, it depends on a sudden change of venous pressure or persistent reflux. In others, it may be an abnormal "angiogenic" response to tissue injury. A hypothetical correlation with hormones is debatable.[23] Matting may spontaneously fade after several months. Alternatively, it may be effectively treated with sclerotherapy, intense pulsed light or various lasers.

Neurological Complications

Local anesthesia may diffuse deeply, causing temporary anesthesia of larger nerves, particularly in the lateral popliteal fold. This may induce a transitory paralysis of the foot. Mobility of the foot must therefore be evaluated before the patient ambulates. Tumescent anesthesia minimizes this possibility.

Intraoperative manipulation of a sensory nerve is painful as it typically remains functional immediately beyond the region of local anesthesia. The immediate patient complaint of a shooting pain distal to the phlebectomy site should be taken seriously and the proposed vein avulsion should be terminated. This will minimize the risk of nerve injury. Under general anesthesia the risk of fracturing a nerve is greater because patient feedback is absent. Small nerve injury is more frequent in patients previously treated with sclerotherapy. Hyper-, hypo- or total anesthesia secondary to nerve injury usually resolves in some weeks or months. Neuroma has been reported but is very unlikely.[23]

Long-term Results

Elimination of reflux, varicose vein ablation and cosmetic results are excellent with ambulatory phlebectomy. Patients can expect many years of few visible veins in the treated area as long as the operative indication was correct and venous reflux definitively treated. Other new varicose veins may develop and the patient has to be warned about the evolution and progressive nature of venous insufficiency in a genetically susceptible individual.

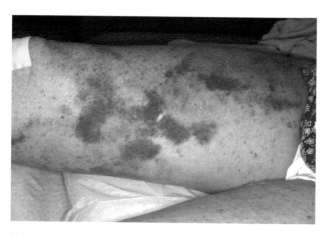

Fig. 7.9. Extensive hematoma in a patient with fragile, actinically damaged skin. These diffuse hematomas disappear completely within few weeks.

References

1. Scholz A. Historical aspects. In: Westerhof W (ed) Leg ulcers. Elsevier, Amsterdam, 1993
2. Muller R. Traitement des varices par la phlébectomie ambulatoire. Bull Soc Fr Phléb 1966; 19:277–9
3. Muller R. Mise au point sur la phlébectomie ambulatoire selon Muller. Phlébologie 1996; 49:335–44
4. Ramelet AA, Monti M. Phlébologie, 3rd edn. Masson, Paris, 1994 (4th edn in press)
5. Ramelet AA. La phlébectomie selon Muller : technique, avantages, désavantages. J Mal Vasc 1991; 16:119–122
6. Fratila A, Rabe E, Kreysel HW. Percutaneous minisurgical phlebectomy. Semin Dermatol 1993; 12:117–22
7. Muller R, Bacci PA. La flebectomia ambulatoriale. Salus editrice internazionale, Roma, 1987
8. Muller R, Joubert B. La phlébectomie ambulatoire: de l'anatomie au geste. Editions Médicales Innothera, Paris, 1994
9. Ramelet AA. Muller Phlebectomy, a new phlebectomy hook. J Dermatol Surg Oncol 1991; 17:814–16
10. Weiss RA, Goldmann MP. Transillumination mapping prior to ambulatory phlebectomy. Dermatol Surg 1998; 24:447–50
11. Larson PO, Ragi G, Swandby M, Darcey B, Polzin G, Carey P. Stability of buffered lidocaine and epinephrine used for local anesthesia. J Dermatol Surg Oncol 1991; 17:411–414
12. Vidal-Michel JP, Arditi J, Bourbon JH, Bonerandi JJ. L'anesthésie locale au cours de la phlébectomie ambulatoire selon la méthode de R. Muller. Phlébologie 1990; 43:305–15
13. Krusche PP, Lauven PM, Frings N. Infiltrationsanästhesie bei Varizenstripping. Phlebol 1995; 24:48–51
14. Sommer B, Sattler G. Tumeszenzlokal Anästhesie. Hautarzt 1998; 49:351–360
15. Smith SR, Goldman MP. Tumescent anesthesia in ambulatory phlebectomy. Dermatol Surg 1998; 24:453–6
16. Ramelet AA. Die Behandlung der Besenreiservarizen: Indikationen der Phlebektomie nach Muller. Phlebol 1993; 22:163–7,
17. Ramelet A-A. Le traitement des télangiectasies: indications de la phlébectomie selon Muller. Phlébologie 1994; 47:377–81
18. Ramelet AA. Une complication rare de la phlébectomie ambulatoire, le granulome silicotique. Phlébologie 1991; 44:865–71
19. Eichlisberger R, Moucka J, Frauchiger B, Jäger K. Ambulante Phlebektomie: das Resultat aus der Sicht des Patienten und des behandelnden Arzt. VASA 1992; 21:453
20. Oesch A. Begleitverletzungen bei den neueren Techniken der Varizenchirurgie. VASA 1988; 17: 18
21. Ramelet AA. Complications of ambulatory phlebectomy. Dermatol Surg 1997; 23:947–54
22. Vion B, Buri G, Ramelet A-A. Necrobiosis lipoidica and silicotic granuloma on Muller's phlebectomy scars. Dermatology 1997; 194:55–58
23. Davis LT, Duffy DM. Determination of incidence and risk factors for postsclerotherapy telangiectatic matting of the lower extremity: a retrospective analysis. J Dermatol Surg Oncol 1990; 16:327–30
24. Deroos KP, Neumann HAM. Traumatic neuroma a rare complication following Muller's phlebectomy. J Dermatol Surg Oncol 1994; 20:681–2

Surgery of the Saphenous Veins

8

John J. Bergan and Jeffrey L. Ballard

The concept that advanced cutaneous changes of chronic venous insufficiency (CVI) are the result of prior deep venous thrombosis continues to inhibit care of limbs with these stigmata. This is true despite the fact that it is known that primary valvular incompetence, not just prior thrombosis, is an important cause of venous ulceration.[1] Dysfunction of the superficial or perforating veins of the legs, alone or in combination, is frequently the only finding in leg ulceration.[2] It is clear, in addition, that the venous leg ulcer occurs mainly from reflux and not usually from persistence of the original obstructive process.[3]

Review of Pathophysiology

When calf muscles contract, there is a rise in pressure in both superficial and deep venous systems. Upon relaxation, pressure in both sets of veins is below that found in the resting muscle. This is due to the protective effects of competent valves preventing downward flow in the venous system. During muscular contraction, pressure in the muscular compartment and the deep venous system rise higher than that in the superficial venous system. During muscular diastole, pressure in the deep venous system falls below that of the superficial venous sytem.[4] The time to refill the veins of the calf after a series of muscular contractions is shortened in patients with valvular insufficiency because of venous reflux. This causes a progressive and sustained increase in calf vein pressure.[5] This pressure, termed ambulatory venous hypertension, is the weight of the blood column from the right atrium transmitted through avalvular abdominal and pelvic veins through dysfunctional limb veins. The peripheral valve dysfunction is often primary and is an important component of venous hypertension. It leads to capillary dilation and increased leakage of plasma, plasma proteins and red cells into subcutaneous tissues. Thus, this has become a target of therapy for limbs with severe chronic venous insufficiency.

The advent of duplex scanning has proven that a majority of limbs with CVI have a marked superficial reflux component. Therefore, correction of this is an essential part of treatment.

Importance of Superficial Reflux

It is an established fact that in limbs with venous ulcers, between 15 and 25% have only superficial reflux[6] (Fig. 8.1). The fact that this can be corrected by a relatively simple outpatient operation allows uncomplicated, effective care. In addition, 20–30% of limbs with CVI have a combined superficial and

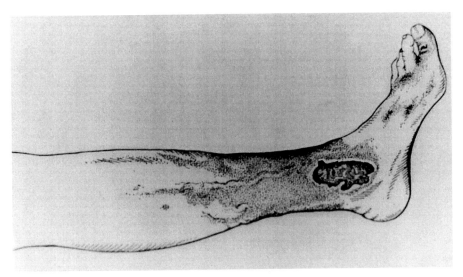

Fig. 8.1. This drawing, from Warren's *Textbook of Surgery*, was used to illustrate the clinical features of the postthrombotic syndrome. Note the accuracy of the artist's depiction of superficial reflux and how this relates directly to the venous ulcer which is the focus of the presentation. Note the accuracy of depiction of hyperpigmentation and the distribution of trophic changes.

deep reflux pattern which can be improved by ablation of the superficial component. It is only a small minority of such limbs, 10–20%, that have isolated deep venous reflux without a superficial component.[7]

Duplex scanning has also contributed to knowledge regarding the interplay of pathologic function of one venous segment upon another. Thus, it has been shown that proximal venous reflux adversely affects distal venous function.[8] This implies that correction of proximal reflux can correct distal venous segment reflux. That fact has been observed clinically after valveplasty.

Another fact has been uncovered by postoperative duplex testing. This is certain to have a profound effect on the care of patients with CVI. This new fact is the discovery that some deep venous reflux is secondary to superficial reflux and that this deep reflux may be abolished by superficial venous stripping.[7] In our experience, in the first 29 limbs with femoral vein reflux which accompanied greater saphenous vein reflux, 27 limbs were found to have the secondary superficial femoral vein reflux abolished after saphenous vein stripping to the knee. An explanation for this is the observation that deep venous reflux is an overload phenomenon secondary to superficial reflux which re-enters the deep circulation through normally functioning perforator veins.[9,10]

Among the first to emphasize the superficial venous system as a cause of chronic venous insuf-

ficiency was Simon Darke of Bournemouth, UK. Over an 8 year period, Darke identified 213 patients with venous ulceration in 232 limbs.[11] These patients were studied by ascending and descending phlebography in addition to hand-held, continuous-wave Doppler ultrasound. Darke found that 39% of the limbs demonstrated only ankle perforator and saphenous incompetence. An additional 35% of limbs had primary deep incompetence usually associated with perforator and saphenous incompetence. The importance of this association in producing the deep venous overload phenomenon is mentioned above. Only 22% of limbs demonstrated post-thrombotic damage and, significantly, 4% of the limbs showed perforator incompetence alone.

Darke's observations made prior to 1992 were remarkably similar to those in the report of the North American Registry of Endoscopic Perforator Surgery.[12] In that report, incompetence of the superficial and perforator system was documented in 98 of 145 limbs (66%). Actual isolated incompetence of the superficial system without deep incompetence was present in 14% of limbs, a figure similar to Darke's observation cited above.

The Middlesex Hospital group has reported on duplex ultrasound examination of 59 consecutive patients with venous ulcers.[1] This revealed that in 42 limbs (53%) there was only superficial venous reflux in either the greater or lesser saphenous systems. In 25 limbs (32%), both superficial and deep venous reflux was present. As indicated above, these limbs, without previous deep venous thrombosis, probably demonstrated secondary reflux and might be expected to have ablation of deep venous reflux after removal of superficial venous incompetence. In this report, there were only 12 limbs (15%) which were probably post-thrombotic, and in which deep venous reflux was the only finding. All of these findings make a strong case for ablation of superficial reflux in conjunction with control of perforating veins.

Obstruction and Superficial Stripping

There is a strongly held belief that limbs with prior deep vein thrombosis (DVT) and presumed obstruction as a cause of chronic venous insufficiency employ the superficial venous system to return extremity blood to the heart. This logic, derived from observations of arterial obstruction and collateral flow, appears to be erroneous in the venous system. Raju observed 137 limbs with well-documented venous obstruction. He found that extensive proximal obstructive lesions could be hemodynamically quite mild. He said, "skin ulceration in the presence of venous obstruction was related to the associated reflux rather than to the hemodynamic severity of the obstruction itself."[13] Raju makes the very important distinction between anatomic and physiologic obstruction. The former is directed by imaging and the latter is difficult to uncover.

The old-fashioned open Linton procedure was done by Raju in 25 of the limbs with severe anatomic venous obstruction. After operation, no worsening of the hemodynamic grade of obstruction occurred during an average follow-up of 15 months. Raju commented on this saying, "…disruption of perforator collateral vessels did not result in a worsening of grade of obstruction." As the operative procedure invariably corrected superficial venous reflux as well as perforator incompetence, there is now hemodynamic proof that ablation of superficial reflux does not worsen limbs with venous obstruction.

Another definitive study by Raju has now validated superficial stripping in the presence of deep venous obstruction. Raju's group compared results of saphenectomy in 51 limbs without anatomic or functional obstruction to saphenous stripping 64 limbs with varying grades of venous documented obstruction.[14] The obstruction was verified by ascending phlebography in all 64 limbs. Functional assessment was based on the Raju technique of arm–foot venous pressure differential; however, preoperatively, the group with obstruction posed a therapeutic dilemma because the saphenectomy and removal of varicose tributaries was indicated, but these veins could have provided collateral flow. Theoretically, saphenectomy could have been contraindicated. Saphenectomy was clinically well tolerated by all patients in both groups. Patients without obstruction, of course, were expected to do well but in fact, objective tests showed that there was no difference in outcome between the two patient groups. Actual improvement in reflux and calf venous pump function was similar in both. When the obstructive grading obtained from arm–foot differential was measured in seven limbs with grade 3 and grade 4, very severe, preoperative venous obstruction, five (70%) had significantly improved obstructive grading after saphenectomy. Presumably, this was the result of elimination of backward reflux flow.

The authors summarized their findings by saying "…no patient in this series, including those with severe preoperative functional obstruction, were made worse clinically in terms of obstructive manifestations after saphenectomy." Furthermore, they added, "the dilation of the saphenous vein, so frequently noted in cases of obstruction, may be related to the reflux reverse flow rather than collateral flow."[14]

In searching for an explanation for the observed fact that ablation of superficial reflux improved obstructive symptomatology, Raju explained that technical factors involved in performing ascending phlebography contribute to the erroneous concept of saphenous systems acting as collateral flow. Deep venous collaterals which are undoubtedly present fail to visualize on ascending phlebography. Contrast material introduced into a dorsal foot vein preferentially flows through the saphenous system. In this way, the contrast fails to adequately opacify the deep system. Clearly, deep collaterals are invariably present in the presence of infrainguinal axial venous obstruction. These collaterals are adequate to withstand the effects of saphenectomy if saphenectomy is indicated.

Saphenous Ligation Versus Stripping

Objectives of treatment of severe CVI should be ablation of the hydrostatic forces of axial reflux and removal of the hydrodynamic forces of perforator vein outward flow. Saphenectomy should be combined with phlebectomy of vein clusters to achieve ablation of high-pressure conduits and excision or obliteration of their target vessels. Fundamentally, only two surgical approaches have been used in treatment of primary venous insufficiency. Discussion of these is appropriate.

In an old Mayo Clinic study, Lofgren examined limbs of patients up to 5 years following high saphenous ligation or complete ankle-to-groin stripping. He reported 94% excellent or good results after stripping compared to 40% after high tie.[15] This, and other old studies,[16] were dismissed by some as being too subjective.[17]

More recently, saphenous vein stripping and stab avulsion was compared to saphenous high tie and mid-thigh perforator interruption.[17] This study found no differences in either patient or physician evaluation of the limbs at 3 years. This report has also been criticized because evaluation was subjective, not objective.[18]

Six prospective studies have compared stripping of the saphenous vein to high ligation.[18–23] The Middlesex group,[18] in their prospective, randomized study, used duplex scanning for postoperative examination of valvular incompetence and photoplethysmography (PPG) as a measure of overall venous physiology. "Both objective tests of venous function as well as subjective assessment suggest that the results 21 months after surgery…are improved by…long saphenous vein stripping from groin to calf."

At Maastricht,[19] stripping and ligation were prospectively randomized. Physician and patient assessment of results at 3 years was supplemented by Doppler ultrasound examination with the conclusion that "…the results remained significantly better for the stripping group.…"

In Copenhagen, Jakobsen's prospective evaluation (confirmed by Carl Arnoldi) concluded that saphenous varices are best treated by radical operation (stripping as compared to high tie) in spite of the fact that the period of disability is significantly longer."[20] In a New Zealand trial, each patient served as his own control, and evaluation was by a single observer at intervals up to 3 to 5 years after operation.[10] Results, judged only by incidence of recurrent varicosities "…were significantly better in limbs from which the long saphenous vein had been stripped." However, saphenous nerve paresthesias biased patient evaluation against ankle-to-groin stripping."

At Lund, conventional subjective and objective evaluation was supplemented by foot volumetry before and after treatment.[22,23] The authors concluded that "this study clearly supports the conclusion that CST (compression sclerotherapy) alone or in combination with high tie cannot replace radical surgery (saphenous stripping, perforator interruption, and stab avulsion) for varicose vein disease with saphenous incompetence."

Only Hammarstein's study concluded "…that the removal of the long saphenous vein *per se* is of no therapeutic value if all perforators have been ligated."[24] However, as he emphasized in a later letter, only "by means of a thorough (ascending and descending) phlebographic mapping of the insufficient perforators…was precise perforator ligation possible."[25] In commenting on this, Darke suggested that with regard to elimination of perforator-induced saphenous recurrences, "…the simplest and least costly and uncomplicated way of eradicating the problem is to remove the saphenous trunk along with the existing and potentially incompetent perforators."[26]

Saphenous Preservation

Despite objective verification of lasting benefit of groin-to-knee stripping, ligation of the saphenous vein at the saphenofemoral junction has been practiced widely. This is being done in the belief that this will control gravitational reflux and preserve vein for subsequent arterial bypass. It is true that the saphenous vein is largely preserved after proximal ligation.[27] However, its reflux continues and hydrostatic forces are not controlled.[28] As stated above:

1. Recurrent varicose veins are more frequent after saphenous ligation than after stripping of the saphenous vein in the thigh.

2. Recurrent varicose veins are more frequent after saphenous ligation and sclerotherapy than after stripping and sclerotherapy.

3. Prospective, randomized trials comparing proximal saphenous ligation and stab avulsion of varices to stripping of the thigh portion of the saphenous vein and stab avulsion of varices has shown superior results of the latter procedure.

In summary, careful duplex evaluation of proximal saphenous vein ligation 2 years following intervention has shown that, "a large group of patients (33%) had developed significant collateral veins at the level of the operative site." Ninety-five percent of the saphenous veins were patent to within 10 cm of ligation and 88% were incompetent.[29]

Finally, in studying recurrent varicose veins, preservation of patency of the saphenous vein and continued reflux in the saphenous vein have been found to be the most frequent elements in varicose recurrence. In patients presenting for surgical relief of recurrent varicosities, it has been found that two-thirds required removal of the saphenous vein as part of the repeat procedure.

Ankle-to-Groin Stripping

Before accurate delineation of site of origin of varicosities by duplex scan, ankle-to-groin stripping of the saphenous vein was considered to be the standard operation which should be done in every operated case. Turn-of-the-century publications had conveyed the belief that reflux was uniformly distributed over the entire length of the saphenous vein.

Now, the object of excision of the saphenous vein is to remove its gravitational reflux and detach its perforator vein tributaries in the thigh (Fig. 8.2). It has been found unnecessary to remove the below-knee portion. Removing the thigh portion detaches perforating veins and communicating veins which enter the saphenous vein.[30] Below the knee, perforating veins enter the posterior arch vein circulation for the most part. There are many venous variations on this general theme of perforator attachments and these variations may be the cause of postoperative recurrent varicosities and persistent perforating veins. However, in legs with severe CVI, the

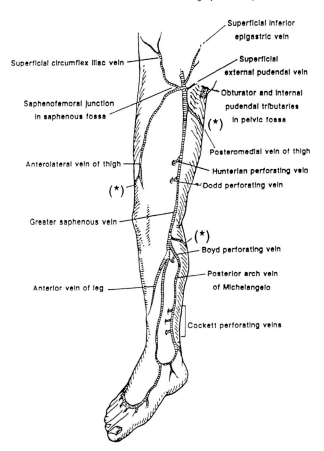

Fig. 8.2. This diagram illustrates the major tributaries to the saphenous vein at the saphenofemoral junction and suggests that simple ligation at this level would leave behind a network of interconnecting veins which would allow reflux into distal veins, thus generating new varicose clusters. The diagram also indicates Hunterian and Dodd perforating veins connected to the saphenous vein in the thigh and how the Cockett veins communicate with the posterior arch vein rather than the saphenous vein below the knee.

perforating veins of the posterior arch system can only be approached subfascially.

Excision of Varicose Clusters

Table 8.1 shows the common patterns of clusters of varicosities and indicates which perforating veins will be detached from the superficial venous circulation by local phlebectomy.

In a significant number of patients, the saphenofemoral junction will be found to be competent and, therefore, can be left intact. When this is true, thigh varicosities often arise from a refluxing anterolateral tributary to the saphenofemoral junc-

Table 8.1. Targets of phlebectomy of varicose clusters

Location of varices	Perforator
Medial thigh, mid-third	Hunterian
Medial thigh, distal third	Dodd
Medial leg, upper third	Boyd
Ankle, posteromedial	Cockett
Ankle, anteromedial	Sherman
Posterolateral knee crease	Unnamed

tion. Judgment will determine whether the saphenous vein should be removed, left intact, or ligated. Stab avulsion of clusters of varicosities derived from reflux from Hunterian or Dodd perforating veins may also remove segments of the greater saphenous vein. Those patients who are found to have lesser saphenous venous incompetence will need to have careful removal or ligation of some or all of that structure.

Superficial Vein Surgery

Following the principle that surgical removal of large varicose veins is superior to sclerotherapy, operation is offered to patients if the findings of CVI are attributable in some way to the varicose veins. Evaluation should indicate that the patient will be likely to benefit from removal of the varicose veins.

As indicated previously, the operation of saphenous vein removal was formerly performed as a stripping procedure from ankle to groin. Often, the intraluminal stripper was placed through the ankle incision. Several problems were encountered using that technique. The most common was saphenous nerve injury due to avulsion of the nerve 7–13 cm below the knee joint crease. Less frequently, the stripper entered the superficial femoral vein through angulated perforating veins. Cases have been reported of stripping of the superficial femoral vein because of this.

As the objective of saphenous vein removal is to detach incompetent perforating veins which transmit venous blood from the deep venous system to the superficial veins, stripping of the saphenous vein need only be done from groin to knee.[30]

Introduction of the stripper can be done, but may be difficult at the medial aspect of the popliteal space where the saphenous vein is relatively constant. However, with preoperative duplex testing confirming saphenous vein reflux, the stripper can usually be placed from above downward to exit at a conveniently placed incision near the knee. Exposure of the saphenous vein at its termination is done through a proximal incision, either in the upper thigh skin fold, or 1 cm above it, where the saphenous vein regularly enters the femoral vein. This incision can be made very short because it is directly over the termination of the saphenous vein. Exposure must allow visualization of the femoral vein 1 cm above and 1 cm below the saphenofemoral junction. This is to verify that no tributaries are entering the femoral vein other than the saphenous vein. Regularly, the epigastric and circumflex iliac tributaries can be seen to enter the saphenous vein and are markers for its location. Less important are the pudendal veins, but of greatest importance are the medial posterior and lateral anterior tributaries. Ruckley advocates dissecting all tributaries to the saphenous junction beyond their primary tributaries in order to avoid leaving a network of veins behind.[31]

Our own practice is to bring each tributary into the incision, avulsing the tributaries as this is done, and applying pressure wherever tributary bleeding is troublesome. While many surgeons advocate clipping or ligating tributaries to the saphenous vein, we find that electrocoagulation is perfectly satisfactory.[32] A good rule is to cannulate, with the internal stripper, each major vein entering the groin incision. In this way, very large lateral anterior tributary veins can be stripped to knee level and even the posteromedial tributary can be stripped to mid-thigh or below. Leaving these large tributaries contributes to recurrent varicosities.[33]

Increasingly, the technique of inversion stripping is being taken up (Fig. 8.3). Our own technique adds a hemostatic pack which has been described elsewhere.[34] If saphenopopliteal incompetence is found, attention must be paid to the short saphenous vein. Because of the specter of sural nerve injury, many surgeons turn to proximal short saphenous ligation rather than stripping. However, the inversion technique described by Oesch[35] has simplified short saphenous stripping and has corrected the problem of sural nerve injury. That injury was found to be associated with an ankle incision and exposure of

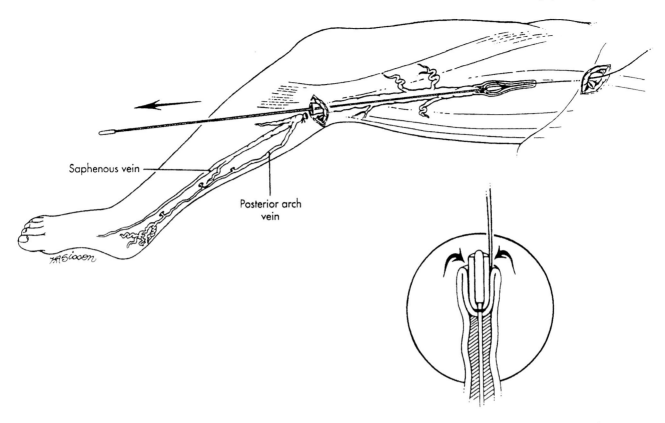

Saphenous vein

Posterior arch vein

Fig. 8.3. In this artist's illustration of the inversion stripping technique, the inversion caused by distal traction on the Codman stripper initiates the maneuver. Although artist's license has allowed the incisions to appear larger than they would in actual surgery, the fact of detachment of thigh perforating veins is illustrated. Note the posterior arch vein and the perforating veins in the leg which do not communicate with the saphenous system.

the short saphenous vein posterior to the lateral malleolus. In any event, imaging and marking of the saphenopopliteal junction must be carried out prior to surgery and, increasingly, duplex scans are favored rather than intraoperative films advocated by Hobbs.[36]

Surgical Technique

In our practice, subfascial endoscopic perforator vein surgery is performed before saphenous stripping. The reason for this is to eliminate any possibility of a subfascial hematoma contributing to postoperative morbidity. The hemostatic tourniquet may be deflated or left inflated during the performance of the saphenous stripping. It has been found that the stripper will pass from above downward under a tourniquet, even one inflated to 300 mmHg. While the stripping procedure has been done with

the tourniquet in place, it is anticipated that most surgeons prefer to deflate the tourniquet first.

The proximal incision is made obliquely in skin lines approximately 1 cm above the inguinal skin crease. Traditionally, the incision is placed in the inguinal skin crease or more distally. However, that placement lacks correlation with the actual saphenofemoral junction. Placing the incision in its proper location proximal to the inguinal skin crease allows a shorter incision to be made. Tributary veins are pulled into the incision beyond their primary and secondary tributaries, and the reason for doing this is that simple flush ligation of the tributaries at the saphenous vein itself allows a profuse network of refluxing interconnecting tributaries to remain. This refluxing network has been found to be an important source of recurrent varicose veins. After complete exposure and excision of the tributaries to the saphenous vein, the femoral vein is exposed proximal and distal to the junction in order to ascertain that there are no major tributaries which enter the saphenofemoral junction or the femoral vein itself.

The saphenous vein is divided and suture ligated flush with the femoral vein. The intraluminal stripper is then placed from above downward. This can usually be done because the saphenous vein in limbs that require correction of superficial reflux has few valves. Valves that remain are incompetent, as proven by preoperative duplex observations. Retrograde introduction of the stripper has the advantage of minimizing the distal incision needed to retrieve the stripper. The distal incision may be placed in the medial aspect of the popliteal space in a convenient skin crease or may pass distally into a cluster of varicosities which will be the site of stab avulsion (Fig. 8.4). Alternatively, the incision used for endoscopic perforator vein interruption may be used as the exit point for the stripper. When introduced from above, the stripping device can be identified when it stops at the first competent valve. Usually, this is in the proximal anteromedial calf. The stripper should be exposed and pulled down so that the vein can be attached to the stripper by heavy ligature. A hemostatic pack can be attached to the stripper at the same location. The hemostatic pack is a two-inch (10 cm) roller gauze. This should be soaked in lidocaine 0.5% with added epinephrine. This is a standard local anesthetic solution available in most operating rooms.

The hemostatic pack has an advantage of acting as a device which prevents vein tearing during the stripping maneuver. As traction is placed, not only on the vein, but also on the pack, the pack serves to bring the inverted saphenous vein into the distal incision. Should the inversion be incomplete, the hemostatic pack acts as an obturator, bringing the accordion-pleated saphenous vein to the distal incision for removal. The saphenous stripping throughout the thigh removes veins tributary to the greater saphenous system. These may be communicating veins on a uniform anatomic layer or perforating veins which penetrate the superficial and deep fascia. Residual communicating or perforating veins would preserve patency of the saphenous vein and preserve reflux within it if the saphenous vein were treated by proximal ligation alone.

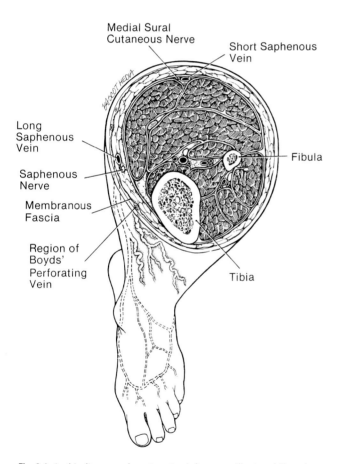

Fig. 8.4. In this diagram, relevant anatomic layers are illustrated. Note that clusters of varicosities appear between the skin and the membranous fascia. These are, for the most part, tributaries to the saphenous system. The saphenous vein itself lies deep to the membranous fascia and superficial to the deep fascia. Note the proximity of the saphenous nerve to the saphenous vein below the knee and how it can be injured either by stripping of the saphenous vein below the knee or stab avulsion of varicose clusters.

Surgery of the Lesser Saphenous Vein

Preoperative determination of the termination of the lesser saphenous vein by duplex scanning must precede surgery of the saphenopopliteal junction. Location of the termination of the lesser saphenous vein is marked on the skin with an indelible marker. Alternatively, if the examination is done at a time remote from the surgery, the termination of the saphenous vein into the popliteal vein must be indicated in the duplex ultrasound report. Should the lesser saphenous vein have an aberrant termination, this must be noted in the report. The lesser saphenous vein may terminate as a femoropopliteal vein, as a vein of Giacomini, or above or below the popliteal skin crease. In any of these events, the termination may be accompanied by a side branch into the popliteal artery or this may be absent.

For surgery of the saphenopopliteal junction, the patient should be intubated and prone or under spinal anesthesia. A generous incision is made, superficial vessels controlled by ligature or electro-coagulation, and the deep fascia opened in the line of the incision. The nerve adjacent to the artery and vein should be identified and carefully preserved. The lesser saphenous vein will be identified between the two heads of the gastrocnemius muscle and gastrocnemius veins identified, ligated and divided. During this maneuver, the knee should be slightly flexed and placed on a pillow or sandbag in order to allow adequate popliteal fossa exploration by relaxing the fascia lata and the gastrocnemius muscles. The vein of Giacomini will be a constant in the upper portion of the incision and this vessel should not only be ligated and divided, but excised as far as is allowed by the popliteal incision. A search for the gastrocnemius veins must be done as these should be ligated and divided.

Opinion is divided on whether the lesser saphenous vein should be stripped or simply ligated. The Oesch technique allows segmental stripping with minimal distal calf incisions. It should be remembered that there is no lesser saphenous vein equivalent to the midthigh Hunterian or distal thigh Dodd perforating veins.

Commentary

While we have subscribed to the theory that all abnormalities should be corrected at the time of initial surgery, not all surgeons have used the same approach.[37] The North American Subfascial Perforator Surgery Registery (NA-SEPS) collected reports from 17 centers in the United States and Canada from 1993 through 1996. In the second report from that registry, the effect of saphenous vein stripping on ulcer healing following subfascial endoscopic perforator surgery could be ascertained.[38] Perforator surgery alone without other concomitant procedures was recorded in 41 operations and SEPS was combined with only avulsion of varicosities in an additional 16. Seventy-nine percent of these limbs had active ulcers and five had healed ulcers. Previous saphenous stripping had been performed in 11 limbs. At 90 days postopera-

tively, 45% of the limbs having perforator surgery alone had healed their ulceration. In contrast, when subfascial endoscopic perforator surgery was combined with stripping, 76% of the limbs had healed by 90 days. This difference was carried out through the first year when 96% of the limbs with stripping and perforator interruption had healed ulceration whereas only 79% of the limbs without superficial stripping had healed ulceration. At 2 years, the results were 100% for the stripping group and 83% for the perforator vein surgery alone group.

References

1. Lees TA, Lambert D. Patterns of venous reflux in limbs with skin changes associated with chronic venous insufficiency. Br J Surg 1993; 80:725–8
2. Labropoulos N, Leon M, Nicolaides AN, Giannoukas AD, Volteas N, Chan P. Superficial venous insufficiency: correlation of anatomic extent of reflux with clinical symptoms and signs. J Vasc Surg 1994; 20:953–8
3. Raju S, Fredericks R. Venous obstruction: an analysis of 137 cases with hemodynamic, venographic, and clinical correlations. J Vasc Surg 1991; 14:305–13
4. Arnoldi CC. Venous pressure in patients with valvular incompetence of the veins of the lower limbs. Acta Chir Scand 1966; 132:427–40
5. Payne SPK, London NJM, Newland CJ, Thrush AJ, Barrie WW, Bell PRF. Ambulatory venous pressure: correlation with skin condition and role in identifying surgically correctable disease. Eur J Vasc Endovasc Surg 1996; 11:195–200
6. Shami SK, Sarin S, Cheatle TR, Scurr JH, Coleridge-Smith PD. Venous ulcers and the superficial venous system. J Vasc Surg 1993; 17:487
7. Walsh JC, Bergan JJ, Beeman S, Comer TP. Femoral venous reflux abolished by greater saphenous vein stripping. Ann Vasc Surg 1994; 8:566–70
8. Walsh JC, Bergan JJ, Moulton SL, Beeman S. Proximal reflux adversely affects distal venous function. Vasc Surg 1996; 30:89–96
9. Gottlob R, May R. Venous valves. Springer-Verlag, Vienna 1986: 150.
10. Bergan JJ. Saphenous stripping and quality of outcome. Leading Article. Br J Surg 1996; 83:1025–7.
11. Darke SG, Penfold C. Venous ulceration and saphenous ligation. Eur J Vasc Surg 1992; 6:4–9.
12. Gloviczki P, Bergan JJ, Menawat SS et al. Safety, feasibility, and early efficacy of subfascial endoscopic perforator surgery (SEPS): a preliminary report from the North American Registry. J Vasc Surg 1997; 25:94–106
13. Raju S, Fredericks R. Venous obstruction: an analysis of 137 cases with hemodynamic, venographic, and clinical correlations. J Vasc Surg 1991; 14:305–13
14. Raju S, Easterwood L, Fountain T, Fredericks RK, Neglen PN, Devidas M. Saphenectomy in the presence of chronic venous obstruction. Surgery 1998; 123:637–44
15. Lofgren KA, Ribisi AP, Myers TT. An evaluation of stripping versus ligation for varicose veins. Arch Surg 1958; 76:310–16
16. Larson RH, Lofgren ED, Myers TT, Lofgren KA. Long-term results after vein surgery. Study of 1,000 cases after ten years. Mayo Clin Proc 1974; 49;114–17
17. Woodyer AB, Reddy PJ, Dormandy JA. Should we strip the long saphenous vein? London, John Libbey & Co., 1986: 151–4
18. Sarin S, Scurr JH, Coleridge-Smith PD. Stripping of the long saphenous vein in the treatment of primary varicose veins. Br J Surg 1994; 81:1455–8

19. Rutgers PH, Kistlaar PJEHM. Randomized trial of stripping versus high ligation combined with sclerotherapy in the treatment of the incompetent greater saphenous vein. Am J Surg 1994; 168:311–15

20. Jakobsen BH. The value of different forms of treatment for varicose veins. Br J Surg 1979; 66:182–4

21. Munn SR, Morton JB, MacBeth WAAG, McLeish AR. To strip or not to strip the long saphenous vein? A varicose veins trial. Br J Surg 1981; 68:426–8

22. Neglen P, Einarsson E, Eklof B. The functional long-term value of different types of treatment for saphenous vein incompetence. J Cardiovasc Surg (Torino) 1993; 34:295–301

23. Neglen P. Treatment of varicosities of saphenous origin: comparison of ligation, selective excision, and sclerotherapy. In: Bergan JJ, Goldman MP (eds). Varicose veins and telangiectasias: diagnosis and treatment. Quality Medical Publishing, Inc., St. Louis, 1993.

24. Hammarsten J, Pedersen P, Cederlund C-G, Campanello M. Long saphenous saving surgery for varicose veins: A long-term follow-up. Eur J Vasc Surg 1990; 4:361–4

25. Hammersten J, Campanello M, Pederson P. Long saphenous vein-saving surgery for varicose veins (letter/comment). Eur J Vasc Surg 1993; 7:763–4

26. Darke SG. Fewer recurrences with stripping. (Letter). Eur J Vasc Surg 1993; 7:764

27. Fligelston L, Carolan G, Pugh N, Minst P, Shandall A, Lane I. An assessment of the long saphenous vein for potential use as a vascular conduit after varicose vein surgery. J Vasc Surg 1993; 18:836–40

28. McMullin GM, Coleridge Smith PD, Scurr JH. Objective assessment of high ligation without stripping the long saphenous vein. Br J Surg 1991; 78:1139–42

29. Fitridge RA, Fronek HS, Dilley RB, Bernstein EF, Benveniste GL. Assessment of reflux in the greater saphenous vein (GSV) two years following high ligation. Cardiovasc Surg 1995; 3:71

30. Papadakis K, Christodoulou C, Christopoulos D et al. Number and anatomical distribution of incompetent thigh perforating veins. Br J Surg 1989; 76:581–4

31. Ruckley CV. A color atlas of surgical management of venous disease. Wolfe Medical Publications, Ltd, London,1988

32. Bergan JJ. Surgical management of primary and recurrent varicose veins. In: Gloviczki P, Yao JST (eds). Handbook of venous disorders. Chapman & Hall, London, 1996

33. Bergan JJ. Common anatomic patterns of varicose veins. In: Bergan JJ, Goldman MP (eds) Varicose veins and telangiectasias: diagnosis and management. Quality Medical Publishing, St Louis, 1993

34. Bergan JJ, Goldman MP, Weiss RA (eds). Varicose veins and telangiectasias: diagnosis and treatment, 2nd edn. Quality Medical Publishing, Inc., St. Louis, 1999

35. Oesch A. Pin stripping: a novel method of atraumatic stripping. Phlebology 1993; 8:171–3

36. Hobbs JT. Perioperative venography to ensure accurate sapheno-popliteal ligation. Br Med J 1980; 2:1578

37. Murray JD, Bergan JJ. Development of open-scope subfascial perforator vein surgery (SEPS): lessons learned from the first 67 cases. Ann Vasc Surg, in press

38. Gloviczki P, Bergan JJ, Rhodes JM, Canton LG, Harmsen S, Ilstrup D. Mid-term results of endoscopic perforator vein interruption for chronic venous insufficiency: lessons learned from the North American Subfascial Endoscopic Perforator Surgery (NA-SEPS) Registry. J Vasc Surg 1999; 29:489–503

Recurrent Varices

9

Simon G. Darke

Introduction: Prevalence of Primary (Previously Unoperated) Varicose Veins and the Incidence of Recurrence

Primary varicose veins affect between 10 and 15% of the adult population of the western countries[1-4] and recurrence after surgery has been reported to occur in 20–30% of cases increasing with time.[5-14] This is found, both in patients being referred for further appraisal, and in patients followed up by systematic review.[8,12-14] This high rate may diminish in the future with improved current techniques in preoperative evaluation and surgical management.

Notwithstanding any anticipated improvement, in practice it is likely that these disappointing results will continue. Unsatisfactory outcomes are distressing and disappointing both for surgeon and patient. In addition, they have important resource implications.[15]

As already implied above, the issue as to how risks of recurrence might be minimized begins with proper primary management. This is addressed in previous chapters. Here the management of established recurrent varicose veins is discussed. These are defined as symptomatic recurrences, for which the patient to seeks further advice. Previous treat-ment is regarded as surgery targeted at the saphenous systems.

Morphology

Rationale and Classification

Management strategy depends on the underlying morphology of recurrence which can be divided into the following categories;[14]

Emergence Through a Second Saphenous System (Either Long or Short)
Strictly speaking, this might not be considered to be "recurrence". It is more accurately regarded as "persistence" or "emergence" in an alternative system. As such, it differs from the categories mentioned below. Nonetheless, it is worthy of note because of the practical implications in its recognition and management. In the author's experience this accounts for about 10% of patients with recurrent varicose veins, the majority of which are from the short saphenous system.[14]

With increasing utilization of continuous wave Doppler and, in selected instances, duplex scanning, preoperative definition of primary patterns of saphenous reflux is now more refined.[16] This has reduced the risk of missing varicosities emanating

79

from a second system, or even worse, operating on the wrong saphenous system. However, these errors can still occur. It is also possible that new reflux can develop after previously appropriate and successful surgery has been directed at the alternative system. It is interesting though that this sequence of events is more likely to occur in the short saphenous system. This is probably because it is this system that poses most of the difficulties at the time of primary evaluation.[16]

Perforating Veins

This pattern of recurrence is characterized by the connection of superficial varicosities to the deep system by incompetent perforating veins. These may arise anywhere in the deep system; the superficial and deep femoral, popliteal vein or calf veins. These connections are frequently multiple. This type of varicosity accounts for about 30% of the total.[14]

Recurrent Saphenofemoral Incompetence

As we shall see, many authors who have studied the morphology of recurrent varicose veins have noticed that persistent or re-established reflux from the saphenofemoral junction is a major cause of recurrence. In one authoritative series it accounted for 90% of cases.[7] A debate still exists, however, as to the mechanism by which this occurs. On one hand there is the view that it is essentially attributable to technical failure at the time of the original surgical procedure. A tributary has been missed, which in due course, enlarges and extends to communicate with distal varicosities (Fig. 9.1).

The alternative explanation is that the junction is actually reconstituted by a process sometimes called "neovascularization" (see Figs 9.2 and 9.3). This concept remains controversial and the distinction is of more than just academic importance because of the implications for the incidence of

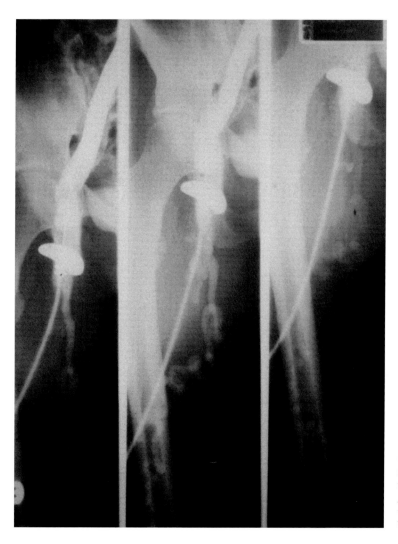

Fig. 9.1. Descending venogram showing recurrence from the saphenofemoral junction. This suggests a missed tributary from the time of original surgery. Reprinted from the European Journal of Vascular Surgery, 6, Darke, SG, The morphology of varicose veins, copyright 1992, by permission of the publisher WB Saunders & Co Ltd, London.

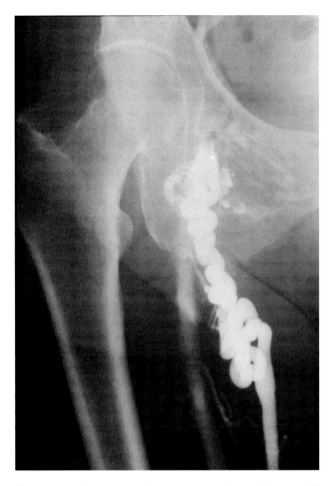

Fig. 9.2. Ascending venogram showing a persistent long saphenous trunk. reconnected to the common femoral vein by multiple mature and serpentine channels typical of neovascularization. Reprinted from the European Journal of Vascular Surgery, 6, Darke, SG, The morphology of varicose veins, copyright 1992, by permission of the publisher WB Saunders & Co Ltd, London.

recurrent varicose veins. If, for instance, the first hypothesis is true, and the major cause of recurrence is due to incomplete saphenofemoral ligation, then meticulous dissection at the junction at the time of primary surgery should eliminate the problem altogether. On the other hand, if neovascularization is the cause, then it may be that no matter how painstaking the primary procedure, some recurrences are inevitable. Let us explore the evidence for these conflicting theories.

The observation that the saphenofemoral junction might reconstitute itself is not new. It was first made by one of the fathers of venous surgery. In 1861 Von Langenbeck wrote:

In one case of very large varix of the great saphena in a young man I had extirpated the enlarged vein in the length of three inches and ligated the upper and lower ends. One

year later I found, in the region of the scar tissue of the extirpation, a new vein channel of the thickness of the quill of a crow's feather, which again joined the both ends of the full functioning remaining saphena.[17]

Subsequently Perthes reported a case on whom he had operated 5 years previously;

A small packet at the site of ligature was extirpated and showed on examination several vessels extending downward from the dilated central end of the saphena. This ended for the most part in a type of blind sac; but one, the thickest, circled closely the site of ligation and communicated with the also dilated peripheral end of the saphena. This, in essence was a renewal of the old observation of Langenbeck, who observed that the trunk of the vena saphena magna regenerated itself after a varix extirpation.[18]

Surgery at the time, of course, was confined to relatively crude saphenous ligation below the groin. Subsequently, Homans introduced accurate and anatomical dissection of the saphenofemoral junction with explicit ligation of all local tributaries.[19] With this came the alternative view that recurrence was largely due to missed veins. This opinion prevailed for many years.[9,20-41]

The possibility that varicose veins might "regrow" was reintroduced by Sheppard in 1978 . He argued that experienced surgeons knew the original groin surgery had been technically complete. This was evident at "redo" surgery by the scarring present at the site of the recurrence. In this large series, many of them operated on personally, he attributed 90% of recurrent varicose veins to further saphenofemoral incompetence in most of whom an adequate flush ligation had been performed previously. On this basis he further postulated the phenomenon of re-recurrence; presented histological data; and made suggestions as to how the problem might be avoided.[7]

Starnes and colleagues in 1984 supported these views based on venography which was stated to show: "...a type of recurrence which can occur even after skilful high ligation, and ascribing all thigh recurrences to a missed venous branch at the time of high ligation is too simple an explanation." In nearly half of the patients the thigh varicosities were communicating with the femoral vein by a new tortuous segment of vein at the site of the previous operation.[42]

Subsequently, Glass has contributed many revealing clinical and animal reports that have shed further light on this problem.[43-46] Among the more interesting of his studies, he describes a series of 10 patients in whom he ligated and excised a segment

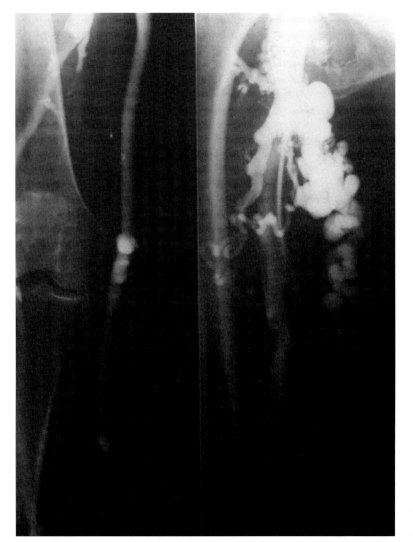

Fig. 9.3. Further example of neovascularization at the saphenofemoral junction with the persistent long saphenous vein.

of incompetent long saphenous trunk in the thigh in order to promote healing of venous ulceration. Once the ulcer had healed, and at a varying time from initial ligation, further surgery with complete excision of the entire saphenous system was undertaken. This included the area previously ligated. The veins were then examined histologically, thus giving the opportunity to harvest serial specimens. This showed that 2 weeks after transection the gap filled with thrombus into which small blood vessels grew. Over ensuing weeks these then aligned themselves (Fig. 9.4). Within a year, they coalesced and enlarged, sometimes into a single trunk with muscle and elastin in their walls resembling mature veins (see Figs 9.2, 9.3 and 9.5).[43]

More recent studies have had the benefits of duplex scanning. Jones and colleagues studied 100 patients with 133 affected limbs with previously unoperated long saphenous varicose veins. These were randomized to flush ligation with and without stripping of the long saphenous trunk. All were operated upon by a single consultant vascular surgeon. When re-assessed by duplex ultrasound 2 years later, neovascularization, defined as serpentine tributaries arising from the ligated saphenofemoral junction was the most common cause of recurrence. This had occurred in 45% of those not stripped and 25% of those that were.[47]

Sarin and colleagues conducted a similar study evaluating the outcome after high saphenous ligation randomized to additional stripping or non stripping. A duplex scan of the saphenofemoral junction was performed preoperatively, at 3 months and then again not less than 18 months after surgery. In 64 limbs comprehensive abolition of saphenofemoral reflux at 3 months after surgery

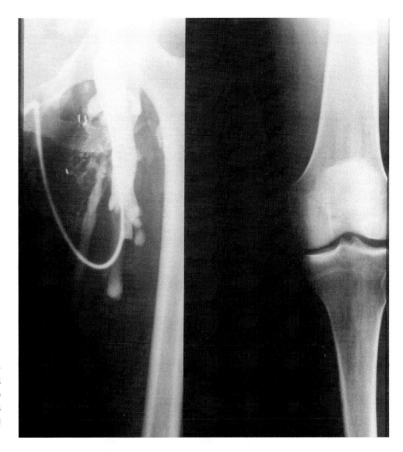

Fig. 9.4. Descending venogram taken 6 months after saphenofemoral ligation with preservation of the long saphenous trunk. Patient referred to author for second opinion due to rapid recurrence of varicose veins. A myriad of tiny channels can already be seen developing between the persistent long saphenous trunk and the common femoral vein.

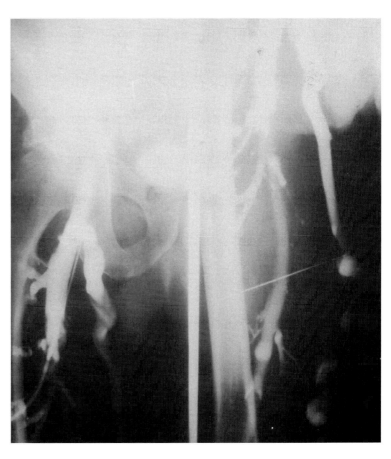

Fig. 9.5. Descending venogram showing a persistent long saphenous trunk and reconstituted saphenofemoral junction. In this instance, several years after surgery, the neovascularized segments have united into a single channel, almost suggestive that the junction had never been ligated. At operation, however, dense scar tissue round the reconstituted junction confirmed that ligation had previously taken place.

was confirmed. In 12 of these duplex scanning showed unequivocal recurrent (neovascularized) reflux at the subsequent 18 month scan. These occurred irrespective of whether or not the saphenous trunk had been stripped.[48]

In summary, the concept that "neovascularization" might occur has been with us for many years, although it lay dormant for nearly a century. The more recent evidence based on clinical observation, histological studies, animal experimentation and now compelling prospective duplex studies would seem to put the issue beyond dispute. In addition, if the "missed tributary" theory is correct then why has it not been possible to demonstrate a reduction in recurrence of saphenofemoral reflux by meticulous groin dissection at primary surgery? Yet this debate has continued. It may seem strange, though commendable, that the surgical profession is more ready to attribute blame to technical inadequacy than to the caprice of nature.

It has to be conceded that both forms of recurrence can occur, and indeed in some patients, there may be a combination of the two (Fig. 9.6). If a tributary or stump of long saphenous is left at the saphenofemoral junction, and with time it expands, becomes tortuous and links by neovascularization with distal varicosities; then an element of both has occurred.

Recurrent Saphenopopliteal Incompetence

Recurrent saphenopopliteal incompetence is more complex. On an anecdotal basis there is evidence that neovascularization can occur in a similar fashion to that described above for the saphenofemoral junction (Figs 9.7 and 9.8). On the basis of the evidence presented above it would be surprising if this were not the case. However, the short saphenous system has significant additional factors which compound the difficulties at the time of primary surgery, thus increasing the risk of inade-

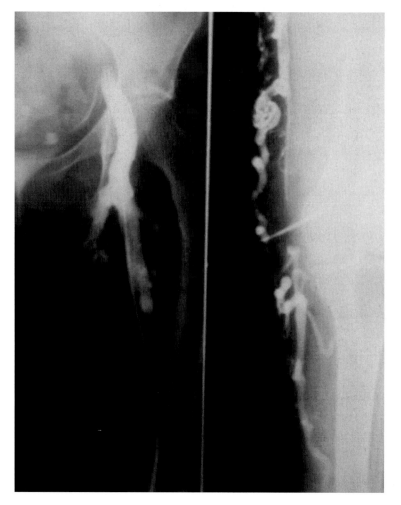

Fig. 9.6. Descending venogram showing a persistent stump of the long saphenous to which are attached a number of serpentine neovascularized segments. At operation the original junction was found to be intact. This therefore would appear to be an example of incomplete previous ligation and neovascularization.

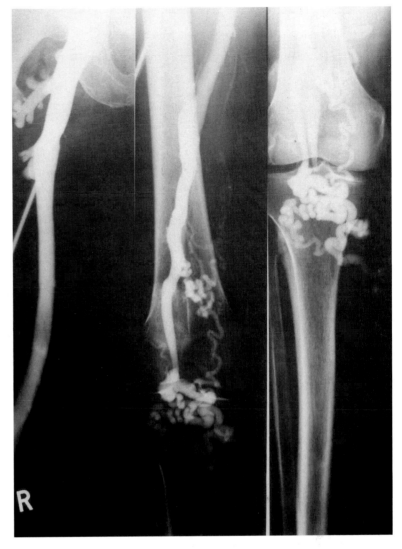

Fig. 9.7. A descending venogram in a patient with recurrent saphenopopliteal reflux and coexistent incompetence in the superficial femoral and popliteal veins. This shows serpentine recurrences of the saphenopopliteal junction strikingly similar to those seen in Figs 9.2 and 9.3. Reprinted from the European Journal of Vascular Surgery, 6, Darke, SG, The morphology of varicose veins, copyright 1992, by permission of the publisher WB Saunders & Co Ltd, London.

quate or incomplete ligation.[49–52] There is considerable anatomical variation at the saphenopopliteal junction. The popliteal vein may be single or double and have varying relations to the calf veins. Furthermore, the saphenopopliteal junction is not always sited in the popliteal fossa but may be above or below it .[51] As a result, there may be difficulties in preoperative as well as operative identification. Additionally, it is not just the short saphenous vein that has to be considered. A variety of veins in the popliteal fossa can be the source for primary or recurrent varicosities. They are the medial and lateral gastrocnemius veins and the vein of the popliteal fossa.[52] For these reasons primary surgical management remains particularly unsatisfactory and poorly investigated.[49–52] There are not even data as to whether or not it is appropriate to strip the short saphenous trunk. Recurrence from the

popliteal fossa remains a significant and largely unresolved problem,[53] and accounts for 10–15% of the total.[14]

Pelvic Recurrence
For completeness it is necessary to mention the occasional case that can recur from a variety of pelvic veins (Fig. 9.9).

Persistent Saphenous Trunk
In addition to the above morphological categories, must be added the question as to whether there is, in addition, a persistent long saphenous trunk. Failure to remove this trunk at the time of primary surgery is known to be a significant contributory factor in the incidence of recurrent varicose veins. A number of prospective clinical trials bear testimony to what is now a widely accepted view.[8,47,48,54] This

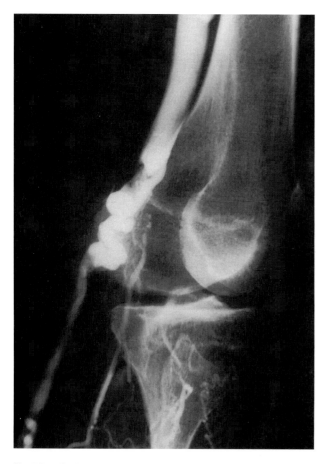

Fig. 9.8. A further example of a reconstituted saphenopopliteal junction with persistent short saphenous trunk.

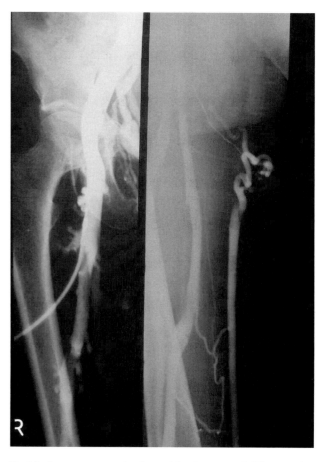

Fig. 9.9. Recurrence emanating from pelvic veins eventually filling a persistent long saphenous trunk.

observation is not surprising from a conceptual standpoint. We have already discussed evidence demonstrating the capacity for recommunication by neovascularization with the femoral vein. To leave the long saphenous vein as a potential link would seem to be a recipe for recurrence. Even if this "recommunication" does not occur, it would also seem likely that the pre-existing perforating thigh or calf veins would form a basis for further varicosities. They may not have been originally removed as a consequence of policy and in some patients there may be an accessory trunk(s). In either event, it is as a vehicle for recurrence.

The position regarding the short saphenous trunk is less clear and it has some important differences. In its upper course it is beneath the deep fascia and could thus be regarded as a "deep" vein.[55] It is not connected to the deep system by perforating veins. The most widely practiced policy is probably not to strip it at the time of primary

surgery because of concerns about injury to the adjacent sural nerve. This problem remains unsolved.

Investigation

Clinical and Hand-held Doppler

Clinical examination can yield some useful information. Clearly, scars may indicate the nature of previous surgery. The distribution of recurrent varices should be noted. Obvious varicosities in the groin region may suggest recurrence from this site, and similarly, perineal veins can indicate reflux from the pelvic veins. Hand-held continuous wave Doppler can give valuable information. The details of its optimal use for detection of persistent or new incompetence from the long or short saphenous system is as for primary examination and has been described in detail elsewhere.[14,16]

The single most important test is to evaluate for the presence of recurrent reflux from the deep system. This is performed by insonating over a convenient and prominent varicosity while the patient is standing. It is advisable to ask him/her to hold onto an adjacent table or chair to minimize body movements that can distort or simulate signals. The patient then gives a brisk cough. A refluxing signal indicates that recurrent groin incompetence is highly likely and that further detailed investigation is usually required. If no evidence of reflux from the deep system is apparent on continuous wave Doppler then the morphology is probably one of multiple perforating veins. Pragmatically, further investigations are not strictly necessary. In terms of operative strategy further information is essentially of academic interest only (see below).

Duplex Ultrasound and Venography

It is outside the scope of this chapter to describe in detail the application of these modes of investigation. In general, however, they provide most of the information required in complex cases with recurrent reflux from the deep system, as demonstrated on continuous wave Doppler.

Skilled duplex scanning can identify the major morphological features classified above and being noninvasive should, therefore, be the next line of investigation. There are a few exceptions that still require venography. The main deficiency of duplex is in identifying obscure and remote points of origin from the deep system. Under these circumstances, signals may be difficult to trace but may be relatively simple with venography. Examples are illustrated in Figs 9.9 and 9.10 which show recurrence from pelvic veins and the distal deep femoral vein, respectively.

A further advantage of venography is that it provides an image easily available and open to

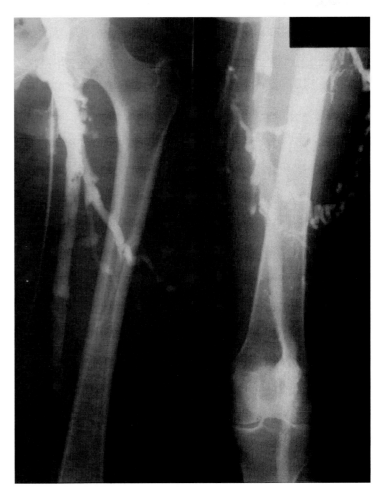

Fig. 9.10. Recurrences from the distal part of the deep femoral vein. Reprinted from the European Journal of Vascular Surgery, 6, Darke, SG, The morphology of varicose veins, copyright 1992, by permission of the publisher WB Saunders & Co Ltd, London.

interpretation by the surgeon. This is an important consideration because a decision may need to be made about the size and significance of a particular communication with the deep system and whether surgical ligation is appropriate. Descending venography is particularly useful in estimating the significance of reconnecting vessels to the femoral vein and the need for re-exploration and ligation.

In some cases where continuous wave Doppler indicates recurrent reflux from the groin it may be assumed that this is due to persistent or neo-vascularized connections at the saphenofemoral junction. There are instances, however, where there is incompetence in the upper valves of the superficial femoral vein and the incompetent cough impulse is transmitted down and out through an incompetent thigh perforator into the superficial varicosity[14] (see Fig. 9.11). It is essential to know this in planning further surgery and it usually requires duplex or descending venography to clarify the situation.

Special Tests of Function

Special tests, such as various forms of plethysmography, are sometimes required in the evaluation of recurrent varicose veins. The principal reason is when previous deep vein thrombosis is suspected and the possibility arises that the superficial "recurrences" are in fact acting as important collateral channels to bypass persisting deep obstruction. Such cases, though uncommon, do occur and it is critical that they be recognized because of the obviously disastrous consequences of injudicious surgical intervention. Details of these techniques are outside the scope of this chapter, but suffice it say that reflux and outflow need to be quantified, with and without a superficial tourniquet, to determine the likely dynamic outcome of surgical ligation of the superficial veins. Impaired outflow, further compromised by the application of a superficial tourniquet, contraindicates any surgical intervention. Although these patients may have a history of deep

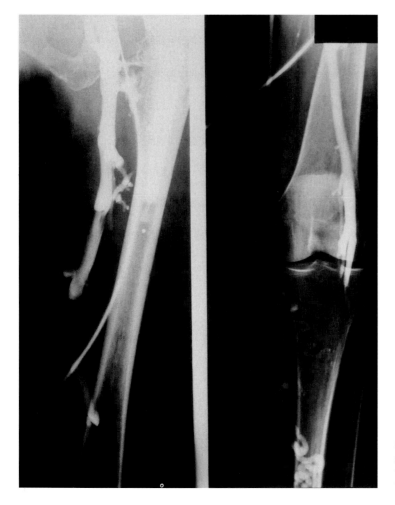

Fig. 9.11. Descending venogram showing an incompetent superficial femoral vein with dye tracking down this and out through a thigh perforator to fill a persistent long saphenous trunk.

vein thrombosis with identifiable changes on their venogram, this is not always the case.

Operative Strategies

Very little has been written about strategies for the operative management of recurrent varicose veins, and even less on the outcome. Therefore, there is minimal evidence on which to base a rationale for treatment. It is necessary to rely on the same basic principles and objectives that have been more widely tested in the management of previously unoperated varicose veins. It is proposed, therefore, that surgery should deliver the following:

1. Removal of superficial varicosities by avulsion.
2. Ligation at source of origins from the deep system.
3. Removal of (residual) saphenous trunks.

To this one might add specific steps to reduce risk of further recurrence. In principle, these would seem sensible objectives but the degree to which they can be realistically delivered will vary in different morphological groups. Furthermore, in some instances, although they may be technically attainable they may not be appropriate. More specifically, the extent and risk of surgery required may be out of proportion to the clinical state and perceived benefits.

We will consider the management in each morphological group.

Emergence Through a Second (Either Long or Short) Saphenous System

This is usually, but not invariably, the short saphenous system. This category is the easiest to treat as the operative strategy is that which would pertain in the nonrecurrent limb. This has been dealt with in Chap. 8.

Perforating Veins

Connections to the deep system, in this form of recurrence, are nearly always deeply situated and in inaccessible sites. The most extreme example might be the distal deep femoral vein. It is seldom, if ever, appropriate to undertake a dissection of such magnitude in order to secure perforating veins at their point of origin from the deep system. It involves large scars, extensive dissection and risk of damage to cutaneous nerves and lymphatics. These perforating veins are often quite small. A conservative view is further underscored by the fact that many such veins have multiple sources from the deep system and run the risk of yet further recurrence. These patients are best treated by simple stab/hook avulsion, which is often a rewarding procedure. However, the patient should be warned that further recurrence is possible, although this may not be for a number of years.

Recurrence from the Saphenofemoral Junction

Missed tributary/inadequate previous ligation. Where this is thought to have truly occurred then the circumstances would seem to be propitious for a satisfactory outcome. A re-exploration of the groin should, by definition, reveal relatively virgin operative territory. The residual untied tributary should be easily identified and secured at its termination on the common femoral vein. Given that, under these circumstances, the patient has no idiosyncratic predisposition to develop further recurrence the longer term outlook should be good. Techniques employed are similar to those described below for the neovascularized groin.

Recurrence from the Saphenofemoral Junction

Neovascularization. This poses potential technical problems of several kinds. The operative procedure may be hazardous. Re-recurrence may occur,[7,14] and there may be little additional that can be done to prevent this from happening.

Dissection of venous structures under these circumstances can certainly be difficult, and on occasion extremely so. There may be dense fibrous tissue around the femoral vein and neovascularized segments may fill the femoral triangle. This obscures vital anatomical landmarks that obviously need to be defined.

This procedure should not, therefore, be undertaken by an inexperienced or unsupervised trainee surgeon. A sucker, vascular instruments and a competent assistant should be available.

A number of maneuvers are possible to facilitate the dissection. A vertical incision has the advantage of proceeding through mainly previously unoperated tissues. This is placed immediately medial to the femoral artery pulsation and extending to just above the inguinal ligament. This does give a less cosmetically satisfactory scar and, thus, if no major difficulties are anticipated, say in a thin patient with a propitious preoperative venogram, then reopening the original scar is reasonable. With a vertical incision, however, the femoral vein can be more easily located immediately adjacent to the artery as it emerges from beneath the inguinal ligament. This is usually above the area of clustered neovascularized veins, thus avoiding the difficulties of bleeding from these before the local anatomy has been fully defined. Once each side of the femoral vein has been displayed it is possible to proceed down to the point at which the reconstituted junction emerges. The key is then to get round this and to define the superficial femoral vein distal to this point. All that now remains is to detach the cluster of veins from the femoral system, either with simple artery forceps or by applying a vascular clamp. Sometimes it is necessary to repair the defect in the femoral vein directly with a vascular suture. The femoral vessel should now be denuded and free from any varicose or other residual connections.

It was first suggested by Sheppard[7] that further recurrence might be inhibited by closing the cribriform fascia with a reflected flap of pectineus fascia, thus covering the femoral vein. Although an attractive concept this has not been shown to confer any advantage in a recent and as yet unpublished study.[56] Forty patients with neovascularized saphenofemoral junctions were prospectively randomized to receive redo surgery for neovascularized saphenofemoral junctions, as described above, with and without the pectineus flap. Clinical follow-up with blind duplex assessment of the saphenofemoral junction at a mean period of 19 months showed no difference in recurrence between the two groups. However, there was a significant incidence of rerecurrence in both groups. In view of this disappointing outcome, other barriers such as the use of Dacron patches[46] are similarly likely to fail, although these have yet to be tested by prospective randomized trials.

This finding is of further significance. It underscores an idiosyncratic tendency in certain patients to reform vein, thus supporting further the theory of neovascularization. At our present state of knowledge we seem powerless to inhibit this. These patients need to be warned and counseled to this effect.

This observation further raises the prospect that in some instances it may not be worth re-exploring the groin at all if further veins are going to develop. This is particularly true where the neovascularized communications are relatively small (see Fig. 9.12). There is, however, an attractive technical alternative to this situation where a significant long saphenous trunk remains (see Fig. 9.4). The site of the distal persistent long saphenous trunk is marked preoperatively with ultrasound. This can then be exposed at surgery and a stripper passed from knee level into the groin where it lodges on the cluster of reformed veins. It is then delivered through the skin with a small stab incision and the residual long saphenous vein stripped up to that point leaving the residual ostensibly trivial connections to the femoral vein *in situ*. If necessary, these can then be oversewn, thus leaving the groin area largely un-

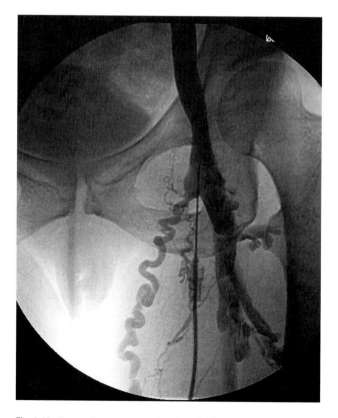

Fig. 9.12. Descending venogram showing trivial reconstituted serpentine veins arising from the common femoral vein.

disturbed. This compromise is a useful variation and can also be applied in the older patient with good results.

Results and Long-term Prognosis

It will be apparent from what has been written above that there is an inevitable recurrence rate in varicose vein surgery; even when the primary procedure has been carried out competently. To a degree this seems to be idiosyncratic. These individuals often have a strong family history and have developed varicose veins at a young age. This should be recognized and the patient counseled accordingly. Notwithstanding this, however, much benefit can be obtained from further carefully planned and executed surgery.

It is also apparent from the above that the patient's future will, to a degree, depend on the morphology of the recurrence. Patients with inadequate primary surgery such as a retained long saphenous trunk or a new or previously missed short saphenous system will do better.

References

1. Coon WW, Willis PW (III), Keller JB. Venous thrombo-embolism and other venous disease: the Tecumseh Community Health Study. Circulation 1973; 48:839–46
2. Widmer LK, Kaufmann L, Hartmann G et al. Organisation der Basler Studie uber Arterier, Venen, und Herz Knankheiker. Schweiz Med Uschr 1967; 97:4–99
3. Widmer LK, Mall T, Martin H. Epidemiology and sociomedical importance of peripheral venous disease. In: Hobbs JT (ed.) The treatment of venous disorders. MTP Press, Lancaster, 1977, 3–12
4. Callam MJ. Prevalence of chronic leg ulceration and severe chronic venous disease in western countries. Phlebology 1992; 7[Suppl. 1] 6–12
5. Hobbs JT. Surgery and sclerotherapy in the treatment of varicose veins. Arch Surg 1974; 109:793–6
6. Doren FSA, White M. A clinical trial to discover if primary treatment of varicose veins should be by Fegan's method or by an operation. Br J Surg 1975; 62:793–6
7. Sheppard M. A procedure for the prevention of recurrent saphenofemoral incompetence. Aust NZ J Surg 1978; 48:322–6
8. Jakobsen BH. The value of different forms of treatment for varicose veins. Br J Surg 1979; 66:182–4
9. Lofgren EP. Treatment of long saphenous varicosities and their recurrence. A long term follow-up. In: Bergan JJ, Yao, JST (eds) Surgery of the veins. Grune & Stratton, London, 1985: 285–300
10. Royle JP. Recurrent varicose veins. World Surg 1986; 10:944–53
11.
12. Berridge DC, Makin GS. Day case surgery: a viable alternative for surgical treatment of varicose veins. Phlebology 1987; 2:103–8
13. Einarsson E. Compression sclerotherapy. In: Eklof B, Giores JE, Thylesius O, Bergqvist D (eds) Controversies in the management of venous disorders. Butterworth, London, 1989: 97–111
14. Darke SG. The morphology of recurrent varicose veins.Eur J Vasc Surg 1992; 6:512–17
15. Campbell WB. Varicose veins. Br Med J 1990; 300:673–764
16. Darke SG, Vetrivel S Foy DMA Smith S, Baker S. A comparison of duplex scanning and continouos wave Doppler in the assessment of primary and uncomplicated varicose veins. Eur J Vasc Endovasc Surg 1997; 14:457–61
17. Von Langenbeck B. Beirtrage zur chirurgischen Pathologie der Venen. Arch Klin Chir 186;1:1–80
18. Perthes G. Ueber die Operatio Unterschenkel varicen nac: Trendelenburg. Deutsche Med Wchnsh 1895; 21:255–7
19. Homans J. The operative treatment of varicose veins and ulcers, based upon a classification of these lesions. Surg Gynecol Obstet 1916; 22:143–58
20. Edwards EA. Anatomical factors of ligation of the great saphenous veins. Surg Gynecol Obstet 1934; 59:916–28
21. Stalker LK, Heyerdale W. Factors in recurrence of varices following treatment. Surg Gynecol Obstet 1940; 71:723–30
22. Glasser ST. An anatomic study of venous variations at the fossa ovalis. The significance of recurrences following ligations. Arch Surg 1943; 46:289–95
23. Wright RB. Some observations on the recurrence of varicose veins after high ligation Glasgow Med J 1949; 30:447–51
24. Foote RR. Varicose veins. Some comments on the repair of surgical failure. Postgrad Med J 1952; 28: 45–51
25. Luke JC. The management of recurrent varicose veins. Surgery 1954; 34:40–4
26. Dodd H, Cockett FB. The pathology and surgery of veins of the lower limb. Edinburgh, E & S Livingstone, 1956
27. Tinnozi EP. Phlebography in the study of recurrence of varices. Minerva Cardioangiol 1956; 4:44–6
28. Elliott JA. Recurrent primary varicose veins. Can Med Ass J 1956; 74:388–9
29. Ross RL. Recurrent primary varicose veins. Calif Med 1957; 87:168–74
30. Brown DB, Graham AG, Toomey WF. Recurrence of varicosity following "high ligation". Scott Med J 1960; 5:88–91
31. Haeger K. Exploration of the fossa ovalis for recurrent varices. Acta Chir Scand 1961; 122:85–92
32. Dodd H. Persistent or recurrent varicose veins. Br J Clin Pract 1963; 17:501–5
33. Nabatoff RA. Reasons for major recurrence following operations for varicose veins. Surg Gynecol Obstet 1969; 128:275–8
34. Lofgren EP, Lofgren KA. Recurrence of varicose veins after the stripping operation. Arch Surg 1971; 102:111–14
35. Li AKC. A technique for re-exploration of the saphenofemoral junction for recurrent varicose veins. Br J Surg 1975; 62: 745–6
36. Tramontano R, Pane G, Passariello F, Aliperta D. Il ruolo delle vene communicanti nella recidiva delle varici post-safenectomia. Minerva Cardioangiol 1983; 38:217–20
37. Corbett CR, McIrvine AJ, Aston NO et al. The use of varicography to identify the sources of incompetence in recurrent varicose veins. Ann Roy Coll Surg Engl 1984; 66:412–15
38. Hoare MC, Royle JP. Doppler ultrasound detection of saphenofemoral and sapheno popliteal incompetence and operative venography to ensure precise sapheno popliteal ligation. Aust NZ J Surg 1984; 54:49–50
39. Lea Thomas M, Posniak HV. Varicography. Int Angiol 1985; 4: 475–82
40. Greaney MG, Makin GS. Operation for recurrent saphenofemoral incompetence using a medial approach to the saphenofemoral junction. Br J Surg 1985; 72:910–11
41. Lofgren KA, Myers TT, Webb WD. Recurrent varicose veins. Surg GynecolObstet 1956; 102:729–36
42. Starnes HF, Vallance R, Hamilton DNH. Recurrent varicose veins. A radiological approach to investigation. Clin Radiol 1984; 35:95–99
43. Glass GM: Neovascularisation in recurrence of the varicose great saphenous vein following transection. Phlebology 1987; 2:81–91

44. Glass GM: Neovascularisation in restoration of continuity of the not femoral vein following surgical interruption. Phlebology 1987; 2:1–6

45. Glass GM: Neovascularisation in recurrent varices of the great saphenous vein in the groin, phlebography. Angiology 1988; 39:577–58

46. Glass GM. Prevention of recurrent saphenofemoral incompetence after surgery for varicose veins. Br J Surg 1989; 76:1210

47. Jones L, Braithwaite BD, Selwyn D Cooke S, Earnshaw JJ. Neovascularisation is the principal cause of varicose vein recurrence. Results of a randomised trial of stripping the long saphenous vein. Eur J Vasc Endovasc Surg 1996; 12:442–5

48. Sarin S, Scurr JH, Coleridge-Smith PD. Stripping of the long saphenous vein in the treatment of primary varicose veins. Br J Surg 1994; 81:1455–8

49. Darke SG. Recurrent varicose veins and short saphenous insufficiency: Evalution and treatment. In: Bergan JJ, Yao JST (eds) Venous disorders. WB Saunders, Philadelphia, 1991: 217–32

50. Darke SG, Foy DMA. Preoperative investigation for uncomplicated varicose veins. In: Greenhalgh RM (ed) Vascular imaging for surgeons. WB Saunders, London, 1995: 401–14

51. Williams AF. The formation of the popliteal vein. Surg Gynaecol Obstet 1953; 97:769–72

52. Dodd H. The varicose tributaries of the popliteal vein. Br J Surg 1965; 52:350–4

53. Tong Y, Royle J. Recurrent varicose veins after short saphenous surgery: a duplex ultrasound study. Cardiovasc Surg 1996; 4:364–7

54. Munn SR, Morton JB, MacBeth WAAG, McLeish AR. To strip or not to strip the long saphenous vein? A varicose vein trial. Br J Surg 1981; 68:426–8

55. Moosman DA, Hartwell SW. The surgical significance of the subfascial course of the lesser saphenous vein. Surg Gynaecol Obstet 1964; 113:761–6

56. Gibbs PG, Smith S, Darke SG. Recurrent neovascularised incompetence at the saphenofemoral junction. A randomised trial of pectineus fascial patching. Submitted 1998

Editors' Commentary

Successful diagnosis and management of primary venous insufficiency requires an organized approach. Thus, it is appropriate that this section begins with a balanced view of the CEAP (clinical, etiologic, anatomic, physiologic) classification. As pointed out by Dr Masuda and colleagues, the classification scheme can be modified to facilitate detailed interchange of data between institutions or to simplify clinical management of patients with a myriad of venous problems. While the general CEAP classification is clinically useful, in fact the details of pathophysiological manifestations of specific anatomic segments have proven to be too unwieldy to enter into patient decisions. Many segments, which enter into classification, are simply not investigated in clinical practice.

One of a number of options for the treatment of severe primary venous insufficiency is described by Sladen and Reid. They represent the many physicians who rely on sclerotherapy to decrease the effects of venous hypertension. They have successfully used compression sclerotherapy to ablate larger calf varicose veins and incompetent perforating veins. Their vast experience, gathered over 20 years, is neatly detailed with technical steps and results well described. It is important to note that successful perforating vein ablation whether by sclerotherapy or endoscopic ligation/division results in similar ulcer healing rates. This fact underscores the importance of perforating vein outflow in the etiology of venous ulceration. We have also noted that recurrent perforating veins or persistent perforating veins may defeat the objectives of surgery when these are detected on long-term follow-up. Sladen emphasizes that saphenofemoral and reflux in axial thigh veins should be controlled surgically and not with sclerotherapy.

Weiss and Ramelet describe principles and technique of ambulatory phlebectomy. Their addition to this volume emphasizes the fact that dermatologists interested in venous pathophysiology can make contributions to care of patients with venous insufficiency. There is no denying the fact that patients and primary care physicians may refer venous problems to dermatologists. The manifestations of CVI are first described in the skin. It is dermatologists who have described the instrumentation of ambulatory phlebectomy.

Discussion of surgical ablation of superficial venous reflux balances the previous chapters on sclerotherapy. This chapter highlights the advantages of complete dissection of all groin tributaries with their ligation well into the periphery, division (not ligation) of the saphenofemoral junction and stripping of the greater saphenous vein to the knee as opposed to the ankle. Inversion stripping of the greater saphenous vein and a hemostatic pack passed into the newly created subcutaneous tunnel greatly decreases the incidence of thigh hematoma. Surgical ablation of lesser saphenous vein reflux completes this chapter.

This section concludes with a thorough discussion of recurrent varices by Mr Darke. Since optimal treatment of this problem first requires an accurate diagnosis and classification, this chapter offers a practical categorization scheme. Clinical examination with a continuous-wave Doppler probe helps to guide the next set of diagnostic studies. Subsequently, surgery can then be specifically directed toward removal of recurrent varices, control of residual saphenous trunks and ligation of persistent perforators. Learning the cause of recurrent varicosities greatly improves the performance of the primary operation. Clearly, the retained saphenous vein in the thigh becomes important to the genesis of recurrent varicosities. Removing the thigh portion of the saphenous vein can prevent this cause, thus decreasing the incidence of recurrent varicose veins.

Section C

CHRONIC SEVERE VENOUS INSUFFICIENCY

Macrosclerotherapy for Patients with Severe Chronic Venous Insufficiency 10

J. Jérôme Guex

Background

Sclerotherapy of severe varicose disease has been discussed but is not fully recognized in many countries, even if it has been successfully used for years in Europe, South America, and more recently, in the USA. The reason for this is the lack of controlled studies leading to a suspicion of poor immediate results and fast recurrences. Potential risks of the method, wich do exist, may also have been overestimated.

Pathophysiology of Chronic Venous Insufficiency

It has been proven that venous valvular incompetence in one or more of the superficial, deep or perforating systems is a factor for venous hypertension (VHT), as are obstruction and poor calf pump function. These latter conditions, which are not commonly observed in primary venous insufficiency, but more often seen in secondary venous insufficiency cannot be cured by sclerotherapy. VHT causes many microcirculatory disorders (such as trapping of leukocytes and fibrin cuffs) leading to skin changes.[1] This is partially compensated by compression therapy, with a correlative efficiency in the cure of skin changes. The decrease of VHT is thought to be associated with a significant improvement of venous ulcer healing because the worst healing conditions are associated with VHT.[2]

Sclerotherapy can decrease VHT in cases of isolated superficial reflux or in cases of deep to superficial reflux. This can be of considerable help in the management of these patients.

Advantages of Sclerotherapy

Sclerotherapy is an ambulatory procedure which does not require much time nor expenses, but a lot of practice. It can be used safely when carried out by a trained physician. Ultrasound guided sclerotherapy (USGS), although criticized in some publications,[3] has been commonly used in the treatment of incompetent saphenofemoral and saphenopopliteal junctions as well as incompetent trunks and perforators.

Some recently presented studies[4] demonstrate efficiency of junctional sclerotherapy with short to medium term follow-up. Regarding recurrences after sclerotherapy, they are *in situ* recurrences, easy to treat again by a simple injection. This usually will not modify the previous venous pattern nor complicate a further surgical treatment.

In practice, two main types of sclerotherapy can be used: proximal (including junctions and main trunks) and distal (including perforators, tributaries, nonsaphenous and periulcerous veins). If the first category of veins can easily be treated by classic surgery (division flush to the deep vein plus stripping plus phlebectomy of tributaries), the second category is more challenging and sclerotherapy must be compared to less simple and more disputed surgical techniques such as stab avulsion, ambulatory phlebectomy, subfascial endoscopic perforator vein surgery (SEPS), etc. But in both cases physician preference for one technique or the other is mainly a personal matter and no controlled study can answer the question, "which one is best?"

Role of the Vascular Laboratory

Patients suffering from chronic venous insufficiency (CVI) must be assessed phlebologically, keeping in mind the possible therapeutic procedures. This explains the growing interest of physicians for duplex technology and the increasing number of such devices in their offices. Availability of duplex ultrasound also allows one to carry out USGS, and this is a major change in the therapeutic approach of these patients.

Duplex scanning is a reliable tool which can accurately assess superficial, deep, perforating and abdominal venous systems.[5] The study provides data on venous patency and competence and allows one to "map" the pattern of varicosities.[6]

Although abnormalities of the superficial, deep and perforating systems can be detected by duplex ultrasound, the respective responsibilities of these networks when several lesions are observed remains difficult to assess. Use of tourniquets during photoplethysmographic (PPG) examination has been successively advocated and then criticized but remains, in our experience, the most simple technique. Air plethysmography (APG) and ambulatory venous pressure (AVP) are favored by some investigators but are much less convenient and not as accurate in the case of lesser saphenous vein insufficiency.

Indications for Proximal Sclerotherapy

The most important criteria in the therapeutic decision is the general status (including age) of the patient. However, the effect of conservative treatment and etiology of venous disease must also be considered.

In young and/or healthy patients, flush ligation and division, plus stripping and phlebectomy of tributaries is an excellent treatment of superficial saphenous incompetence when the deep system is not the main problem. However, in elderly patients where sclerotherapy may be particularly effective because of venous wall sensitivity to sclerosing agents, and where the risk of late recurrence is not a problem, sclerotherapy must be considered, because it can avoid postoperative morbidity.

Very few contraindications to sclerotherapy exist and these are certainly less than those for surgery. For example, ambulatory patients with congestive heart failure, diabetes mellitus or respiratory insufficiency can tolerate a few sclerotherapy sessions better than an operation, even carried out under local anesthesia.

Regarding the response of the patient to conservative treatment and the importance of etiology, it is quite obvious that if a patient with chronic severe venous insufficiency is well controlled with compression therapy, and has no ulcer reccurrence, there may be no use for surgery or sclerotherapy for the superficial incompetence. Respective influences of the superficial and deep venous systems are not always easy to demonstrate and the role of perforators is even more delicate. Indications for sclerotherapy (USGS) are actually similar to those of surgery, with a preference for surgery on large veins and in young patients, and a preference for sclerotherapy for smaller veins and elderly patients.

Importance of reflux should be considered but at the present time we have not found a satisfactory method to accurately quantify superficial venous reflux. Neither peak flow velocity, nor duration of reflux are reliable; however, calculations of volume are reliable because blood flow varies with lumen size.

Indications for Distal Sclerotherapy

Sclerotherapy is the ideal tool for removing the residual veins after surgery, but this must not be its main use. Nonsaphenous networks, perforators and isolated truncular reflux have been successfully treated by sclerotherapy. Periulcerous sclerotherapy has been used for years with excellent immediate results with regard to pain and healing speed. Sclerotherapy of prehemorrhagic telangiectasias (blebs) is of great interest to prevent massive bleeding. A limited distal sclerotherapy can be undertaken in emergency in case of skin changes related to local VHT, even if proximal treatment has already been done. However, cure of proximal reflux must be planned and carried out as soon as possible.

Sclerotherapy of incompetent perforating veins has been presented by Thibault[7] and Schadeck[8] with good results. Results can be quite dramatic when saphenous reflux has been suppressed or does not exist.

Technique and Complications

Guidelines for Sclerotherapy

Details of the technique have been described elsewhere.[9] However, particularities of sclerotherapy deserve emphasis. For instance, concentration of sclerosant must be carefully chosen and progressively increased if the desired result is not obtained after the first injection. It is better to have one more session than too much at one session.

Sclerotherapy of incompetent saphenous veins (greater or lesser) begins at the respective incompetent junction (preferably around 10 cm under the inguinal crease) with 1 or 2 ml of 3% Sotradecol (or the same quantity of Lauromacrogol 400, which is not yet Food and Drug Administration (FDA) approved) with addition during the same session of two or three injections of 1 ml of 1% sclerosing agent along the incompetent trunk. Here, USGS is recommended to accurately define the incompetent junction. According to some authors,[10] it is important to observe venospasm which is associated with an immediate good result.

Main tributaries, such as the anterior saphenous vein of the thigh or posterior arch vein, can be injected with 1% sclerosing agent. The volume injected will vary according to vein diameter, and preferably be split in a number of small injections along the course of vein. In this case, venospasm can be observed without ultrasound and is a reliable indication of the sclerosing effect.

In these dilated, tortuous, pseudoaneurysmal varices, postsclerotherapy intraluminal thrombosis occurs very often and compression cannot avoid it. These thrombi (actually they do not have the same nature as spontaneous thrombi) will naturally soften by the lytic process after 3 to 5 weeks and can be painlessly punctured at that time. Earlier mini-thrombectomies are sometimes necessary if localized pain is severe or if skin viability is threatened.

Sclerosing treatment of nonsaphenous varicose patterns is probably the easiest and most gratifying. It must be organized according to the principle that the largest and most proximal varicosities are treated first. The technique described for tributaries applies for these varices.

Sclerotherapy of incompetent perforating veins must not be carried out before duplex assessment after successful treatment of overlying varicose networks. It has been indeed observed very often a dramatic involution of perforators after surgery[11] or sclerotherapy of refluxing junctions and trunks; probably due to their previous role of drainage of the varicose network. When incompetence of the perforating vein(s) has been established (this point remains to be defined, but reflux longer than 1 s is a necessary criteria[12]) and a sclerosing injection has been decided, it can be carried out under manual or better under ultrasound guidance, for the vein is very often difficult to puncture. A typical treatment dose is 0.5–1 ml of 3% Lauromacrogol 400 or Sotradecol. As indicated previously, compression with semielastic bandage and foam pelotte must be applied.

Periulcerous sclerotherapy is more simple and should be considered in all cases of venous ulcer. This form of sclerotherapy requires a low concentration (0.5%) of injectate. All varices can be injected after appropriate skin preparation, including varices situated inside the ulcer. This technique, which has not been reported as causing to any septic complication, increases healing speed and avoids ulcerous hemorrhage. After injections, the ulcer dressing can be made as usual (we prefer paraffin gauze dressings and/or gentamicin ophthalmic ointments).

Compression

We do not use much compression for sclerotherapy of patients with mild venous insufficiency because we think that accurate concentration and dosage will avoid most post-sclerotherapy problems. However, we strongly recommend the use of compression during sclerotherapy of C4–6 patients. The first reason is that, because of their disease extent, they need compression regardless of the treatment just carried out. The second reason is that compression will help to mollify the postsclerotherapy inflammatory reaction that the patients' inefficient venolymphatic system will not be able to deal with. For example, sclerotherapy of varicose veins included in a lipodermatosclerotic plate (canyon varice) can be challenging, with the risk of a significant recurrent inflammatory process. Sclerotherapy near such a plate will potentially extend it. In these cases, we use a semi-elastic or inelastic bandage with latex foam pads to reduce the curve radius above lesions.

Complications of Sclerotherapy

Specific sclerotherapy complications are related to edema and skin changes. Extravasation of sclerosing agents (especially Lauromacrogol 400; Sotradecol is even more aggressive) during an injection usually causes no trouble in normal skin (except pain). However, in patients with severe CVI, the risk of blisters and skin necrosis is greater. Regarding edema and the fact that the sclerosing reaction is more or less an inflammatory reaction, intrinsic inflammatory edema will not be controlled by physiological mechanisms and must be prevented by compression.

Another complication to keep in mind is venous thrombosis. Some patients with severe CVI have had a previous deep venous thrombosis (DVT). This, in itself, is a risk factor for DVT recurrence.

The cause of the first DVT, if it still exists, is another. In patients with an acquired or primary coagulopathy, the risk of DVT after sclerotherapy has been conjectured[13] but not yet proven.

Finally, the exceptional but severe and feared complications of sclerotherapy are arterial injection leading to skin and/or muscle necrosis and general allergy with risk of anaphylaxis.

Conclusion

Sclerotherapy of lower extremity varicose veins in patients with severe chronic venous insufficiency is a tool whose potential must not be underestimated. Whether it is used to treat the entire varicose network or simply to avoid the bleeding of a telangiectasia, it is of great utility to physicians in charge of these fragile patients. Sclerotherapy is easily available, inexpensive, ambulatory and is quite harmless if carefully indicated and carried out. Main drawbacks are that it has not been validated in randomized clinical trials nor rigorously compared to reference techniques. However, few surgical procedures used in these C4–C5–C6 patients have been evaluated that way and reference techniques are currently in evolution.

References

1. Saharay M, Shields DA, Porter JB, Scurr JH, Coleridge Smith PD. Leukocyte activity in the microcirculation of the leg in patients with chronic venous disease. J Vasc Surg 1997; 25:265–73
2. Nicolaides AN, Sumner DS. Ambulatory venous pressure measurements. In: Nicolaides AN, Sumner DS (eds) Investigations of patients with deep vein thrombosis and chronic venous insufficiency. Med-Orion Publishing Company, London, Los Angeles, Nicosia, 1991: 29–31
3. Goren G, Yellin AE. Hemodynamic principles of varicose vein therapy. Dermatol Surg 1996; 22:657–60 (Letter)
4. Kanter A, Thibault PK. Saphenofemoral incompetence treated by ultrasound-guided sclerotherapy. Dermatol Surg 1996; 22:648–52
5. Myers KA. Exploration ultrasonique echodoppler duplex dans le diagnostic et l'evaluation des pathologies veineuses chroniques. Artères et Veines 1997; 16(5):190–203
6. Guex JJ, Hilbrand B, Bayon JM, Henri F, Allaert FA, Perrin M. Anatomical patterns in varicose vein disease. Phlebology 1995; 10:94–7
7. Thibault PK, Lewis WA. Recurrent varicose veins, Part 2: injection of incompetent varicose veins using ultrasound guidance. J Dermatol Surg Oncol 1992; 18:895–900

8. Schadeck M. Sclérothérapie des perforantes jambières. Phlébologie 1997; 50(4):683–8

9. Cornu-Thénard A, Boivin P. Treatment of varicose veins by sclerotherapy: an overview. In: Bergan JJ, Goldman M (eds) Varicose veins and telangiectasias. Diagnosis and treatment. Quality Medical Publishing, St Louis, MO, 1993: 189–207

10. Marley WA. Ultrasound directed sclerotherapy: 90% closure one year after treating truncal varices with junctional incompetence. Presentation 11th Annual Meeting NASP, Palm Desert, CA (Abstract)

11. Campbell WA, West A. Duplex ultrasound audit of operative treatment of primary varicose veins. Phlebology 1995; Suppl 1: 407–9

12. Laroche JP, Guex JJ, Coupe M, Muller G, Dauzat M, Janbon C. Exploration par echo-doppler des perforantes jambieres. Phlébologie 1997; 50(4):669–77

13. Thiollet M, Lajou J. Thrombose veineuse profonde sclerose et thrombophilie: a propos de deux observations. Acta Med Int Angiol 1998; 242:4854–6

Surgery of Perforating Veins

Jeffrey M. Rhodes and Peter Gloviczki

Few topics have attracted as much attention on venous disease as ligation of incompetent perforator veins. Debate has intensified in the past decade because of the introduction of a new, minimally invasive technique to interrupt incompetent perforators. Subfascial endoscopic perforator vein surgery (SEPS) has advantages over open techniques of perforator ligation. Wound complications are less, hospitalization is not required and a better operation can be performed under visual control of the endoscope, placed in the subfascial space. SEPS has emerged as a useful tool to fight venous ulceration, a disabling condition, that nonoperative management has failed to control effectively.

This chapter will review evidence supporting the role of perforators in chronic venous disease. Surgical indications, preoperative patient evaluation and review of open and endoscopic techniques for interruption of perforators are discussed. Finally, available data on efficacy of perforator vein interruption is summarized.

Pathophysiology of Perforating Veins

Thorough knowledge of the anatomy of perforating veins[1] is essential to understand their hemodynamic effects. The reader is referred to Chap. 4 for a complete review of pertinent venous anatomy. Although pathophysiology of chronic venous insufficiency (CVI) is also reviewed by Bergan and Ballard in this volume (Chap. 3), points specific to the hemodynamic effects of incompetent perforating veins will be emphasized here.

While the pathophysiology CVI at the cellular level remains controversial, and several theories have expert supporters, most authors agree that ambulatory venous hypertension is the most important factor responsible for signs and symptoms of chronic venous disease. Reflux of venous blood due to valvular incompetence and calf muscle pump failure are the two most important causes of venous hypertension. Linton,[2] and later Cockett,[3,4] emphasized the key role incompetence of calf perforating veins had in the genesis of ambulatory venous hypertension. Perforator vein incompetence can raise pressures in the supra-malleolar venous network well above 100 mmHg during calf muscle contraction, a phenomenon described by Negus using the analogy of a "broken bellows".[5] The importance of incompetent perforators is supported by the observation, that skin changes and venous ulcers almost always develop in the gaiter area of the leg, above the medial malleolus, where large incompetent medial perforating veins are located.

Most patients with CVI have multisystem venous incompetence.[6–10] In the North American Subfascial

Endoscopic Perforator Surgery (NASEPS) registry, 72% of the patients with advanced CVI had associated deep venous reflux or obstruction.[11] In one fourth of patients, however, only perforator and/or superficial incompetence was observed, with a normal deep system. The role of the superficial system is important and it is emphasized in a much quoted report from the Middlesex Hospital, where 53% of 79 limbs with venous ulcers had normal deep veins, without any incompetence.[12] Unfortunately, the role of perforating veins in this study was not investigated.

Presence of incompetent perforating veins in most patients with venous ulcers is acknowledged even by those who do not attribute much hemodynamic significance to them.[13] In three reports, that included a variety of medical and surgical patients with venous ulcers, the prevalence of incompetent perforating veins, investigated with duplex, was between 56 and 63%.[8,10,14]

The presence of incompetent perforators, however, does not necessarily mean that they primarily contribute to the pathogenesis of venous ulcers; a key point of much controversy. Evidence, however, has accumulated to support those who favor perforator interruption. Using Doppler ultrasound and ambulatory venous pressure measurements to assess functional significance of incompetent perforating veins, Zukowski and Nicolaides found that 70% of incompetent perforators were of moderate or major hemodynamic significance.[15] These authors also confirmed that hemodynamic deterioration caused by incompetent perforators correlated with the severity of CVI. Using duplex scanning, Labrapoulos in a recent report also found good correlation between the number and size of incompetent perforating veins and severity of CVI. Data on hemodynamic improvement following perforator ligation, an important aspect to prove efficacy, will be discussed later in this chapter.

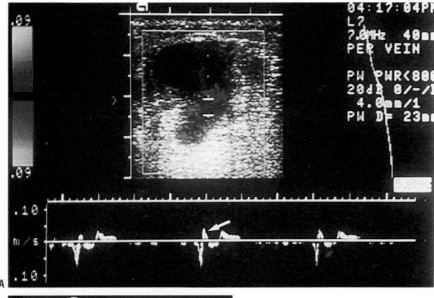

Fig. 11.1. A Color Doppler and spectral tracing of an enlarged incompetent perforating vein. Spectral analysis demonstrates bidirectional flow (arrow). Color Doppler image shows blue indicating superficial to deep flow with augmentation. **B** With release of augmentation perforator valve incompetence is shown by the color change to red. (From Gloviczki P, Lewis BD, Lindsey JR, McKusick. Preoperative evaluation of chronic venous insufficiency with Duplex scanning and venography. In: Gloviczki P, Bergan JJ (eds) Atlas of endoscopic perforator vein surgery, Springer-Verlag, London, 1998: 81–91 with permission.)

Indications for Perforator Interruption

In good risk patients with clinical class 4, 5 or 6 disease (lipodermatosclerosis, healed or active ulceration), the presence of incompetent perforators are an indication for surgical treatment. Contraindications include nonambulatory or high-risk patients, associated chronic arterial occlusive disease, infected ulcer or morbid obesity. Diabetes, rheumatoid arthritis or scleroderma are relative contraindications. Patients with previous perforator interruption, extensive skin changes or large legs may not be suitable for SEPS.

Preoperative Evaluation

Potential candidates for perforator interruption should undergo preoperative duplex scanning to document incompetence of perforator veins in addition to incompetence or obstruction of the deep system (Fig. 11.1A, B).[16] Incompetence of the greater or lesser saphenous vein should also be confirmed during the same examination. We reserve contrast phlebography (Fig. 11.2) for patients with underlying occlusive disease or for those who are candidates for deep venous reconstruction. Preoperative mapping of incompetent medial perforators is performed the day before surgery. This test is done with the patient on a tilted examination table at a 60° upright position with nonweight bearing of the affected extremity. Perforator incompetence is defined by outward flow that is greater than 0.5 s during the relaxation phase after release of manual compression. Using color duplex scanning, the change in blood flow direction can be easily confirmed by change in color. Duplex scanning will miss small perforating veins, but it has 100% specificity and the highest sensitivity of all diagnostic tests to predict the site of incompetent perforating veins.[17,18]

The advantage of strain gauge or air plethysmography in addition to duplex ultrasound is that it helps to define degree of overall incompetence and exclude any venous outflow obstruction. These modalities are also suitable to assess calf muscle

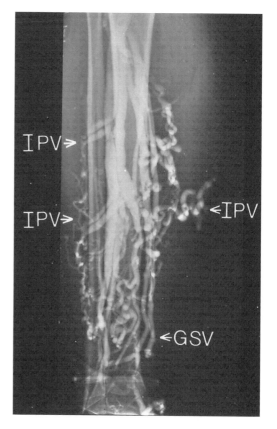

Fig. 11.2. Ascending venogram in anteroposterior projection of the right calf of a 41-year-old female with nonhealing venous ulcer due to primary valvular incompetence. Note medial and lateral incompetent perforators (IPV) filling the superficial system with contrast. GSV, greater saphenous vein. (From Gloviczki P, Lewis BD, Lindsey JR, McKusick. Preoperative evaluation of chronic venous insufficiency with duplex scanning and venography. In: Gloviczki P, Bergan JJ (eds) Atlas of endoscopic perforator vein surgery, Springer-Verlag, London, 1998: 81–91 with permission.)

pump function and to confirm hemodynamic improvement following SEPS.

Surgical Techniques

Open Technique of Perforator Interruption

The classic Linton operation that included a long medial, anterolateral and posterolateral calf incision, is not performed anymore.[2] Indeed, Linton, himself, in an article published in 1953 advocated the use of a long medial skin incision from the ankle to the knee only to interrupt the medial and the posterior perforating veins.[19] His original operation also included stripping of the greater and lesser saphenous veins and excision of a portion of the deep fascia. He also suggested, for treatment of valvular incompetence of the deep veins, ligation of the proximal superficial femoral vein. Wound complications caused by the long medial incision, however, were frequent and hospitalization of these patients was prolonged. In addition, ligation of the superficial femoral vein increased the risk of acute deep venous thrombosis.

Modification of the classic open technique focused on using shorter skin incisions to decrease wound complications.[20–24] Unfortunately, this resulted in less complete interruption of incompetent perforators and still did not significantly decrease the degree of wound problems. Another modification, suggested by Cockett,[3,4] was interruption of perforating veins above the deep fascia, a technique that is distinctly different from subfascial ligation suggested by Linton. DePalma reported the best results by using multiple, parallel incisions placed along skin lines of the calf to access and ligate perforating veins at different levels above and below the fascia (Fig. 11.3).[22,25] This operation was combined with stripping of the greater saphenous vein, removal of varicose veins ulcer, excision and skin grafting.

To further decrease wound complications, additional techniques have been developed to interrupt incompetent perforating veins from incisions made at sites remote from diseased skin. Edwards, in 1976,[26] designed a device called a phlebotome, which was inserted through a short incision made just distal to the knee into the subfascial space (Fig. 11.4). The instrument was advanced to the level of the medial malleolus and medial perforating veins were blindly divided. While DePalma reported good results using this technique, it is obvious that paratibial perforating veins that lie close to the tibia or that are positioned under the fascia of the deep posterior compartment cannot be interrupted using this technique.

Additional techniques of open perforator ligation include the use of stab wounds and blind avulsion using hooks. Accuracy of this operation can be improved if preoperative duplex scanning is used for mapping. Another technique that has been suggested to interrupt perforating veins without skin incisions is to place sutures around the perforator and ligate them through the skin guided by preoperative mapping. The technique of perforator

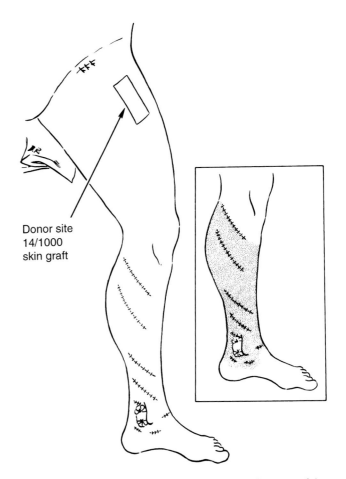

Donor site
14/1000
skin graft

Fig. 11.3. Linton operation modified by DePalma. Note the extent of the area which is dissected as shown in the shaded inset. Also note the submalleolar skin line incisions, used for interruption of the Cockett I perforator. (From DePalma RG, Surgical therapy for venous stasis ulcers. Surgery 1975; 76:910–17, with permission.)

occlusion using sclerotherapy to ablate perforating veins is discussed in Chap. 6.

Technique Of Subfascial Endoscopic Perforator Vein Surgery

SEPS originated from Germany and was reported first in 1985 by Hauer.[27] Since its introduction, two main techniques for SEPS have emerged. The first followed the original work of Hauer,[27] Fischer and Sattler[28,29] and was further developed by Wittens and Pierik[30,32] and in the United States by Bergan and his group.[33–35] This technique, which is discussed further in Chap. 13, uses a single scope for both viewing and for working (Figs 11.5 and 11.6). Perforating veins are either electrocauterized or they are clipped and divided. Until recently, instru-

Fig. 11.4. Excision and dissection of a deep ulcer prior to extrafascial shearing operation. Note the submalleolar access incisions which allow division of the most distal perforating veins below the malleolus. (From DePalma RG, Surgical therapy for venous stasis ulcers. Surgery 1975; 76:910–17, with permission.)

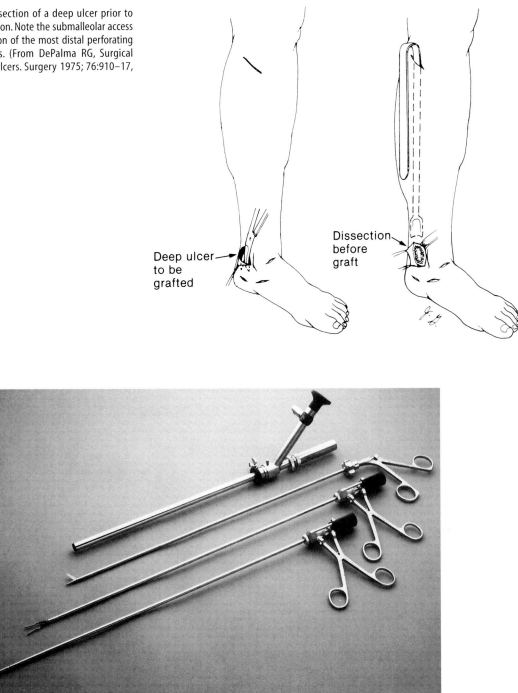

Deep ulcer to be grafted

Dissection before graft

Fig. 11.5. This photograph shows the Storz instrumentation used for endoscopic perforator vein interruption. The straight tube indicates the working channel while the angulated port displays the attachment of the video camera. Instruments utilized include the angulated scissors and small and large bipolar electrocoagulation forceps. (From Bergan JJ, Ballard JL, Sparks S. Subfascial endoscopic perforator vein surgery. The open technique. In: Gloviczki P, Bergan JJ (eds) Atlas of endoscopic perforator vein surgery, Springer-Verlag, London, 1998: 141–9 with permission.)

mentation for this technique has not allowed carbon dioxide insufflation into the subfascial plane and most reported series using the open SEPS technique have not used gas insufflation (Fig. 11.7) Advantage of the open, single scope technique is that manipulation with one endoscopic port is easier than with two scope, placed into the subfascial space. The single scope can be turned around easily to go upwards to the level of the knee and interrupt the Boyd perforating vein (Fig. 11.8).

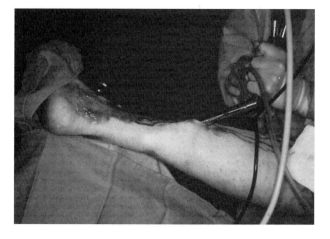

Fig. 11.6. This operative photograph illustrates distal insertion of the scope to the level of the malleolus and suggests that the scope can be manipulated as far posteriorly as the middle and as far anteriorly as the edge of the tibia to create adequate operative space. (From Bergan JJ, Ballard JL, Sparks S. Subfascial endoscopic perforator vein surgery. The open technique. In: Gloviczki P, Bergan JJ (eds) Atlas of endoscopic perforator vein surgery, Springer-Verlag, London, 1998: 141–149 with permission.)

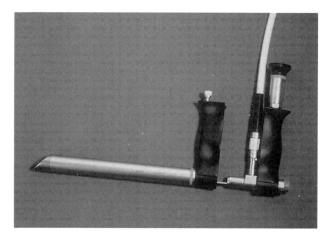

Fig. 11.7. Olympus endoscope for subfascial perforating vein interruption. The scope can be used with or without CO_2 insufflation. It has an 85° field of view and the outer sheath is either 16 or 22 mm in diameter. The working channel is 6×8.5 mm, with a working length of 20 cm. (From Bergan JJ, Ballard JL, Sparks S. Subfascial endoscopic perforator vein surgery. The open technique. In: Gloviczki P, Bergan JJ (eds) Atlas of endoscopic perforator vein surgery. Springer-Verlag, London, 1998: 141–9 with permission.)

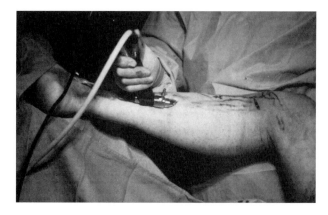

Fig. 11.8. After distal exploration, electrocoagulation, clipping, and division of perforating veins has been accomplished, the scope is reversed to inspect the proximal third of the leg where the Boyd perforating vein is expected to be found. (From Bergan JJ, Ballard JL, Sparks S. Subfascial endoscopic perforator vein surgery. The open technique. In: Gloviczki P, Bergan JJ (eds) Atlas of endoscopic perforator vein surgery, Springer-Verlag, London, 1998: 141–9 with permission.)

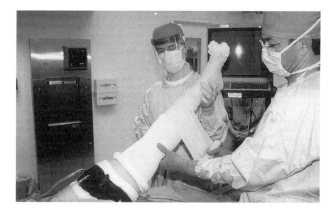

Fig. 11.9. Endoscopic perforator division is performed in a bloodless field, placing a pneumatic tourniquet on the thigh and exsanguinating the extremity with an Esmarch bandage. (From Gloviczki P, Canton LG, Cambria RA, Rhee RY. Subfascial endoscopic perforator vein surgery with gas insufflation. In:Gloviczki P, Bergan JJ (eds) Atlas of endoscopic perforator vein surgery. Springer-Verlag, London, 1998: 125–38 with permission.)

The second technique utilizes instrumentation from laparoscopic surgery and is performed with two laparoscopic port sites. This technique was initiated by O'Donnell[25] and was further developed by our group at the Mayo Clinic[11,36,39] and also by Conrad[40] in Australia. As in the technique described above, a bloodless field is assured by a thigh tourniquet (Fig. 11.9). We use two 10-mm diameter endoscopic ports that are placed 6–10 cm from each other, always proximal to the diseased skin in the medial calf (Fig. 11.10A). We prefer the use of a 10-mm scope, although 5- and 2-mm scopes are also available. Skin incisions are limited to less than 12 mm in size to avoid air leak, since the fascia does not provide a strong seal around the ports (Fig. 11.10B). The 10-mm laparoscopic port is inserted with the help of a blunt obturator to avoid placement of the port in the calf muscles.

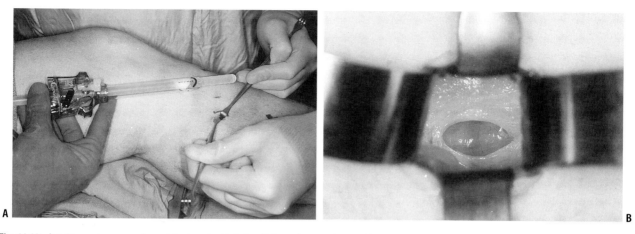

Fig. 11.10. **A** A 10-mm laparoscopic port is placed with help of blunt obturator into subfascial space. **B** Incision of the fascia of the superficial posterior compartment. Note the small skin incision to permit air seal round port. (From Gloviczki P, Cambria RA, Rhee RY, Canton LG, McKusick MA. Surgical technique and preliminary results with endoscopic subfascial division of perforating veins. J Vasc Surg 1996; 23:517–23 with permission.)

Fogarty has designed a dissecting balloon that can also be placed at this point into the subfascial space[41,42] (Fig. 11.11A–C). Carbon dioxide is insufflated into the subfascial space to obtain a pressure of 30 mmHg[43] (Fig. 11.12). The video camera is inserted first through the incision closer to the edge of the tibia and the second port is used for instrumentation. The veins are dissected and clipped using a 5-mm Allport clip applier or a 10-mm clip applier (Ethicon-Endosurgery, Inc.)

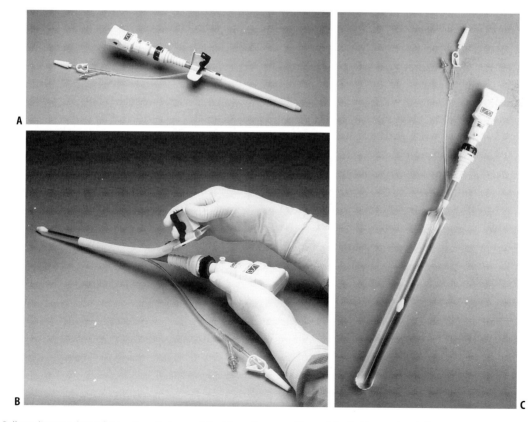

Fig. 11.11. Balloon dissector device for creation of a large subfascial working space (General Surgical Innovations, Palo Alto, CA). **A** Before and **B** during cover removal. **C** Balloon dissector filled with saline. (From Kulbaski MJ, Lumsden AB. Technical armamentaria for endoscopic perforator vein surgery. In: Gloviczki P, Bergan JJ (eds) Atlas of endoscopic perforator vein surgery. Springer-Verlag, London, 1998: 117–22 with permission.)

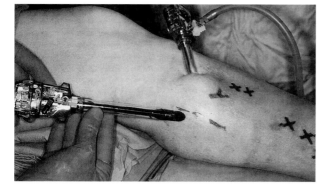

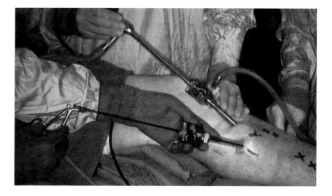

Fig. 11.12. Carbon dioxide is insufflated through first port, that is used for the video camera. Placement of a second 10-mm port is performed under video control. Note that incompetent perforators were marked with an X preoperatively using duplex scanning. (From Gloviczki P, Cambria RA, Rhee RY, Canton LG, McKusick MA. Surgical technique and preliminary results with endoscopic subfascial division of perforating veins. J Vasc Surg 1996; 23:517–23 with permission.)

Fig. 11.13. Clipping and division of perforators is performed with laparoscopic instruments placed through the second port; first port is used for video control. (From Gloviczki P, Cambria RA, Rhee RY, Canton LG, McKusick MA. Surgical technique and preliminary results with endoscopic subfascial division of perforating veins. J Vasc Surg 1996; 23:517–23 with permission.)

(Figs 11.13 and 11.14A,B). More recently we have been using the harmonic scalpel (Fig. 11.15A–D) for ultrasonic coagulation of smaller perforating veins with good results. The dissection can be extended distally a couple of centimeters proximal to the medial malleolus, posteriorly towards the midline and medially to the edge of the tibia. The fascia of the deep posterior compartment should be opened close to the tibia to dissect the paratibial perforator veins, but avoid injury to the posterior tibial vessels and tibial nerve. As discussed in the chapter of Mozes et al., it is important to dissect the

Cockett II perforating vein, which is frequently located within an intramuscular septum under the fascia of the deep compartment. Paratibial fasciotomy (incision of the deep posterior compartment fascia close to the tibia) is a routine part of our operation. Perforator vein interruption is followed by stripping of the greater saphenous vein, usually from the groin to below the knee, frequently using the incision of one of the endoscopic ports for the distal endpoint of stripping. Avulsion of varicose veins is performed at the end of the procedure.

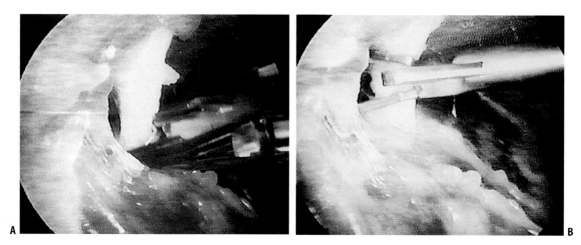

Fig. 11.14. **A** Clipping of a medial calf perforator with a 10-mm clip applier. **B** Division of the perforator with endoscopic scissors after placement of vascular clips. (From Gloviczki P, Cambria RA, Rhee RY, Canton LG, McKusick MA. Surgical technique and preliminary results with endoscopic subfascial division of perforating veins. J Vasc Surg 1996; 23:517–23 with permission.)

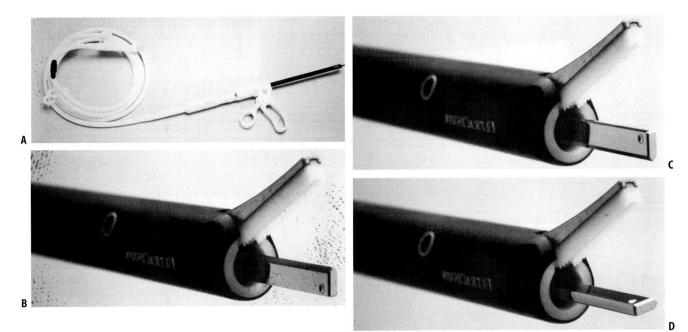

Fig. 11.15. A–D Ultrasonic scalpel. **A** Ultrasonic scalpel (Ultracision, Smithfield, RI) with handset and cable. **B–D** Shows the 10-mm shaft with its adjustable oscillating arm. As the contact surface increases from **B** to **D**, the time and energy required to divide tissues increases as does the security of hemostasis. (From Iafrati MD, O'Donnell TF. Subfascial dissection and perforating vein ablation. In: Gloviczki P, Bergan JJ (eds) Atlas of endoscopic perforator vein surgery. Springer-Verlag, London, 1998: 165–73 with permission.)

Results of Surgical Technique

Clinical Results of Perforator Interruption

Initial clinical experience of Linton[2] and Cockett[3,4] has been stimulating and improvement following perforator ligation was reported subsequently by several investigators.[5,20–24] In nine of the largest series of open perforator ligation, venous ulcers recurred in 22% (range 0–55%)[5,21,24,30,44–48] (Table 11.1). Negus, in a study that included 108 limbs with venous ulcer, reported a 15% ulcer recurrence up to 6 years after the operation.[5]

However, wound complications following open perforator vein ligation were frequent, ranging from 12 to 53%. The most disappointing results following perforator ligation were reported by Burnand et al.[48] who noted 100% ulcer recurrence in a group of 23 patients who had post-thrombotic damage of the deep veins. It was notable in this series, however, that those patients who had normal deep veins had a recurrence of only 6%.

Data have been accumulating on the advantage of SEPS over open ligation of perforating veins. In a prospective, randomized study, that included 39

Table 11.1. Results of open perforator interruption for the treatment of advanced chronic venous disease

Reference	No. of limbs treated	Wound complications (%)	Ulcer recurrence* No. (%)	Mean follow-up (years)
Silver,[21] 1971	31	14	10	1–15
Thurston,[44] 1973	102	12	13	3.3
Bowen,[45] 1975	71	44	34	4.5
Burnand,[48] 1976	41	–	55	–
Negus,[5] 1983	108	22	15	3.7
Wilkinson,[46] 1986	108	24	7	6
Cikrit,[24] 1988	32	19	19	4
Bradbury,[47] 1993	53	–	26	5
Pierek,[30] 1997	19	53	0	1.8
Total: no. of limbs (%)	565 (100)	113/468 (24)	97/443 (22)	–

*Recurrence calculated for Class 5 and 6 limbs only, where data available and percentage accounts for patients lost to follow-up.

patients, wound complications occurred in 53% in the open ligation group versus 0% in those patients who underwent endoscopic perforator ligation.[30] Clinical results regarding ulcer recurrence, however, were similar with no ulcer recurrence noted in either group during a mean follow-up at 21 months.

We recently presented the Mayo Clinic experience that included 57 consecutive SEPS procedures, performed in 48 patients[6] (Fig. 11.16A,B). In this series, concomitant ablation of saphenous reflux was performed in 41 patients. Minor wound complications occurred in 5% and one patient had deep venous thrombosis within 30 days. Another patient with protein C deficiency developed recurrent deep venous thrombosis at 2 months after the operation. In this patient acute deep venous thrombosis early after the operation was excluded by duplex scanning. All ulcers healed at a median of 36 days after surgery (Fig. 11.17). Recurrent or new ulceration

developed in 9% of all patients. However, when we calculated ulcer recurrence or new ulcer development in preoperative Class 5 and Class 6 patients, the rate was 12%. Cumulative ulcer recurrence at 2 years for the entire group was 18% and all recurrence occurred in post-thrombotic patients (Fig. 11.18). Follow-up in this series averaged 17 months and extended up to 52 months after the operation. These results were similar to those reported by others using a variety of SEPS techniques[6,11,30,32,33,49,50,51] (Table 11.2).

The safety of endoscopic perforator ligation was also confirmed in the North American (NASEPS) Registry.[11,36] In this series where results of 146 patients were followed an average of 24 months after the operation, wound complications occurred in 6% and deep vein thrombosis occurred in one patient 2 months after surgery. Cumulative ulcer healing at 1 year was 88% with median time to

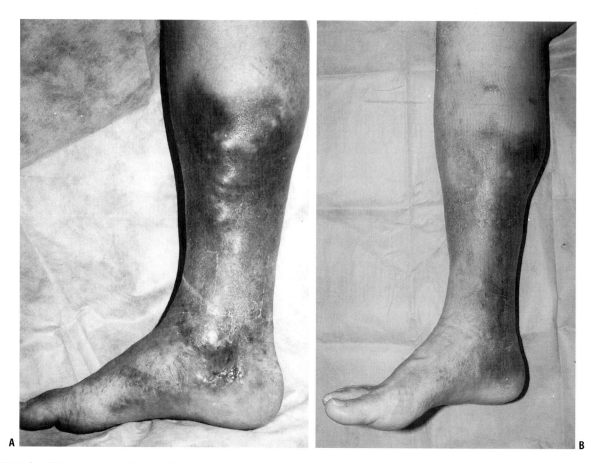

Fig. 11.16. **A** Right leg of a 64-year-old male with a 2-year history of ulcer and severe syndrome. **B** Postoperative picture at 6 weeks shows healed ulcer and incisions following SEPS, stripping and avulsion of varicose veins. Three years later the patient is asymptomatic, does not use elastic stockings and has had no ulcer recurrence. (From Gloviczki P, Canton LG, Cambria RA, Rhee RY. Subfascial endoscopic perforator vein surgery with gas insufflation. In: Gloviczki P, Bergan JJ (eds) Atlas of endoscopic perforator vein surgery, Springer-Verlag, London, 1998: 125–138 with permission.)

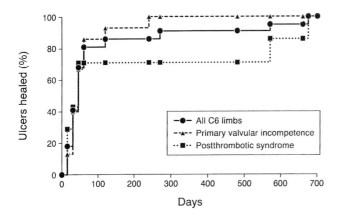

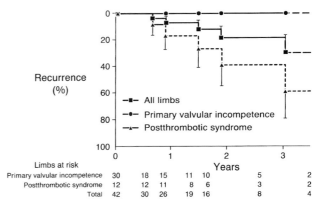

Fig. 11.17. Cumulative ulcer healing. (From Rhodes JM, Gloviczki P, Canton LG, Rooke T, Lewis BD, Lindsey JR. Factors affecting clinical outcome following endoscopic perforator vein ablation. Am J Surg 1998; 176:162–7 with permission.)

Fig. 11.18. Cumulative ulcer recurrence. (From Rhodes JM, Gloviczki P, Canton LG, Rooke T, Lewis BD, Lindsey JR. Factors affecting clinical outcome following endoscopic perforator vein ablation. Am J Surg 1998; 176:162–7 with permission.)

Table 11.2. Results of SEPS for the treatment of advanced chronic venous disease

Reference	No. of limbs treated	Wound complications (%)	Ulcer healing (%)	Ulcer recurrence* (%)	Mean follow-up (months)
Jugenheimer,[49] 1992	103	3	94	0	27
Pierek,[32] 1995	40	8	100	2.5	46
Bergan,[33] 1996	31	10	100	0	–
Wolters,[50] 1996	27	7	96	8	12–24
Padberg,[54] 1996	11	–	†	0	16
Pierek,[30] 1997	20	0	85	0	21
Rhodes,[6] 1998	57	5	100	12	17
Gloviczki,[11] 1998	146	6	84	21	24
Total: No. of limbs (%)	435 (100)	23/424 (5)	197/218 (90)	34/303 (11)	–

*Recurrence calculated for Class 5 and 6 limbs only, where data available and percentage accounts for patients lost to follow-up.
† Only Class 5 (healed ulcer) patients were admitted in this study.

healing of 54 days. Ulcer recurrence at one year was 16% and at 2 years it was 28% with a standard error less than 10%. Post-thrombotic limbs did worse than those with primary valvular incompetence. Post-thrombotic patients had a 46% 2 year cumulative ulcer recurrence rate versus 20% for those with primary valvular incompetence. One hundred twenty two patients had active (C6) or healed ulceration (C5) in the registry. Twenty-eight (23%) of these patients had new or recurrent ulcers at last follow-up. Although these recurrence rates are high, they still compare favorably to results of nonoperative management.

Hemodynamic Results of Perforator Interruption

In a recent review, we studied the hemodynamic consequence of incompetent perforator vein interruption, using strain gauge plethysmography to assess calf muscle pump function, venous incompetence and outflow obstruction before and within 6 months following endoscopic perforator vein surgery.[52] Strain gauge plethysmography demonstrated improved calf muscle pump function following surgery that was significantly better than calf muscle pump

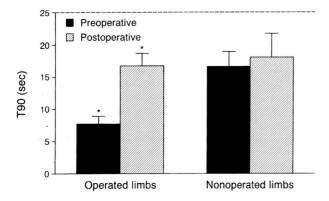

Fig. 11.19. Venous incompetence measured by time to refill 90% of calf blood volume (T_{90}) following exercise, both pre and postoperatively in operated ($n = 28$) and non-perated contralateral limbs ($n = 18$). (* = $p < .01$; — indicates normal $T_{90} \geq 5$ s). (From Rhodes JM, Gloviczki P, Canton LG, Heaser TV, Rooke TW. Endoscopic perforator vein division with ablation of superficial reflux improves venous hemodynamics. J Vasc Surg 1998; 28:839–47 with permission.)

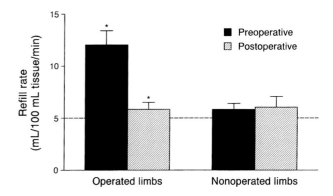

Fig. 11.20. Venous incompetence (refill rate) measured following passive drainage both pre and postoperatively in operated ($n = 30$) and non-operated contralateral limbs ($n = 20$). * = $p < 0.001$; — indicates normal refill rate ≥ 5.0 ml/100 ml tissue/minute). (From Rhodes JM, Gloviczki P, Canton LG, Heaser TV, Rooke TW. Endoscopic perforator vein division with ablation of superficial reflux improves venous hemodynamics. J Vasc Surg 1998; 28:839–47 with permission.)

function before the operation. Venous incompetence also improved as evidenced by prolonged duration to refill following exercise and by a decrease in refill volume following passive drainage (Figs 11.19 and 11.20). Most importantly, improved refill rates correlated with clinical improvement of our patients.

When we analyzed hemodynamic changes in patients with primary valvular incompetence and compared those to patients who have post-thrombotic syndrome, we noted that hemodynamic improvement was significantly better only in limbs with primary valvular incompetence. Similar to findings of Burnand et al.[53] and Stacy et al.,[54] we were not able to show significant hemodynamic improvement in post-thrombotic patients. It is important to note, however, that the number of patients studied in this subgroup has been low. In our series[52] it included seven patients, while the study reported by Stacy et al.[54] included eight patients

Conclusions

Level 1 evidence of clinical and hemodynamic improvement directly related to interruption of incompetent perforators is currently not available. This can only be achieved by expensive multicenter prospective studies, with follow-up that must be between 2 and 4 years. Since the surgical arm has to be stratified

into two groups, ablation of superficial reflux, with and without perforator ligation, the key question on perforators will be difficult to answer. The NASEPS registry experience and reports from larger centers however, provide impressive data on rapid ulcer healing, low morbidity and decreased wound complications from perforator interruption, performed together with ablation of the superficial reflux, when indicated. A prospective randomized study also confirmed the advantage of SEPS over open surgical ligation of perforators. Ulcer recurrence at 2 years after SEPS is 10–15% in series from single institutions and, expectedly higher, 22% in the multicenter NASEPS registry, independent of patient compliance. These results compare favorably to series of nonoperative management, where noncompliant patients had 100% ulcer recurrence. SEPS, together with ablation of superficial reflux should be offered at present to surgical candidates with advanced chronic venous insufficiency. While improvement in all patients may be modest, those with primary valvular incompetence will have a predictably good clinical outcome and improved hemodynamic result.

References

1. Mozes G, Gloviczki P, Menawat SS, Fischer DR, Carmichael SW, Kadar A. Surgical anatomy for endoscopic subfascial division of perforating veins. J Vasc Surg 1996; 24:800–8

2. Linton RR. The communicating veins of the lower leg and the operative technique for their ligation. Ann Surg 1938;107:582-32.

3. Cockett FB, Jones BD. The ankle blow-out syndrome: a new approach to the varicose ulcer problem. Lancet 1953; i:17–23

4. Cockett FB. The pathology and treatment of venous ulcers of the leg. Br J Surg 1956; 44:260–278

5. Negus D, Friedgood A. The effective management of venous ulceration. Br J Surg 1983; 70:623–7

6. Rhodes JM, Gloviczki P, Canton LG, Rooke TW, Lewis BD, Lindsey JR. Factors affecting clinical outcome following endoscopic perforator vein ablation. Am J Surg 1998; 176:167

7. van Rij AM, Solomon C, Christie R. Anatomic and physiologic characteristics of venous ulceration. J Vasc Surg 1994; 20:759–64

8. Labrapoulos N, Leon M, Geroulakos G, Volteas N, Chan P, Nicolaides AN. Venous hemodynamic abnormalities in patients with leg ulcerations. Am J Surg 1995; 169:572–4

9. Labrapoulos N, Mansour MA, Kang SS, Gloviczki P, Baker WH. New insights into perforator vein incompetence. J Vasc Surg 1998 in press

10. Hanrahan LM, Araki CT, Rodriguez AA, Kechejian GJ, LaMorte WW, Menzoian JO. Distribution of valvular incompetence in patients with venous stasis ulceration. J Vasc Surg:1991; 13:805–12

11. Gloviczki P, Bergan JJ, Rhodes JM, Canton LG, Harmsen WS, Ilstrup DM, North American Study Group. Mid-term results of endoscopic perforator vein interruption for chronic venous insufficiency: lessons learned from the North American Subfascial Endoscopic Perforator Surgery (NASEPS) registry. J Vasc Surg 1999; 29:498–502

12. Shami SK, Sarin S, Cheatle TR, Scurr JH, Coleridge Smith PD. Venous ulcers and the superficial system. J Vasc Surg 1993; 17:487–90

13. Darke SG, Penfold C. Venous ulceration and saphenous ligation. Eur J Vasc Surg 1992; 6:4–9

14. Lees TA, Lambert D. Patterns of venous reflux in limbs with skin changes associated with chronic venous insufficiency Br J Surg 1993; 80:725–8

15. Zukowski AJ, Nicolaides AN, Szendro G et al. Haemodynamic significance of incompetent calf perforating veins. Br J Surg 1991; 78:625–9

16. Gloviczki P, Lewis BD, Lindsey JR, McKusick MA. Preoperative evaluation of chronic venous insufficiency with Duplex scanning and venography. In: Gloviczki P, Bergan JJ (eds) Atlas of endoscopic perforator vein surgery. London, Springer-Verlag, 1998: 81–91

17. O'Donnell TF, Burnand KG, Clemenson G, Thomas ML, Browse NL. Doppler examination vs clinical and phlebographic detection of the location of incompetent perforating veins. Arch Surg 1977; 112:31–3

18. Pierik EGJM, Toonder IM, van Urk H, Wittens CHA. Validation of duplex ultrasonography in detecting competent and incompetent perforating veins in patients with venous ulceration of the lower leg. J Vasc Surg 1997; 26:49–52

19. Linton RR. The post-thrombotic ulceration of the lower extremity: its etiology and surgical treatment. Ann Surg 1953; 138:415–32

20. Dodd H, Cockett FR. The management of venous ulcers. In: Dodd H, Cockett F (eds) The pathology and surgery of the vein of the lower limbs. Churchill-Livingstone, New York, 1976: 269–96

21. Silver D, Gleysteen JJ, Rhodes GR, Georgiade NJ, Anylan WG, Durham NC. Surgical treatment of the refractory postphlebitic ulcer. Arch Surg 1971; 103:554–60

22. De Palma RG. Surgical therapy for venous stasis: results of a modified Linton operation. Am J Surg 1979; 137:810–13

23. Schanzer H, Pierce EC. A rational approach to surgery of the chronic venous stasis syndrome. Ann Surg 1982; 195:25–9

24. Cikrit DF, Nichols WK, Silver D. Surgical management of refractory venous stasis ulceration. J Vasc Surg 1988; 7:473–8

25. O'Donnell TF. Surgical treatment of incompetent communicating veins. In: Bergan JJ, Kistner RL (eds) Atlas of venous surgery. WB Saunders, Philadelphia, 1992: 111–24

26. Edwards JM. Shearing operation for incompetent perforating vein. Br J Surg 1976; 63:885–6

27. Hauer G. The endoscopic subfascial division of the perforating veins: preliminary report. VASA 1985; 14:59–61

28. Fischer R, Schwahn-Schreiber C, Sattler G. Conclusions of a consensus conference on subfascial endoscopy of perforating veins in the medial lower leg. Vasc Surg 1998; 32:339–47

29. Fischer R, Sattler G, Vanderpuye R. The current status of endoscopic treatment of perforators (in French). Phlebologie 1993; 46:701–7

30. Pierik EGJM, van Urk H, Hop WCJ, Witten CHA. Endoscopic versus open subfascial division of incompetent perforating veins in the treatment of venous leg ulceration: A randomized trial. J Vasc Surg 1997; 26:1049–54

31. Wittens CHA. Comparison of open Linton operation with subfascial endoscopic perforator vein surgery In: Gloviczki P, Bergan JJ (eds) Atlas of endoscopic perforator vein surgery. Springer-Verlag, London, 1998: 177–85

32. Pierik EGJM, Wittens CHA, van Urk H. Subfascial endoscopic ligation in the treatment of incompetent perforator veins. Eur J Vasc Endovasc Surg 1995; 5:38–41

33. Bergan JJ, Murray J, Greason K. Subfascial endoscopic perforator vein surgery: a preliminary report. Ann Vasc Surg 1996; 10:211–19

34. Bergan JJ, Ballard JL, Sparks S. Subfascial endoscopic perforator surgery: the open technique. In: Gloviczki P, Bergan JJ (eds) Atlas of endoscopic perforator vein surgery. Springer-Verlag, London, 1998: 141–49

35. Sparks SR, Ballard JL, Bergan JJ, Killeen JD. Early benefits of subfascial endoscopic perforator surgery (SEPS) in healing venous ulcers. Ann Vasc Surg 1997; 11:367–373

36. Gloviczki P, Bergan JJ, Menawat SS et al. Safety, feasibility, and early efficacy of subfascial endoscopic perforator surgery: a preliminary report from the North American Registry. J Vasc Surg 1997; 25:94–105

37. Gloviczki P, Cambria RA, Rhee RY et al. Surgical technique and preliminary results of endoscopic subfascial division of perforating veins. J Vasc Surg 1996; 23:517–523

38. Gloviczki P. Endoscopic perforator vein surgery: Does it work? (Editorial) Vasc Surg 1998; 32:303–5

39. Gloviczki P, Bergan JJ (eds). Atlas of endoscopic perforator vein surgery. Springer-Verlag, London, 1998

40. Conrad P. Endoscopic exploration of the subfascial space of the lower leg with perforator vein interruption using laparoscopic equipment: a preliminary report. Phlebology 1994; 9:154–7

41. Allen RC, Tawes RL, Wetter A, Fogarty TJ. Endoscopic perforator vein surgery: creation of a subfascial space. In: Atlas of Endoscopic Perforator Vein Surgery, eds. Gloviczki P, Bergan JJ. London, Springer-Verlag, 1998:153-162.

42. Kulbaski MJ, Lumsden AB. Technical armamentaria for endoscopic vein surgery. In: Gloviczki P, Bergan JJ (eds) Atlas of endoscopic perforator vein surgery. Springer-Verlag, London, 1998: 117–22

43. Gloviczki P, Canton LG, Cambria RA, Rhee RY. Subfascial endoscopic perforator vein surgery with gas insufflation. In: Gloviczki P, Bergan JJ (eds) Atlas of endoscopic perforator vein surgery. Springer-Verlag, London, 1998: 125–38

44. Thurston OC, Williams HTG. Chronic venous insufficiency of the lower extremity. Arch Surg 1973; 106:537–9

45. Bowen FH. Subfascial ligation of the perforating leg veins to treat post-thrombophlebitic syndrome. Am Surg 1975; 148–51

46. Wilkinson GE, Maclaren IF. Long-term review of procedures for venous perforator insufficiency. Surg Gyn Obs 1986; 163:117–20

47. Bradbury AW, Stonebridge PA, Callam MJ, Ruckley CV, Allen PL. Foot volumetry and duplex ultrasonography after saphenous and subfascial perforating vein ligation for recurrent venous ulceration. Br J Surg 1993; 80:845–8

48. Burnand KG, O'Donnell T, Thomas ML, Browse NL. Relation between postphlebitic changes in the deep veins and results of surgical treatment of venous ulcers. Lancet 1976; 1:936–8

49. Jugenheimer M, Junginger T. Endoscopic subfascial sectioning of incompetent perforating veins in treatment of primary varicosities. World J Surg 1992; 16:971–5

50. Wolters U, Schmitz-Rixen T, Erasmi H, Lynch J. Endoscopic dissection of incompetent perforating veins in the treatment of chronic venous leg ulcers. Vasc Surg 1996; 30:481–7

51. Padberg FT, Pappas PJ, Araki CT et al. Hemodynamic and clinical improvement after superficial vein ablation in primary combined venous insufficiency with ulceration. J Vasc Surg 1996; 24:711–18

52. Rhodes JM, Gloviczki P, Canton LG, Heaser TV, Rooke TW. Endoscopic perforator vein division with ablation of superficial reflux improves venous hemodynamics. J Vasc Surg 1998; 28.

53. Burnand KG, O'Donnell TF, Thomas ML, Browse NL. The relative importance of incompetent communicating veins in the production of varicose veins and venous ulcers. Surgery 1977; 82:9–13

54. Stacey MC, Burnand KG, Layer GT, Pattison M. Calf pump function in patients with healed venous ulcers is not improved by surgery to the communicating veins or by elastic stockings. Br J Surg 1988; 75:436–9

Single-Port Open-Scope Perforator Vein Surgery

12

John J. Bergan, Jeffrey L. Ballard, Jay Murray and Steven Sparks

As detailed throughout this volume, venous ulceration of the leg is a severe and debilitating outcome of chronic venous insufficiency. While it has been termed the post-thrombotic syndrome, it is now known that primary valvular dysfunction, not just prior thrombosis, is an important cause of leg ulcer. This is important because primary valvular dysfunction is eminently treatable while post-thrombotic dysfunction is not.

Primary venous dysfunction develops upon an hereditary hormonal substrate and is promulgated by gravitational venous hypertension and pressure from muscular contraction transmitted through failed perforating vein–valves. It is assumed that repeated pulses of high venous pressure generated by muscular contraction apparently drive leukocytes into the expanded endothelium of unsupported subcutaneous and intracutaneous postcapillary venules. There, activation occurs and free oxygen radicals and other toxic products are released. The result is an inflammatory reaction which leads to the clinical manifestations of chronic venous insufficiency. Clinical diagnosis is confirmed by ultrasound examination and treatment can be applied through compression therapy assisted by pharmacologic management and surgery. Compression reduces existing edema and decreases tendency for edema formation. Pharmacologic manipulations are designed to increase noradrenaline activity and improve stimulation of lymphatic contraction. However, no such agents are available in the United States. Surgery is targeted at eliminating superficial reflux and high-pressure perforating vein outflow. The latter is markedly enhanced by minimally invasive endoscopic techniques which may be performed on an outpatient basis.

As early as the 1930s, perforating veins with outward flow were implicated in the pathogenesis of this condition.[1] Recognition that such outward flow promotes leukocyte adhesion and activation as the principal microcirculatory cause for cutaneous changes has explained the importance of perforating vein interruption[2,3]. Because of disability of chronic venous insufficiency in the past, surgeons and patients reluctantly tolerated the open operation with its morbid knee-to-ankle incision because of the efficacy of the procedure.[4,5] Modifications done to reduce the morbidity of the procedure at first eliminated two of the three incisions used in the explorations of the 1930s.[6] Other modifications followed.[7] However, the most significant modern alteration was to utilize endoscopic techniques introduced by Fischer[8] and Hauer[9] (Fig. 12.1). Very quickly it was learned that this technique minimized postoperative complications.[10] Application of endoscopic perforator interruption to varicose vein surgery validated the safety of the procedure but did not contribute to knowledge about treating chronic venous insufficiency.[11]

From the beginning of our experience in July 1993, we have worked toward the development of a single-port, open-scope approach[12] (Fig. 12.2).

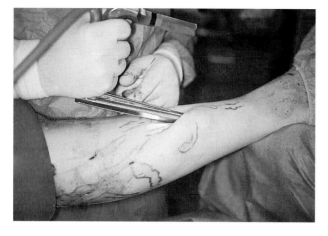

Fig. 12.1. The open mediastinoscope technique illustrated here opened the door to subfascial endoscopic perforator vein interruption.

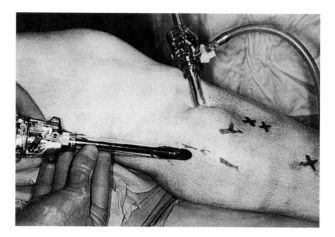

Fig. 12.3. The multiple-port technique using laparoscopic instrumentation is shown here. Gas insufflation and simultaneous instrumentation is possible using this method.

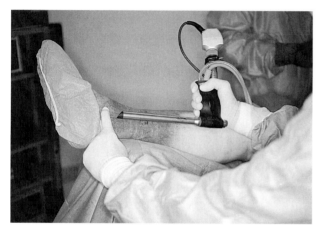

Fig. 12.2. The development of dedicated endoscopes for perforator vein interruption allows more efficient operative technique. This photograph illustrates the Olympus scope connected to a videocamera, gas insufflation, and light source. The working channel can be used for instrumentation and is occluded manually by the right hand of the surgeon during the expanded or cave view of the subfascial space.

Simultaneously, another approach using multiple ports, gas insufflation, and disposable equipment was developed by Gloviczki, Conrad, and others[13-15] (Fig. 12.3). These procedures, using single or multiple ports, had the same objective; that is, elimination of perforator vein outflow. This was to minimize leukocyte adherence and activation in the enlarged subdermal endothelial pool.[16]

Perforating Veins

Medial calf perforating veins have been the subject of considerable research. In the study by the Middlesex group, direction of blood flow within medical calf perforator veins was seen to be both inward and outward, even in limbs without evidence of venous disease.[17] Outward flow could be demonstrated in 21% of perforators in normal limbs. However, only limbs with superficial or deep venous insufficiency demonstrated flow in the perforating veins during the relaxation phase after distal compression. When compression was applied proximal to the perforating vein being observed by ultrasound, a significant number of perforating veins demonstrated outward flow, particularly those limbs with deep venous insufficiency. Comparison of the number of perforators allowing inward flow and outflow during compression and relaxation showed a statistical difference between the results after proximal and distal compression.

Careful observation of the location of perforating veins seen through the endoscope was documented by Fischer.[18] His careful study measured the location of perforating veins according to the distance from the sole of the foot. This is commonly done when referring to the clinical location of Cockett perforating veins. His conclusion was:

"in contrast to reports of the authors mentioned (Cockett, Haeger, Kubik, and May), we did not find any predilection levels even when the perforator heights found by means of the lower leg length (radiological patients) or the height (surgical patients) were corrected or made relative."

Fischer's conclusion is that one cannot presuppose the location of Cockett or 24 cm perforating veins.

In 1995, Hauer described the open endoscope technique of dividing perforator veins in the calf.[19] His contribution was addition of video to the endoscope. This produced a new method of subfascial division of perforating veins. With this technique, he was able to obtain secure division of the veins after electrocoagulation or clip ligation. Hauer stressed that this method combined the advantages of single-access port with entry through an area of unimpaired skin (Fig. 12.4). Furthermore, he stressed the rapidity and reliability of the division of all perforating veins of the medial lower leg with a guarantee that hemorrhage would not occur. His experience was described in 80 legs and suggested a further exploration of the method.

By 1992, Fischer was able to detail his experiences using the open, nonvideo, single-port technique.[20] He reported on experience over a 5 year period, in which he developed accessory instrumentation for dissection of veins, division of veins, and performance of prograde and retrograde fasciotomies. Endoscopy was done under direct vision with the patient supine, hip in outward rotation, slightly flexed, and the knee slightly flexed. Fischer described use of the Esmarch bandage to obtain a bloodless leg and an orthopedic pneumatic tourniquet. Later, he employed the relatively bloodless state achieved by the help of the Löfqvist tourniquet.

In Fischer's experience, the skin incision was 18 mm long, placed a few centimeters behind the dorsal edge of the tibia in the proximal part of the leg. The endoscope was introduced through the incision with endoscope light on and the room lights off so that the exact location of the end of the endoscope could be seen through the skin. He pointed out that the connective tissue between the fascia and the underlying flexor muscles was so loose that this space could easily be opened up and inspected with the endoscope without need for other instrumentation, gas or liquid irrigation. Fischer performed the endoscopic portion of the operation during withdrawal of the instrument while performing pendulum-like, sideward movements to completely open the subfascial space. He described normal and normally functioning perforating veins as being thin-walled and often double-barreled, passing obliquely. In contrast, incompetent perforating veins were thick-walled, appeared to be single-barreled, and tended to pass transversely through the space seen with the endoscope. Fischer is unique in advocating severing of perforating veins bluntly, either with a spatula or with a hook. He stressed that the ends of the severed perforating veins bled very little, especially after blunt division. He stressed that the endoscopic fasciotomy, if necessary, could be done under direct vision through the short 18-mm incision.

During the time period from the spring of 1991 until the fall of 1995, a total of 1,280 legs were operated upon by Fischer for varicose veins. Endoscopy was done in 463 of them and in only one was the endoscopy impossible because of fascial adhesions due to severe chronic venous insufficiency. In 354 of 462 successful cases, incompetent perforating veins were found and sectioned. A total of 480 perforating veins were divided. As 108 legs were explored without perforator veins being found, it appears that perforators were identified and sectioned in only 75% of the limbs. Possibly, this was because video endoscopy was not used. After this, the term SEPS (subfascial endoscopic perforator surgery) was accepted by interested surgeons.

Indications for the endoscopic perforating vein procedure in Fischer's experience included varicose veins and venous ulcer without limitation to classes 4, 5, and 6 of the new CEAP classification. Therefore, Fischer was unable to provide observations on rapidity of healing of venous ulcerations or prevention of recurrence of venous ulcers, but instead focused on recurrence of varicose veins.

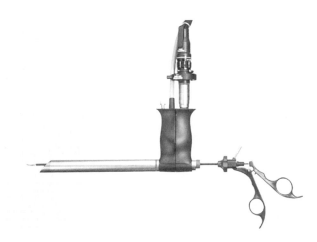

Fig. 12.4. The Olympus endoscope and its working channel are illustrated here.

Open-Scope Experience with SEPS

Other groups in central Europe have had experience with subfascial perforating vein division using the open, single-port scope. In Hamburg, Sachs treated 85 patients and performed subfascial perforator vein division on 100 legs.[21] In most of the cases, the subfascial portion of the procedure was combined with standard superficial vein stripping, although in a few cases it was done in an isolated fashion. Sachs used the Löfqvist roller cuff, used a small medial leg incision much like Fischer, and tabulated a very small number of complications, including two cases of venous thrombosis, 11 of hematoma, and one of tibial nerve injury.

Jugenheimer reported similar results from Aachen in the Federal Republic of Germany.[11] He described 72 patients (103 limbs) with delayed wound healing in three limbs, two patients with complaints of dysesthesias in the distribution of the sural nerve, hematoma in six limbs, and dysesthesia in the saphenous nerve territory in 10 limbs. At follow-up examination at a mean time of 27 months postoperatively, only two incompetent perforating veins were identified by ultrasound. New varices were seen in nine limbs.

A summary statement of the art of perforator vein interruption using open techniques was made in 1996.[22] This noted that there were four techniques of subfascial perforator vein interruption. These included the single scope, direct vision technique of Fischer, the single-scope video-assisted method of Hauer, the variation of this technique using a directed fascial view with gas insufflation, and the multiple port gas insufflation method using laparoscopic instruments.

The available SEPS instruments are summarized in Table 12.1.

Instrumentation

ETB Berlin (Hauer[23])

Description
Surgical shaft 183.3 mm in length overall with a usable length of 170 mm. Working channel 7.5×13.0 mm with an integrated suction port. Surgical optical system 16 mm in diameter with an angle of view of 30°. A shaft sleeve protects the lens from fogging and blurring, and all standard fiberoptics and cameras can be attached at the handle.

Advantages
The cold light and camera attachment are located at the end of the handle which simplifies manipulation. The strong handle allows mechanical enlargement of the subfascial space without employing additional techniques. Standard endoscopic instrumentation with diameters up to 7.5 mm can be used. Such instruments may include the angled, original Fischer-designed instrumentation, Allport clip appliers, and ultrasonic surgical knives Fasciotomy under direct vision is easy even despite large areas of lipodermatosclerosis.

Table 12.1. Instruments for subfascial endoscopy of perforating veins in the medial lower leg

Company	ETB Berlin	Storz	Wolf	Ethicon	Storz	Olympus
Authors	Hauer	Sattler/Lang	Langer	Gloviczki, et al.	Fischer	Wittens
Visualization	Monitor	Monitor	Monitor	Monitor	Monitor	Monitor
Size of endoscopic field	Excellent	Good	Good	Big	Small	Good
CO_2 insufflation	Possible	Possible	Possible	Yes	No	Possible
Suction of smoke integrated	Yes	Yes	Yes	Possible	No	Yes
Handling	Good	Good	Good	Difficult	Easy	Good
Swiftness	Good	Good	Good	Poor	Very good	Good
Clipping possible	Yes	Soon	Yes	Yes	Yes	Yes
Autoclaving possible	Soon	Soon	Yes	Yes	Yes	Yes
Number of ports	1	1	1	2–3	1	1
Costs	Normal	Normal	Normal	High	Low	Normal

Modified from: Fischer R, Schwahn-Schreiber C, Sattler G. Conclusions of a consensus conference on subfascial endoscopy of perforating veins in the medial lower leg. Vasc Surg 1998; 32(4):343.

Disadvantages

The instrument is large in diameter and short for long limbs.

Storz (Sattler[24])

Description

Endoscopic shaft 300 mm, outer diameter 10 mm, and working channel 5.5 mm with two optical light carriers. Lens system angle of view, 0°. Operation may be done through a 15-mm incision. Diagnostic and therapeutic manipulations can be done with a 360° rotating scissors as well as 1-mm and 3-mm bipolar clamps designed especially for this scope. Angled instruments designed by Fischer may be used as well. Enlargement of the subfascial space must be done by lifting the skin with strong curved needles or sutures.

Advantages

After the surgeon is fully trained, the technique is fast and relatively simple because of an excellent visual field. The instrument easily reaches the full length of the leg, both proximally and distally.

Disadvantages

The length of the instrument occasionally makes its manipulation somewhat difficult. Problems with the knee and tourniquet have been encountered.

Wolf (Langer[25])

Description

This is an Hauer-modified mediastinoscope with a working shaft 180 mm long and with an inner diameter of 20 mm (Fig. 12.5). The ergonomically styled handle of the endoscope has a sharp angle

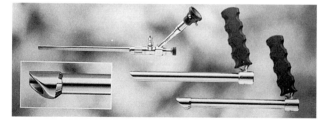

Fig. 12.5. The Wolf endoscope with its rugged design and angulated handle are illustrated in this photograph.

toward the shaft. This allows lifting of the fascia and enlargement of the subfascial space. The optical system is angled 5° and there is a working channel of 5 mm with an integrated suction channel. Simple guiding devices allow 400- and 600 nm fibers to be used for laser instrumentation.

Advantages

This is a very solid instrument with simple orthograde manipulations due to the excellent position of the handle. Easy enlargement of the subfascial space is possible and the optical system is quite good.

Disadvantages

The shaft is too short for long legs and for limbs with a large area of severe trophic damage. The viewing angle is oriented toward the calf muscle rather than toward the fascia.

Ethicon (Laparoscopy Instruments[13-15])

Description

These are standard laparoscopic instruments from Ethicon and require multiple incisions, 10–15 mm in length (Fig. 12.3). Prechanneling with a plexiglass trocar is done and this is followed by insertion of the 10-mm diameter endoscopic shafts. A space-making device is often used. Insufflation is achieved through a second 10-mm port at pressures of 30–40 mmHg. A large endoscopic area is created and the second port can be used for trocar and instrument manipulation. A tourniquet is used to prevent gas embolization.

Advantages

There is an outstanding view and large endoscopic working area. Instruments are readily available.

Disadvantages

Increased surgical effort is needed because of the greater invasiveness of two or three ports. There is a problem with CO_2 leaks. As the instruments are disposable, there is greater cost. The space-making balloon also adds cost.

Storz (Fischer[26])

Description

A 17-mm endoscopic tube with beveled tip and separate inner shaft light carrier. Outer diameter

13 mm, inner diameter 10 mm, incision length 18 mm. The handle is located in an obtuse angle and contains the light channel. Diagnostic and therapeutic manipulation with angled instruments is possible.

Advantages
The advantages are simplicity, reasonable price, and that it is fast and efficient; it is beautifully designed.

Disadvantages
A perfect view and exactly adapted monofocal glasses are required for the surgeon. Details cannot be detected clearly. Protection of accompanying nerve and artery is not possible.

Olympus (Wittens[27])

Description
A 21 cm endoscopic tube with hooded tip (Fig. 12.6). There are 16-mm or 22-mm sheaths which allow 5.0–5.4 mm instruments. The direction of view is 8° with a field of view of 80–85°. Gas insufflation is possible.

Advantages
There is a proper orientation of view toward fascia. Insufflation to enlarge view is possible. There is a large working channel.

Disadvantages
The scope is short and the large sheath is too large.

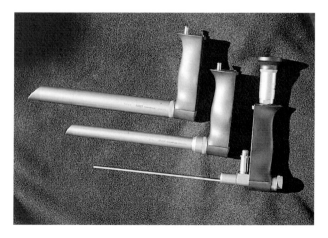

Fig. 12.6. The Olympus scope has two sheaths to allow a larger working channel to be employed during endoscopic manipulations.

Clinical Experience

Our own explorations into the development of a single-scope, open subfascial perforator vein operation have been published.[27–30] In San Diego, in the most recent experience, a total of 67 operations were accomplished in 60 patients in the period from July 1993 to March 1998.[31] During this period, instrumentation and surgical practice changed. Ultimately, nearly all operations were done on an entirely outpatient basis using ambulatory surgicenters without any in-hospital care. Because an aggressive policy of anticoagulation prophylaxis was used, this was responsible for nearly all of the in-hospital days for operations that were followed by hospital admission. At the present time, outpatient deep venous thrombosis prophylaxis is done using low-molecular-weight heparins which were introduced into clinical practice in America more recently than in Europe. This has eliminated the need for in-hospital care following SEPS.

The objective of the subfascial perforator vein interruption was to prevent recurrent ulceration in 20% of limbs. In these patients, outpatient conservative care had allowed healing of ulcerations or amelioration of lipodermatosclerosis. Clinically, it was difficult to detect improvement in these patients, and insufficient time has passed to determine the incidence of recurrent ulceration. However, when the objective was to achieve ulcer healing, this occurred in 80% of limbs. In these cases, the ulcers had been present intermittently from one to five years prior to operation. Without changing ulcer care, all but five ulcers healed within four weeks of the surgical intervention. Four more healed within 8 weeks. One ulcer healed at 6 months, and another required further interventions including left iliac vein stenting and ulcer excision to achieve complete healing. In two limbs, venous ulcers had been present for a very short time, and both of these healed within 4 weeks of the operation.

Technique of Open-Scope SEPS

In developing the operation, varying techniques were used by various surgeons. Observations have now guided the selection of the order of the procedures.

First, the most limiting postoperative complication was a subfascial hematoma. This caused excessive pain and limited ambulation in some patients operated on early in the experience. Second, experience with surgery of the superficial venous system taught that stripping of the saphenous vein from groin to knee caused a tremendous proximal venospasm. This, in turn, caused distal venous hypertension and excessive bleeding during stab avulsion of varices. Third, release of the tourniquet caused hyperemia and bleeding from transected and uncontrolled vessels.

With these observations in mind, we currently perform the procedure in the following order. First, an Esmarch bandage and tourniquet exsanguinate the limb and control inflow. Second, the subfascial exploration is done choosing a site for an entrance of the scope which will coincide with maximum mobility of instrumentation and possible use of the incision for removing clusters of varicosities or terminating saphenous stripping. No space expander is used. After perforator interruption (Figs 12.7 and 12.8) and fasciotomy, the subfascial exploration wound is left open and the procedure continues with ablation of superficial reflux. The groin incision and passage of the stripping device can proceed with the tourniquet in place. However, with careful and complete ligation of perforating veins, this is not mandatory as bleeding is minimal after release of the tourniquet. While this is done, the stab avulsion portion of the procedure can continue and, if necessary, the saphenous vein can be cannulated at the ankle for removal of the leg portion of the vein if it is thought to be the source of varicosities or in any way contributes to the severe chronic venous insufficiency. After all else is done, the tourniquet is released, the saphenous vein stripped, the subfascial space thoroughly irrigated, and skin closure begun. The last closure is the one in which subfascial exploration was done (Fig. 12.9).

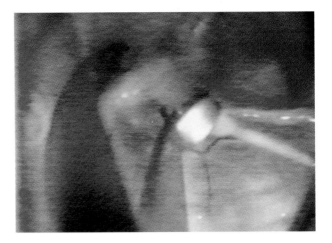

Fig. 12.8. This operative photograph shows a perforating vein exiting from the muscular compartment to the left and entering the fascia to the right. The 5-mm Ethicon clip is illustrated as well as the scissors which sever the perforating vein.

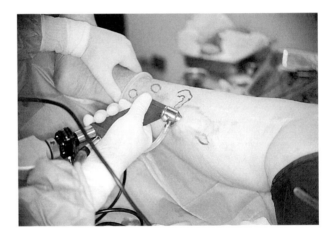

Fig. 12.9. Use of the single-scope technique allows reversal of the field of view so that the Boyd perforating vein and even the lesser saphenous vein can be clipped and divided.

Wound closures are effected with monofilament absorbable suture. The wound is reinforced with Steri-Strips and infiltrated with 0.25% Marcaine local anesthesia. The local anesthesia allows comfort in the recovery room, early mobilization of the patient, and the possibility of discharge home within 1 hour of the termination of the procedure.

Discussion

The subfascial perforator vein interruption surgery performed by the open technique has proven to be an

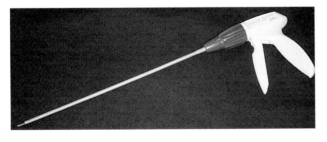

Fig. 12.7. The Ethicon 5-mm clip applier has proven to be eminently useful in single-scope endoscopic perforator vein interruption.

operation well within the capabilities of general surgeons and interested vascular surgeons. Availability of nondisposable instrumentation and simplicity of the procedure itself makes the operation extremely cost effective. Because operative morbidity is decreased by the small size of the incision, the absence of serious septic complications, and the prevention of subfascial hematomas, even overnight hospitalization has been found to be unnecessary in nearly all cases.

As the procedure has proven itself to be effective in control of severe chronic venous insufficiency, it is clear that more complex procedures such as valveplasty and valve transplantation can be held in reserve for those few cases in which the ablation of superficial reflux and control of perforators has proven to be ineffective.

References

1. Linton RR. The communicating veins of the lower leg and the operative technique for their ligation. Ann Surg 1938; 107:582–93
2. Arnoldi CC. Venous pressure in patients with valvular incompetence of the veins of the lower limbs. Acta Chir Scand 1966; 132:427–30
3. Coleridge Smith PD, Thomas P, Scurr JH, Dormandy JA. Causes of venous ulceration: A new hypothesis. Br Med J 1988; 296;1726–7
4. Wilkinson GE, Maclaren IF. Long-term review of procedures for venous perforator insufficiency. Surg Gynecol Obstet 1986; 163:117–20
5. Field P, Van Boxel P. The role of the Linton flap procedure in the management of stasis, dermatitis, and ulceration in the lower limb. Surgery 1971; 70:920–26
6. Linton RR. The post-thrombotic ulceration of the lower extremity: its etiology and surgical treatment. Ann Surg 1953; 138:415–32
7. DePalma RG. Surgical therapy for venous stasis: results of a modified Linton procedure. Am J Surg 1979; 137:810–13
8. Fischer R. Die chirurgische Behandlung der Varizen-Grundlagen und heutiger Stand. Schweiz Rundsch Med Prax 1990; 79:155–67
9. Hauer G. Operationstechnik der endoskopischen subfaszialen Diszision der Perforansven. Chirurg 1987; 58:172–5
10. Gloviczki P, Bergan JJ, Menawat SS et al. Safety, feasibility, and early efficacy of subfascial endoscopic perforator surgery: a preliminary report from the North American Registry. J Vasc Surg 1997; 25:94–105
11. Jugenheimer M, Junginger Th. Endoscopic subfascial sectioning of incompetent perforating veins in treatment of primary varicosis. World J Surg 1992; 16:971–5
12. Bergan JJ, Murray J, Greason K. Subfascial endoscopic perforator vein surgery (SEPS): a preliminary report. Ann Vasc Surg 1996; 10:211–19
13. Gloviczki P, Cambria RA, Rhee RY, Canton LG, Mikusic MA. Surgical technique and preliminary results of endoscopic subfascial division of perforating veins. J Vasc Surg 1996; 23:517–23
14. Conrad P. Endoscopic exploration of the subfascial space of the lower leg with perforator vein interruption using laparoscopic equipment: a preliminary report. Phlebology 1994; 9:154–7
15. Tawes RL, Wetter LA, Hermann GD et al. Endoscopic technique for subfascial perforating vein interruption. J Endovasc Surg 1996; 3:414–20
16. Scott HJ, Coleridge Smith PD, Scurr JH. Histological study of white blood cells and their association with lipodermatosclerosis and venous ulceration. Br J Surg 1991; 78:210–11
17. Sarin S, Scurr JH, Coleridge Smith PD. Medial calf perforators in venous disease: the significance of outward flow. J Vasc Surg 1992; 16:40–6
18. Fischer R, Füllemann HJ, Alder W. Zum phlebologischen dogma der prädilektionstellen der Cockettschen venae perforantes. Phlebol u Proktol 1987; 16:184–7
19. Hauer G. Die endoskopische subfasziale diszision der perforansvenen – vorläufige mitteilung. VASA 1995; 14:59–61
20. Fischer R. Erfahrungen mit der endoskopischen perforantensanierung. Phlebology 1992; 21:214–58
21. Sachs G, Thiele H, Gai H. Erste erfahrungen mit der endoskopisch subfaszialen dissektion der perforansvenen (ESDP) nach 100 eingriffen. Zentralbl Chir 1994; 119:501–5
22. Fisher R, Schwahn-Schreiber C, Sattler G. Conclusions of a consensus conference on subfascial endoscopy of perforating veins in the medial lower leg. Vasc Surg 1998; 32(4):339–47
23. Hauer G, Wisser I, Deiler S. Subfasziale endoskopische Diszision der Perforansvenen. In: Brunner U (ed.) Der Unterschenkel. Aktuelle Probleme in der Angiologie. Huber, Bern, 1988: 187–92
24. Sattler G, Mössler K, Hagedorn M. Prophylaxe und Therapie des Ulcus cruris: Endoskopische Perforantenen diszision und antegrade paratibiale faszcitome. In: Mahrle G, Schulze Hospitalization, Krieg T (eds) Wundheilung-Wundverschluss, Fortschritte der operativen und onkologischen Dermatologie, Band 8. Springer Verlag, Berlin, 1994: 225–9
25. Langer C, Vorpahl U. Endoskopische Fasziotomie und Perforansdissektion in Phlebologie. In: Berlien P, Müller GJ (eds) Angewandte Lasermedizin. Lehr-und Handbuch für Praxis und Klinik, 8, Erg. Lfg. Ecomed Landsberg Lech, 1994
26. Wittens CHA, Pierik RGMJ, van Urk H. The surgical treatment of incompetent perforating veins. Eur J Vasc Endovasc Surg 1995; 9:19–23
27. Juhan C et al. Angiotechniques. Chirurgie particularly voie endoscopique des veines perforantes de jambe et chirurgie des veines jumelles. Abstract: Phlébologie 1996; 9:358, Livre des Communications de la Réunion du 2 Février 1996; Prof. Claude Juhan, Hôpital Nord, Marseille, France, 104 pp
28. Bergan JJ, Ballard JL, Sparks S, Murray JS. Chirurgie subfasciale des veines perforantes. Phlébologie 1996; 49:467–72
29. Sparks SR, Ballard JL, Bergan JJ, Killeen JD. Early benefits of subfascial endoscopic perforator vein surgery (SEPS) in healing venous ulcers. Ann Vasc Surg 1997; 11:367–73
30. Bergan JJ, Ballard JL, Sparks S. Subfascial endoscopic perforating surgery: the open technique. In: Bergan JJ Gloviczki P (eds) Atlas of endoscopic perforator vein surgery. Springer-Verlag, London, 1997: 141–52
31. Murray JA, Bergan JJ, Riffenburg RH. Development of open-scope SEPS: lessons learned from the first 67 cases. Ann Vasc Surg in press

Management of Venous Ulceration: Excision, Skin Grafting and Microsurgical Flaps

13

Raymond M. Dunn, Michael J. Rohrer and Adam J. Vernadakis

A regimen of leg elevation, compression bandaging and local wound care is successful in healing the majority of venous ulcers. Failure of a venous ulcer to heal with appropriate wound care or recurrence despite these measures leaves the physician with a challenge in which multiple factors must be addressed in order to achieve long-term wound closure. Most surgical interventions employed to address refractory venous ulceration have been directed at correcting underlying venous hypertension with the assumption that this would lead to resolution of the ulcer. However, even if successful control of venous hypertension in the extremity is achieved, a chronically scarred wound with compromised healing capacity may remain and require surgical reconstruction. Thus, the approach to reconstruction of the tissue defect associated with chronic venous ulceration is the subject of this chapter.

Characterization of the Chronic Venous Ulcer Wound

Venous ulcers are typically found on the medial and lateral perimalleolar areas. Extent of involvement in an individual patient may vary from discrete foci of ulceration to extensive bi-malleolar or even circumferential ulceration.[1] Though unusual, we have seen ulceration on the dorsum of the foot and toes as well. As the extent and duration of ulceration and liposclerosis progress, further involvement of the extremity can occur which may further limit already compromised wound healing ability. Scarring of the leg may also progress to involve the lymphatic system,[2] resulting in lymphedema. This predisposes the patient to recurrent infection and additional skin and tissue damage.

Chronic venous ulceration leads to a protracted inflammatory and fibroplastic phase of wound healing which results in the deposition of excessive scar tissue in the area of the wound, termed liposclerosis or lipodermatosclerosis. The deposition of collagen, fibrinogen and hemosiderin results in a complex nutritional deficiency with respect to wound healing.[3-5] As demonstrated in Chap. 3, an appropriation of the complexity of the pathogenesis of venous ulceration is important to understand the limitations of current surgical management of the chronic venous ulcer wound.[6-13]

Chronic Venous Ulcer Wound Reconstruction

When the area of venous ulceration is localized and underlying tissue involvement is limited, wound care and control of venous hypertension by elevation and external compression bandaging almost always allows ulcer healing to occur[14]. Compliant use of elastic support usually prevents recurrence in most of these patients. When the tissue defect is sufficiently large or combined with severe underlying scar (liposclerosis), healing of the wound may not be possible without tissue replacement. The tendency of venous ulcer disease to remain localized to one region (the medial and lateral lower leg) and to be chronic or recurrent in the same area in an individual patient provides a distinct opportunity for limited tissue replacement to accomplish very good long-term results in properly selected and executed cases.

Measures employed in the pursuit of tissue replacement began with skin grafting over 100 years ago[15-18] and have evolved as new reconstructive techniques have been developed. Each technique of soft tissue reconstruction involves many of the same basic principles. Appropriate application of these principles will determine the type of reconstruction employed and substantially influence the likelihood of a successful outcome.

Techniques of tissue replacement can be divided into two broad categories. The first encompasses all forms of skin grafting and tissue engineered replacements, which depend on the revascularization or "take" of the graft by the recipient site. The second category includes all types of flap transfers, where the tissue replacement is supported by its own blood supply and does not depend upon deriving vascular supply from the recipient site. These latter forms of reconstruction may actually add vascularity to the area being grafted. Skin grafts require a healthy, well vascularized recipient site, while flaps may be applied to areas where scar tissue, tendon or bone require tissue coverage.

Excision and Skin Grafting

Skin grafting is the most common technique of tissue replacement utilized for the treatment of venous ulcers because of its relative simplicity and low morbidity. There is wide variation in published recommendations for excision of venous ulcer tissue at the time of skin grafting, which makes a critical assessment of results very difficult. It is our opinion that results of any type of skin graft reconstruction for venous ulceration may be as much

dependent on the type of wound excision performed as the type of skin graft used. This illustrates the critical importance of the condition of the ulcer bed in supporting the grafted skin. Discussion regarding the approach to chronic venous ulcer excision assumes the patient has undergone thorough investigation of underlying venous hemodynamic abnormalities as well as evaluation of any related medical disorders. Remedial conditions should have been addressed and corrected whenever possible. It is very important to identify and treat peripheral arterial occlusive disease as a contributing cause of impaired ulcer healing.[19] Removal of grossly nonviable wound tissue prior to reconstruction is presumed throughout this discussion.

Biology of Skin Grafts

The biology of skin graft healing has been investigated carefully in both experimental and clinical studies.[20-26] Skin grafts heal by attachment to the tissues onto which they are placed. Initially, grafts attach by a fibrin clot and are nourished by diffusion from the underlying wound bed. This diffusional nutrition was initially referred to as "plasmatic circulation" and was first described 100 years ago in 1888.[27] Subsequent investigational work proposed a more accurate description of this phase of healing as serum imbibition,[28,29] referring to the diffusional nutrition of the graft prior to actual revascularization, which begins to occur at 48–72 hours. The importance of the fibrin clot for initial graft adhesion cannot be underestimated since the presence of excessive endogenous or exogenous fibrinolysins such as those produced by certain bacterial strains of *Staphylococcus*, *Streptococcus* or *Pseudomonas* can impair initial graft adherence and interfere with adequate serum imbibition, leading to failure of the skin graft.[30,31]

An understanding of the process of skin graft healing helps one to understand the importance of appropriate preparation of the graft recipient site at the time of surgery and its significance to graft survival. In an initially stable graft, "inosculation" to existing graft blood vessels begins between 48–72 h, with capillary ingrowth soon occurring to existing and newly formed microvessels within the grafted skin.[32,33] The process of healing of epithelial, split thickness and full thickness grafts is similar, but there are important differences which relate to the healing of different types of grafts as well as the amount of available donor sites for such grafts. These areas will be discussed further in the following sections.

Techniques of Skin Grafting

Skin grafts can be classified as allografts or autografts. Each of these graft types can be employed as a split thickness or full thickness graft and can be placed as either a meshed or sheet graft.[34,35] Allografting refers to the use of human skin grafts from an unrelated donor. Although this technique does not provide permanent wound closure because of eventual immunologic graft rejection, it can be used to promote intrinsic healing of the underlying wound in selected cases.[36]

Essentially, all reports discussing skin grafting of venous ulcers utilize some form of split thickness skin graft. Split thickness skin grafting refers to the use of a "split" portion of dermis, which includes the epithelial layers of skin. Split thickness skin grafts can easily be harvested in sheets with modern dermatomes. Skin grafts also can be harvested using the "pinch" graft technique, where grafts are raised by pinching the piece of skin to be used and cutting it off beneath the pinched area. This technique is rarely used, except for the treatment of small wounds. Donor sites will heal spontaneously from residual epithelial elements in the remaining dermis in roughly 10–14 days, depending upon the site selected for donor skin and the thickness of the split graft.

The thickness of the split thickness skin graft will determine the proportion of epithelial remnants which are left at the donor site to regenerate epithelial wound closure as well as the proportion of these which are transferred to the graft site. This ratio will influence the quality of skin in both the residual donor site as well as the recipient grafting site. The initial "take" or healing of a split thickness skin graft is inversely proportional to the thickness of the graft, since the thickness determines the nutritional and metabolic needs of the graft during the initial period of plasmatic imbibition.[37,38] Once initial healing of the skin graft occurs, a maturation process begins with rapid epithelial growth and desquamation, with substantial loss and turnover of collagen in healing skin grafts over the first several months.[39,40] Survival

and growth of skin appendages, such as sebaceous and sweat glands, is dependent on the thickness of the graft and sympathetic reinnervation, which is important for the long-term stability of grafted areas. Skin appendages in split thickness skin grafts mimic recipient sites in function but lack the same density, thereby providing an improved albeit imperfect tissue replacement. This fact may play a role in the limited long-term stability of skin grafts and subsequent recurrent ulceration.

Meshing of skin grafts is an additional technique which may be employed in ulcer treatment. The technique of meshing involves mechanically cutting multiple small windows into the harvested graft. These "windows" allow the drainage of any serous fluid that might otherwise lift the graft from the wound bed and limit its take. Meshing also increases the surface area of the graft, reducing the size of the donor site. As no components of the dermis exist in these small "windows", healing occurs by epithelialization from the adjacent skin graft.

Wound Excision in Conjunction with Skin Grafting

Nonexcisional Grafting
A chronic venous ulcer with granulation tissue provides the minimal acceptable condition for skin grafting. Application of a split thickness skin graft to a granulating ulcer is a simple and minimally invasive option for the surgical management of chronic venous ulceration. However, there are several clinical limitations which are important to consider. A favorable microbiologic wound environment is crucial for healing of the transferred skin graft.[31,41–43] Determination of the extent of bacterial colonization of granulation tissue without quantitative tissue culture is subjective and difficult to determine by clinical judgment alone. More importantly, no alteration in the pathogenesis of the underlying tissue disorder which produced ulceration will have been made, predisposing the patient to ulcer recurrence. Despite these limitations, this approach has been successfully employed in certain circumstances, and it may be considered appropriate in patients who are otherwise poor candidates for more thorough excision of their ulcers because of its low morbidity.

Results of simple grafting of ulcers without ulcer excision come predominantly from the dermatology literature where there are multiple reports of grafting using various types of split thickness skin grafts and "pinch" grafts, some of which were meshed[44-60] (Table 13.1). A thorough analysis of this work is limited by the failure of most of these reports to carefully document an objective hemodynamic assessment of the ulcerated extremity, making the role of this simple technique difficult to determine. Millard et al.[46] reported on 75 patients who underwent pinch grafting of leg ulcers. Most of the patients had wounds that were described as "gravitational" ulcers, but diagnostic criteria were not outlined, nor were any concomitant medical problems noted. They reported a 75% initial ulcer healing rate and 68% success at 2 years in this group. Additional reports using similar techniques of split thickness skin grafting, all without any ulcer excision, report healing rates from 80%[49] to 90%[50] at 1 year to 64%[53] at 6 weeks. Each of these reports relates little or no information on patient evaluation or more extended follow-up, both of which are critically important to objectively evaluate efficacy of this grafting technique, particularly as it relates to venous ulcer treatment. Ruffieux et al.[61] reported on a cohort of 188 patients with mixed but predominantly venous ulcers. Again, there was no objective data on the diagnostic criteria. They noted a 44% ulcer recurrence rate with split thickness skin grafting versus 45% ulcer recurrence in a non randomized group who did not undergo grafting. The nongrafted group had substantially smaller ulcers than the group that underwent skin grafting. Other studies using similar techniques show generally similar results.[62-64]

Tangential Ulcer Excision and Grafting

Tangential excision in the fatty layer immediately beneath the ulcer removes a greater amount of surrounding scar tissue. This approach has the advantage of removing some amount of bacterial colonization in the overlying granulation tissue. However, this superficial excision fails to remove the adjacent liposclerotic tissue and accomplishes nothing with respect to changing the underlying hemodynamic or tissue abnormality. The value of this approach is found in its low morbidity and blood loss. However, review of results in which partial ulcer excision was performed[65-67] (Table 13.1) reveals very little difference from those in which no ulcer excision was done. Descriptions of the technical aspects of ulcer excision suggest a range of excision from a minor excision of granulation tissue to more extensive excision into the fatty tissue beneath the ulcer. Wide variability in techniques makes it difficult to draw conclusions about the role ulcer excision has in reported results.

Table 13.1. Results of skin graft reconstruction of chronic venous ulcers

Author (year)	No. patients/no. ulcers	Follow-up (mean)	Failure/recurrence	Vascular evaluation
Non-excision STSG/pinch graft				
Millard (1977)	33/33	24 months	49%	None described
Kirsner (1995)	29/36	11 months	48%	Mixed pathology
Ceilley (1977)	75	12 months	20%	None described
Berretty (1979)	12/12	14 months	11%	None described
Poskitt (1987)	25/53	3 months	26%	Noninvasive testing
Ruffieux (1997)	188/144	?	44%	None described
Vesterager (1980)	34	13 months	41%	None described
Wood (1995)	10	?	80%	2 patients evaluated
Wide-excision/skin graft				
Lofgren clinical (1965)	129/129	(87%) 3–12 years	30%	Limited/good criteria
Andersen (1963)	33/40	12 months	15%	Venograms
	37/40		(5% if minor dermatitis excluded)	
Silver (1971)	28/311	58% (5 years)	10%+	"Postphlebitic" *simultaneous perforator ligation
Harma (1994)	21	?	19%	None described
Teplitsky (1948)	21	(50%) 24 months	? 20%	None described
Cikrit (1988)	27	6 months–10 years	22%	22 venograms
Porter (1984)	14	4 years	20%	

Subfascial Excision and Grafting

The high rate of recurrence of venous ulceration after either nonoperative management[61] or split thickness skin grafting without ulcer excision has led surgeons to focus on control of venous hypertension transmitted to the skin, with the goal of decreasing the rate of ulcer recurrence after surgical intervention. This approach, originally advocated by Cockett,[68] Linton[69] and others,[70-74] involved ligation of perforating veins and superficial vein tributaries even beyond the area of actual ulcer involvement. However, even with contributions to the correction of venous hypertension in the extremity, these surgical modalities may not be successful[75] if tissue damage (liposclerosis/ ulceration) has progressed to a point where skin loss is replaced by fibrotic scar that cannot reliably support thin epithelial coverage, a function provided by the dermis.[7] By performing resection of ulcer tissue at the subfascial level, the surgeon is obligated to combine some degree of ligation of perforating veins in the base of the ulcerated area. Closure of the resulting wound with a skin graft may then result in an area less

prone to ulcer recurrence (Figs 13.1 and 13.2) and may play a role in the improved results reported employing this type of grafting. Numerous reports advocate either suprafascial or subfascial excision of a venous ulcer at the time of planned skin grafting or shortly before. Although difficult to compare studies because of differences in technique, results of this approach have been reported by various authors[76-83] (Table 13.1). Those reports attribute improvement in ulcer recurrence rates to wider excision of compromised tissue. One common observation in each of these reports is the description of recurrent ulceration at the margins of previous ulcer excision within areas of residual lipodermatosclerosis. Andersen[78,84] reported a 15% ulcer recurrence after wide excision and grafting, but two-thirds of these were not actual ulceration. Instead, they were minimal psoriatic breakdown of skin grafts, which can in part be attributed to limitations of graft biology itself and not to underlying venous disease. Excluding these cases yields a 95% success of wide excision and grafting in the study group. Of note, no comments were made regarding

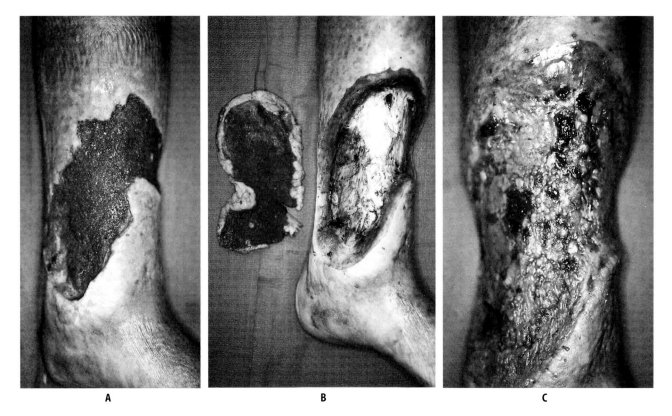

A   **B**   **C**

Fig. 13.1. A Extensive venous ulceration with severe lipodermatosclerosis with failure of healing after 6 months of compression therapy. **B** Conservative subfascial ulcer excision with beveled cutaneous margins and adjacent ulcer specimen. **C** Skin grafted ulcer 2 weeks postoperatively, with overall good "take". Compression therapy and small secondary skin graft has allowed complete ulcer healing.

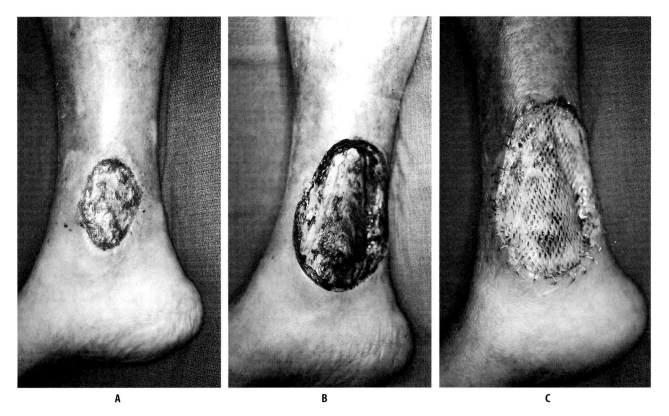

A   **B**   **C**

Fig. 13.2. A Refractory venous ulceration in an elderly patient. Ideally this wound would be reconstructed with a free flap after subfascial resection but the patient's age and medical problems prompted a lesser procedure to be undertaken. **B** Ulcer is resected widely, and in a supra- and subfascial plane, being careful to avoid exposure of tendon or bone, leaving paratenon and periosteum intact. **C** Simple meshed split-thickness skin graft. With meticulous postoperative care including application of compression therapy, initially biweekly starting at postoperative day 5, and then weekly for 6 weeks, this patient has experienced complete ulcer healing.

ulcer recurrence in an area outside the original area of ulceration and surrounding scar bed. It is interesting that in 1917 Homans[85] advocated an approach much the same as described by these authors above with respect to resection of venous ulcers.

Early ulcer recurrence after skin grafting is more likely a failure of complete skin graft "take".[86] Several months of diligent postoperative care of the grafted ulcer may be required for the graft to hypertrophy and develop stable adherence to the underlying tissue.

Tissue Engineering Skin Equivalents

The need for skin substitutes to treat burns, trauma or other injury, as well as venous ulceration has led clinicians to use skin substitutes for decades.[87–90] Initially these grafts were porcine xenografts or human allografts. Historically, these have had very little application in the treatment of venous ulcer disease since they provide only temporary wound coverage. More recently, advances in biotechnology have extensively explored a class of products called living skin equivalents (LSE), although other nomenclature has been employed such as biologic wound dressings (BWD). These products have been developed for use in three areas; to replace the dermal component of skin, to replace the epidermal component of skin, or to replace both dermal and epidermal elements as a true bioengineered skin substitute.

Dermal and epidermal tissue elements have complex cellular and acellular tissue components which serve complex immunologic, barrier and mechanical functions. The development of LSE/BWD has focused on the barrier and mechanical functions of skin. Currently available bioengineered products have used either bovine, porcine or human collagen, all of which have been extensively tested to exclude infectious or communicable diseases. One example of the dermal substitutes is Biobrane™ (Dow B. Hickam, Sugarland, TX). This product, which is used as a temporary wound dressing, is derived from porcine collagen covered with silastic.[91] The addition of neonatal fibroblasts to a polygalactin or polyglycolic substrate with subsequent cryopreservation and maintenance of cellular viability as a construct for dermal substitution is found in Dermagraft Transitional Coverage (Advanced Tissue Sciences, La Jolla, CA).[92,93] Integra (Integra Life Sciences Corporation, Plainsboro, NJ) employs bovine collagen with chrondroitin-6-sulfate covered with silastic, which is followed several weeks later by the placement of an epidermal autograft. Alloderm (LifeCell Corporation, The Woodlands, TX), which uses a human dermal matrix that preserves basement membrane and ground substance elements, also requires an epidermal overlay as a second procedure.

In May of 1998, a bioengineered skin substitute composed of bovine collagen, human fibroblast and keratinocytes known as Apligraf (Organogenesis, Inc, Canton, MA) was specifically approved for treatment of chronic venous ulceration. In a comparative study using Apligraf, a statistically significant improvement in venous ulcer healing was demonstrated in the early data, particularly in patients with venous ulcers that were present for greater than 1 year compared to control patients treated with compression bandaging.[5]

In summary, each of the LSE/ BWD provide temporary coverage of a wound where tissue replacement ultimately occurs by autologous cellular turnover of the bioengineered matrix. An important observation is that investigations with all these products have shown utility (i.e., enhanced healing), without long-term data on wound or ulcer recurrence. It would seem reasonable to postulate that the best possible healing results would be similar to those obtained in studies that have used nonexcisional autografts as described earlier. However, assessment of long-term results is ongoing. The advantage that these bioengineered products may offer is the minimal morbidity associated with their use since the LSE/BWD do not require an autologous tissue donor site or wound debridement. However, one area of concern that may become apparent is the potential preferential use of these products because of their convenience when a more significant surgical intervention is actually indicated.

Flap Reconstruction of Chronic Venous Ulceration

Surgeons over the last century recognized the advantage of removing all severely scarred tissue associated with venous ulceration but were faced with the need for more extensive tissue reconstructive needs when this type of resection was performed. Radical excision of ulcers in the distal leg often resulted in exposure of bony areas of the tibia and malleolus which were highly prone to reulceration with minor trauma when simple skin grafts were applied (Fig. 13.1). In addition, the "take" of grafts was more difficult in these locations because of limited ability of bone to provide the initial diffusional nutrition to support the graft as well as critical neovascularization for full healing. These facts led surgeons to employ composite tissue grafts that carry their own blood supply for use in closure of ulcers which involve structures not suitable for simple skin grafts. These flap grafts can be divided into two categories, "local" and "free." Local flaps include those grafts that are transferred from the region of the leg near the area of ulceration. The flap must have a blood supply which will allow it to be rotated into an ulcer defect without disruption of arterial and venous circulation. Free flaps are composite tissue grafts that have an anatomically specific and reliable arterial and venous circulation. This flap can be taken from one area of the body and transferred "free" of any attachment and then connected to a remote arterial and venous blood supply for immediate revascularization. This type of flap is not dependent on the site of grafting for any nutritional or metabolic requirements and only requires presence of the vessels needed for the anastamoses. Free flaps have the advantage of being flexible in dimension to specifically correct or close any wound in any location within defined size limitations.

Local Flaps

Utility of local flaps is very limited in the distal one-third of the leg, which is the most common site of venous ulcers requiring reconstruction. These flaps are derived from local tissues, and there is very often some degree of liposclerosis in the skin, fat and fascia which are used for a component of the flap. This fact may limit the size of the flap which would be used

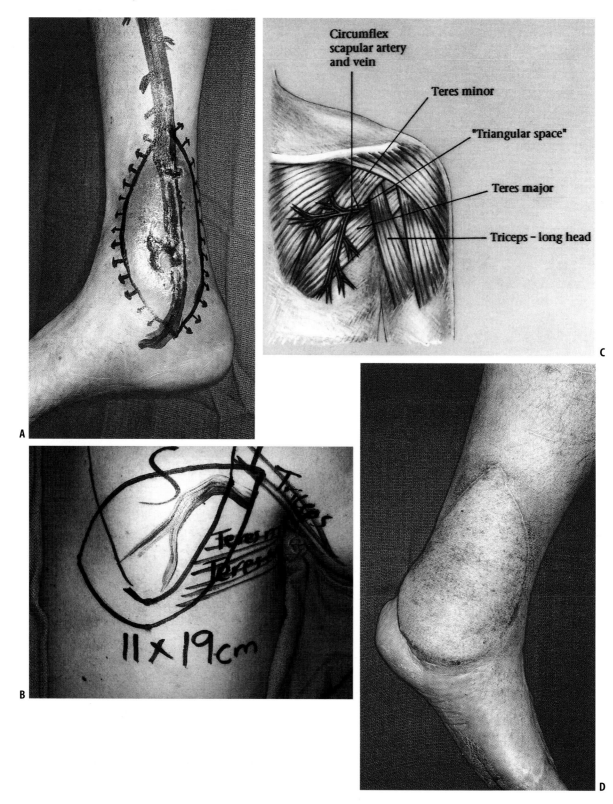

Fig. 13.3. A Healthy active patient with recurrent ulceration and deep venous valvular insufficiency failing multiple attempts at compressive therapy. Two areas of ulceration and liposclerosis are present, which are amenable to wide excision. Posterior tibial vessels are outlined in red and blue and are examined preoperatively via duplex exam to locate incompetent perforating veins and assure normal arterial flow and adequate venous outflow. **B** Outline and dimensions of the donor flap with the patient placed in the lateral decubitus position. **C** Schematic outline of the typical vascular anatomy of the circumflex scapular vessels and tributaries exiting the triangular space of the back and supplying the skin overlying the vessels and in fact the entire upper and mid back skin territory. **D** Patient 5 years after free scapular flap reconstruction of a recurrent chronic venous ulcer. He has no ulcer recurrence either in the flap or in any portion of the leg. He wears elastic stockings.

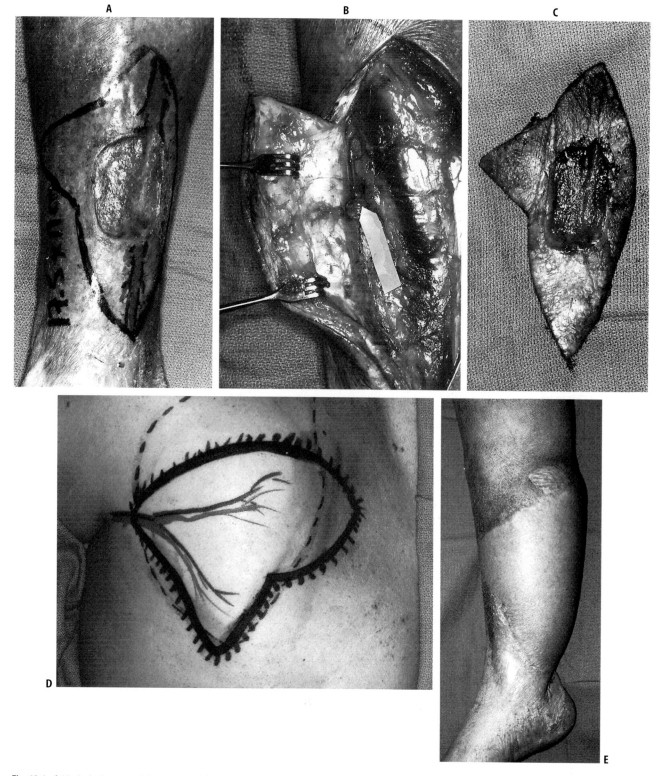

Fig. 13.4. A Moderately overweight woman with 17-year history of refractory venous ulceration and liposclerosis. Multiple attempts at compression therapy were unsuccessful. The area of proposed ulcer resection is outlined, encompassing the most severe tissue disease. **B** At the time of subfascial ulcer resection, several perforating veins from the anterior tibial venous system were noted (arrow) and ligated. **C** Ulcer and surrounding liposclerotic skin. This patient's extensive liposclerosis could not be resected in its entirety. **D** Outline of flap on the back showing a *fleur-de-lis* pattern, allowing a larger flap to be harvested and still obtain primary closure of the donor wound. **E** Flap reconstruction 4.5 years postoperatively. Note the small skin graft in the upper medial leg which was placed over fatty tissue of the flap at the initial operation. This small skin graft has remained as soft and pliable as the flap itself. This patient suffered a delayed area of healing at the "crotch" of the *fleur-de-lis* pattern on both the leg and the back, each of which healed secondarily without further operative intervention. The patient faithfully wears elastic stockings and has had no recurrence of ulceration even in the areas of unresected liposclerotic skin.

for wound closure. Muscle flaps, such as those derived from the gastrocnemius and soleus muscles, occasionally may be used. Although muscle flaps are not subject to liposclerosis, they are limited in size and by their arc of rotation. Therefore, they primarily provide coverage of areas in the more proximal lower leg which are less commonly involved with venous ulceration. Despite these limitations, if the area of liposclerosis and ulceration is finite, local flaps may be a good choice for a very select number of cases. Because of their limited applicability, there are only a few clinical reports of the reconstruction of venous ulcers using local/regional leg flaps.[94,95]

Microsurgical Free Flaps

The advent of principles and instrumentation for microvascular surgery in the 1970s eventually led pioneering microsurgeons to attempt reconstructive procedures in many areas of the body where previous reconstructive efforts were performed in multiple stages, or not at all. Initially, there was a reluctance to perform these procedures on patients with venous ulcer disease because of the perception that wound severity could be made worse by flap failure. In addition, a free microvascular flap requires good quality venous outflow and patients with venous ulcer disease have underlying venous hypertension. As experience in microsurgery grew and results improved, indications for employing this technique expanded. Descriptive case reports of patients undergoing free flap reconstruction for chronic venous ulcers were published, demonstrating the potential utility of this technique.[96–98] Assessment of the success of these early series was limited by short follow-up. Furthermore, patients had limited or no preoperative hemodynamic evaluation and determination of the role of this technique for reconstruction of venous ulcer disease was still pending clarification. In 1994, we reported on a series of patients with documented deep venous insufficiency and chronic venous ulceration who underwent microvascular fasciocutaneous flap reconstruction.[99] Postoperative photoplethysmographic (PPG) refill time measurements on the flap areas revealed improvement to the normal range over the reconstructed areas, as well an absence of histologic evidence of liposclerotic changes in the flap tissue over a 2–7 year period. There were no ulcer recurrences in the limited patient series reported.

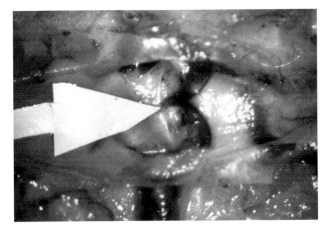

Fig. 13.5. Approximately 1 mm. bicuspid valve in the circumflex scapular vein of the scapular flap shown at the tip of the arrow. Our morphologic studies have shown numerous valves to be present in an average flap transfer.

Ours and other subsequent anatomic studies have documented the presence of multiple valves (Fig. 13.5) in the venous system of the transferred flaps, representing the hemodynamic equivalent of a combined tissue and valve transplantation.[100–102] Subsequent work has revealed *in-vivo* evidence of competency of the transferred valve segments.[103] In one patient who underwent amputation because of unreconstructable ulceration of the forefoot and toes, the amputation specimen showed continued valve competency and integrity of the flap tissue (Fig. 13.6).

There have been additional reports of free flap reconstruction in patients with chronic venous ulceration using predominantly muscle flaps.[104,105] One of these reports[106] revealed a 90% flap success rate and a 95% ulcer-free rate at a mean of 32 months postoperatively in 18 patients. In this study, there were no recurrent ulcerations within the territory of the transplanted flap. Recurrent ulcerations were noted to be present at the flap margin in some patients where residual liposclerotic tissue might remain. An additional study[43] showed a much higher rate of ulcer recurrence, but upon careful review, the recurrences were noted to be at the margins of the flaps. These reports demonstrate the value of wider debridement margins, since ulcer recurrence could potentially be prevented by excising the involved liposclerotic tissue at the time of flap reconstruction. However, resection of ulcer tissue and surrounding liposclerotic scar may be limited since each flap has a somewhat defined anatomical size limitation.

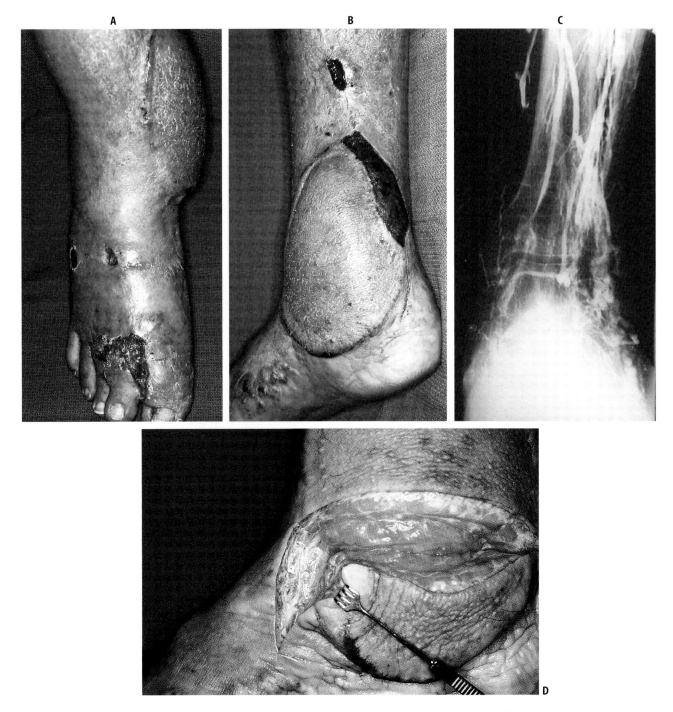

Fig. 13.6. **A** Patient shown following flap transfer with severe recalcitrant ulceration in the foot in multiple locations. **B** The same patient is shown with additional ulceration in an old perforator ligation incision as well as at the margin of his flap reconstruction where incomplete resection of liposclerosis was accomplished. **C** The patient elected to undergo a below the knee amputation after 1 year of compression therapy failed to heal the ulceration. At the time of specimen removal a retrograde venogram through the posterior tibial vein was performed and is shown. The flap is on the left side of the photo. The posterior tibial vein and venous system of the foot fill readily via retrograde injection illustrating the magnitude of venous valvular insufficiency present. The flap vein fails to fill as a result of a readily visible vein valve which is competent in the flap, shown on the upper left adjacent to the tibia. **D** The leg specimen, including the previous flap transfer shows no gross evidence of any morphologic changes of liposclerosis as clearly visible in the adjacent tissues.

Review of our recent results in 20 patients with 23 flaps with an average 49 month follow-up with the use of fasciocutaneous flaps in reconstruction of refractory venous ulcers has shown an 18% ulcer recurrence. Each of these recurrences presented at the margin of the flaps adjacent to liposclerotic skin.[103] No ulceration occurred within the flap.

Experience has taught us that the critical aspect of successful free flap reconstruction is adequate resection of the venous ulcer and the surrounding liposclerotic tissue area. At this time, the ability to determine what constitutes an adequate soft tissue resection remains subjective and defined by clinical judgment. We currently make every effort to resect the ulcer and liposclerosic tissue back to an area of soft pliable skin and subcutaneous tissue. Ulcer resection should be performed in a subfascial plane so that simultaneous ligation of perforating veins in the region of tissue resection and several centimeters beyond this margin may be performed. When the free flap covers the wound in this area, this effectively "cures" the region of resection and immediately adjacent tissue from the likelihood of ulcer recurrence. Microvenous valves in flap transfers may provide limited protection within the flap from the overall venous hypertension of the abnormal extremity in which the reconstruction is performed.

Amputation

Some recurrent ulcerations have not been amenable to reconstructive attempts, or the aforementioned treatment modalities have been unsuccessful. For these unfortunate patients, amputation may be the only reasonable alternative to alleviate the pain and disability associated with the recurrent ulcerations.

Summary

Review of the literature on reconstruction of recurrent venous ulceration illustrates several principles. Readily treatable venous abnormalities should be corrected to improve venous hemodynamics. Assessment of the location, extent and severity of the ulcer and liposclerotic tissue involvement should be made in patients with severe tissue damage who require grafting. These findings will determine extent of required ulcer excision as well as the suitability of skin grafting or flap reconstruction to accomplish wound closure. If only the

superficial venous system is involved and there is a limited extent of ulceration with no involvement of joint, tendon or bone, then, saphenous stripping with varicose vein excision and possible skin grafting can be performed with an expectation of excellent healing and long-term stability. If venous ulceration extends to an area such that ulcer resection will result in exposure of bone, tendon or joint or if the scar tissue is severe, then free flap reconstruction should be considered. If the area of ulceration and liposclerosis extends substantially beyond the dimensions that a flap can reconstruct then a combination of flap reconstruction and skin grafting may be employed.

References

1. Hallbook T. Leg ulcer epidemiology. Acta Chir Scand Suppl 1988; 544:17–20
2. Collins PS, Villavicencio JL, Abreu SH et al. Abnormalities of lymphatic drainage in lower extremities: a lymphoscintigraphic study. J Vasc Surg 1989; 9(1):145–52
3. Gingrass P, Grabb WC, Gingrass RP. Skin graft survival on avascular defects. Plast Reconstr Surg 1975; 55(1):65–70
4. Michel CC. Oxygen diffusion in oedematous tissue and through peri-capillary cuffs. Phlebology 1990; 5:223–30
5. Falanga V, Kirsner R, Katz MH et al. Pericapillary fibrin cuffs in venous ulceration. Persistence with treatment and during ulcer healing. J Dermatol Surg Oncol 1992; 18(5):409–14
6. Fagrell B. Local microcirculation in chronic venous incompetence and leg ulcers. Vasc Surg 1979; 13(4):217–25
7. Burnand K, Thomas ML, O'Donnell T et al. Relation between post-phlebitic changes in the deep veins and results of surgical treatment of venous ulcers. Lancet 1976; 1(7966):936-8.
8. Burnand KG, Whimster I, Naidoo A, et al. Pericapillary fibrin in the ulcer-bearing skin of the leg: the cause of lipodermatosclerosis and venous ulceration. Br Med J (Clin Res Ed) 1982; 285(6348):1071–2
9. Burnand KG. The aetiology of venous ulceration. Acta Chir Scand Suppl 1988; 544:21–4
10. Burnand KG. Aetiology of venous ulceration [see comments]. Br J Surg 1990; 77(5):483–4
11. Cornwall JV, Dore CJ, Lewis JD. Leg ulcers: epidemiology and aetiology. Br J Surg 1986; 73(9):693–6
12. Angel MF, Ramasastry SS, Swartz WM et al. The causes of skin ulcerations associated with venous insufficiency: a unifying hypothesis. Plast Reconstr Surg 1987; 79(2):289–97
13. Labropoulos N, Delis K, Nicolaides AN et al. The role of the distribution and anatomic extent of reflux in the development of signs and symptoms in chronic venous insufficiency. J Vasc Surg 1996; 23(3):504–10
14. Fegan G. Skin-grafting leg ulcers. Lancet 1970; 1(7643):416
15. Reverdin JL. Greffe épidermique. Bull Imp Soc Chir Paris 1869; 10:511
16. Reverdin JL. Sur la greffe épidermique. Compt Rend Acad Sci (Paris) 1871; 73:1280
17. Thiersch C. Ueber hautverpflanzung. Zentralbl Chir 1886; 13:17
18. Wolfe JR. A new method of performing plastic operations. Br Med J 1875; 2:360
19. Gilliland EL, Nathwani N, Dore CJ et al. Bacterial colonisation of leg ulcers and its effect on the success rate of skin grafting. Ann R Coll Surg Engl 1988; 70(2):105–8

20. Hauben DJ, Baruchin A, Mahler A. On the history of the free skin graft. Ann Plast Surg 1982; 9(3):242–5
21. Ratner D. Skin grafting. From here to there. Dermatol Clin 1998; 16(1):75–90
22. Chick LR. Brief history and biology of skin grafting. Ann Plast Surg 1988; 21(4):358–65
23. Kirsner RS, Falanga V, Eaglestein WH. The biology of skin grafts. Skin grafts as pharmacologic agents [see comments]. Arch Dermatol 1993; 129(4):481–3
24. Smahel J. The healing of skin grafts. Clin Plast Surg 1977; 4(3):409–24
25. Mir y Mir, L. Biology of the skin graft: New aspects to consider in its revascularization. Plast Reconstruct Surg 1951; 8(5):378–89
26. Wright JK, Brawer MK. Survival of full-thickness skin grafts over avascular defects. Plast Reconstr Surg 1980; 66(3):428–32
27. Huebscher W. Beitrage zur hautverpflanzung nach thiersch. Beitr Klin Chir1888; 4:395
28. Converse JM, Ballantyne DL Jr., Rogers BO et al. "Plasmatic circulation" in skin grafts. Transpl Bull 1957; 4:154
29. Converse JM, Uhlschmid GK, Ballantyne DL Jr. "Plasmatic circulation" in skin grafts. The phase of serum imbibition. Plast Reconstr Surg 1969; 43(5):495–9
30. Dahlstrom KK, Weis-Fogh US, Medgyesi S et al. The use of autologous fibrin adhesive in skin transplantation. Plast Reconstr Surg 1992; 89(5):968–72; discussion 973–6
31. Krizek TJ, Robson MC, Kho E. Bacterial growth and skin graft survival. Surg Forum 1968; 18:518
32. Birch J, Branemark PI, Nilsson K. The vascularization of a free full thickness skin graft. 3. An infrared thermographic study. Scand J Plast Reconstr Surg 1969; 3(1):18–22
33. Birch,J, Branemark PI, Lundskog J. The vascularization of a free full thickness skin graft. 2. A microangiographic study. Scand J Plast Reconstr Surg 1969; 3(1):11–17
34. Fifer TD, Pieper D, Hawtof D. Contraction rates of meshed, nonexpanded split-thickness skin grafts versus split-thickness sheet grafts. Ann Plast Surg 1993; 31(2):162–3
35. Converse JM. Reconstructive plastic surgery, 2nd edn. WB Saunders, Philadelphia, 1977: 182–191, 3522–3525
36. Leigh IM, Purkis PE, Navsaria HA et al. Treatment of chronic venous ulcers with sheets of cultured allogenic keratinocytes. Br J Dermatol 1987; 117(5):591–7
37. Vistnes LM. Grafting of skin. Surg Clin North Am 1977; 57(5):939–60
38. Birch J, Branemark PI. The vascularization of a free full thickness skin graft. 1. A vital microscopic study. Scand J Plast Reconstr Surg 1969; 3(1):1–10
39. Rudolph R, Klein L. Healing processes in skin grafts. Surg Gynecol Obstet 1973; 136(4):641–54
40. Hinshaw JR, Miller ER. Histology of healing split-thickness, full-thickness autogenous skin grafts and donor sites. Arch Surg 1965; 91(4):658–70
41. Teh BT. Why do skin grafts fail? Plast Reconstr Surg 1979; 63(3):323–32
42. Robson MC, Krizek TJ. Predicting skin graft survival. J Trauma 1973; 13(3):213–7
43. Steffe TJ, Caffee HH. Long term results following free tissue transfer for venous stasis ulcers. Ann Plast Surg 1998; in press
44. Michaelides P, Camisa C. The treatment of ulcers on legs with split-thickness skin grafts: report of a simple technique. J Dermatol Surg Oncol 1979; 5(12):961–5
45. Townsend J. Skin-grafting leg ulcers. Lancet 1970; 1(7636):39
46. Millard LG, Roberts MM, Gatecliffe M. Chronic leg ulcers treated by the pinch graft method. Br J Dermatol 1977; 97(3):289–95
47. Kirsner RS, Falanga V. Techniques of split-thickness skin grafting for lower extremity ulcerations [see comments]. J Dermatol Surg Oncol 1993; 19(8):779–83
48. Kirsner RS, Mata SM, Falanga V et al. Split-thickness skin grafting of leg ulcers. The University of Miami Department of Dermatology's experience (1990–1993). Dermatol Surg 1995; 21(8):701–3
49. Ceilley RI, Rinek MA, Zuehlke RL. Pinch grafting for chronic ulcers on lower extremities. J Dermatol Surg Oncol 1977; 3(3):303–9
50. Berretty PJ, Neumann HA, de Limpens AM et al. Treatment of ulcers on legs from venous hypertension by split-thickness skin grafts. J Dermatol Surg Oncol 1979; 5(12):966–70
51. Mol MA, Nanninga PB, van Eendenburg JP et al. Grafting of venous leg ulcers. An intraindividual comparison between cultured skin equivalents and full-thickness skin punch grafts [see comments]. J Am Acad Dermatol 1991; 24(1):77–82
52. Picascia DD, Roenigk HH Jr. Surgical management of leg ulcers. Dermatol Clin. 1987; 5(2):303–12
53. Poskitt KR, James AH, Lloyd-Davies ER et al. Pinch skin grafting or porcine dermis in venous ulcers: a randomised clinical trial. Br Med J (Clin Res Ed) 1987; 294(6573):674–6
54. van den Hoogenband HM. Treatment of leg ulcers with split-thickness skin grafts. J Dermatol Surg Oncol 1984; 10(8):605–8
55. Wheeland RG. The technique and current status of pinch grafting. J Dermatol Surg Oncol 1987; 13(8):873–80
56. Dzubow LM. Skin grafts [comment]. Dermatol Surg. 1995; 21(3):202
57. Dinner MI, Peters CR. Surgical management of ulcers on the lower limbs. J Dermatol Surg Oncol 1978; 4(9):696–9
58. Field LM. Grafts for ulcers on legs [letter]. J Dermatol Surg Oncol 1980; 6(3):164–5
59. Macadam R, Berridge DC. Use of split-skin grafting in the treatment of chronic leg ulcers [letter; comment]. Ann R Coll Surg Engl 1995; 77(6):463–4
60. Rivlin S. Skin-grafting leg ulcers. Lancet 1969; 2(7633):1310
61. Ruffieux P, Hommel L, Saurat JH. Long-term assessment of chronic leg ulcer treatment by autologous skin grafts. Dermatology 1997; 195(1):77–80
62. Vesterager L. Split-skin grafting for ulcers on legs. J Dermatol Surg Oncol 1980; 6(9):739–41
63. Wood MK, Davies DM. Use of split-skin grafting in the treatment of chronic leg ulcers [see comments]. Ann R Coll Surg Engl 1995; 77(3):222–3
64. Monk BE, Sarkany I. Outcome of treatment of venous stasis ulcers. Clin Exp Dermatol 1982; 7(4):397–400
65. Lofgren KA, Lofgren EP. Extensive ulcerations in the postphlebitic leg. Surg Clin North Am 1969; 49(5):1033–42
66. Brown, JB, Byars, LT, and Blair, VP. A study of ulcerations of the lower extremity and their repair with thick split skin grafts. *Surg Gynec Obstet* 1936; 63:331–40
67. Lofgren, KA. Surgical management of chronic venous insufficiency. *Acta Chir Scand Suppl* 1988; 544:62–8
68. Cockett, FB. the pathology and treatment of venous ulcers of the leg. *Br J Surg* 1956; 43(179):260–78
69. Linton, RR. The post-thrombotic ulceration of the lower extremity: its etiology and surgical treatment. *Ann Surg* 1953; 138:415
70. De Palma, RG. Surgical therapy for venous stasis. *Surgery* 1974; 76(6):910–7
71. Negus, D, Friedgood, A. The effective management of venous ulceration. *Br J Surg* 1983; 70(10):623–7
72. Hansson, LO. Venous ulcers of the lower limb: A follow-up study five years after surgical treatment. *Acta Chir Scand* 1964; 128:269–277
73. Jamieson, WG, DeRose, G, Harris, KA. Management of venous stasis ulcer: long-term follow-up. *Can J Surg* 1990; 33(3):222–3
74. Field, P, Van Boxel, P. The role of the Linton flap procedure in the management of stasis dermatitis and ulceration in the lower limb. *Surgery* 1971; 70(6):920–6
75. Robison, JG, Elliott, BM, Kaplan, AJ. Limitations of subfascial ligation for refractory chronic venous stasis ulceration. *Ann Vasc Surg* 1992; 6(1):9–14
76. Silver, D, Gleysteen, JJ, Rhodes, GR et al. Surgical treatment of the refractory postphlebitic ulcer. *Arch Surg* 1971; 103(5):554–60
77. Harma, M, Asko-Seljavaara, S, Lauharanta, J. Surgical treatment of chronic leg ulcers [letter]. *Acta Derm Venereol* 1994; 74(6):484–5
78. Andersen, MN, McDonald, KE. Results of surgical therapy of severe stasis ulceration of the legs. *Ann Surg* 1963; 157(2):281–6
79. Teplitsky, D, Shapiro, RN, and Robertson, GW. radical excision and skin grafting of leg ulcers. *Plast Reconst Surg* 1948; 3(2):189–96
80. Cikrit, DF, Nichols, WK, Silver, D. Surgical management of refractory venous stasis ulceration. *J Vasc Surg* 1988; 7(3):473–8

81. Porter, JM, Griffiths, RW, McNeill, DC. The surgical management of intractable venous ulceration in the lower limbs: excision, decompression of the limb and split-skin grafting. *Br J Plast Surg* 1984; 37(2):179–83

82. Lofgren, KA, Lauvstad, WA, Bonnemaison, MF. Surgical treatment of large stasis ulcer: review of 129 cases. *Mayo Clin Proc* 1965; 40:560–3

83. Julian, OC, Dye, WS, Schneewind, J. Surgical management of ulcerative stasis disease of the lower extremities. *Arch Surg* 1954; 68:757–68

84. Andersen, MN, Stephens, JG. A controlled study of surgical treatment and pathogenesis of stasis ulcers. *Ann Surg* 1959; 150(1):57–62

85. Homans, J. The etiology and treatment of varicose ulcer of the leg. *Surg Gynecol Obstet* 1917; 24:300–11

86. Trier, WC, Peacock, EE, Jr., Madden, JW. Studies on the effectiveness of surgical management of chronic leg ulcers. *Plast Reconstr Surg* 1970; 45(1):20–3

87. Burke, JF, Yannas, IV, Quinby, WC, Jr et al. Successful use of a physiologically acceptable artificial skin in the treatment of extensive burn injury. *Ann Surg* 1981; 194(4):413–28

88. Heimbach, D, Luterman, A, Burke, J et al. Artificial dermis for major burns. A multi-center randomized clinical trial. *Ann Surg* 1988; 208(3):313–20

89. Gallico, GGd, O'Connor, NE, Compton, CC et al. Permanent coverage of large burn wounds with autologous cultured human epithelium. *N Engl J Med* 1984; 311(7):448–51

90. Mahajan, R, Mosley, JG. Use of a semipermeable polyamide dressing over skin grafts to venous leg ulcers. *Br J Surg* 1995; 82(10):1359–60

91. Woodruff, EA. Biobrane, a biosynthetic skin prosthesis. In: DL Wise (ed.), *Burn Wound Coverings.* New York, NY; CRC, Inc, 1984

92. Purdue, GF, Hunt, JL, Still, JM, Jr et al. A multicenter clinical trial of a biosynthetic skin replacement, Dermagraft-TC, compared with cryopreserved human cadaver skin for temporary coverage of excised burn wounds. *J Burn Care Rehabil* 1997; 18(1 Pt 1):52–7

93. Cooper, ML, Hansbrough, JF, Spielvogel, RL et al. In vivo optimization of a living dermal substitute employing cultured human fibroblasts on a biodegradable polyglycolic acid or polyglactin mesh. *Biomaterials* 1991; 12(2):243–8

94. Lees, V, Townsend, PL. Use of a pedicled fascial flap based on septocutaneous perforators of the posterior tibial artery for repair of distal lower limb defects. *Br J Plast Surg* 1992; 45(2):141–5

95. Browse, NL, Burnand, KG, Thomas, ML. *Diseases of the Veins,* 2nd ed. London, Edward Arnold,1988: 424–7

96. Swartz, WM. Presented at the Proceedings of the Annual Meeting of the American Association of Plastic Surgeons. Scottsdale, AZ, 1989

97. Ramirez, OM. The effectiveness of the free muscle flap in the treatment of the recalcitrant venous stasis ulceration. *Plast Surg Forum* 1992; 15:77–78

98. Allen, RJ, Celentano, R, Dupin, C et al. Management of chronic venous insufficiency ulcers with free flaps: case study. *Wounds* 1989; 1:193–7

99. Dunn, RM, Fudem, GM, Walton, RL et al. Free flap valvular transplantation for refractory venous ulceration. *J Vasc Surg* 1994; 19(3):525–31

100. Aharinejad, S, Dunn, RM, Nourani, F et al. Morphological and clinical aspects of scapular fasciocutaneous free flap transfer for treatment of venous insufficiency in the lower extremity. *Clin Anat* 1998; 11(1):38–46

101. Aharinejad, S, Dunn, RM, Fudem, GM et al. The microvenous valvular anatomy of the human dorsal thoracic fascia. *Plast Reconstr Surg* 1997; 99(1):78–86

102. Shimizu, T, Ohno, K, Michi, K et al. Morphometric examination of the free scapular flap. *Plast Reconstr Surg* 1997; 99(7):1947–53

103. Dunn, RM, Fudem, GM, Vernadakis, AJ et al. The American Society of Reconstructive Microsurgery, Kamuela, Hawaii, 1999 (Accepted for presentation)

104. Weinzweig, N, Schlechter, B, Baraniewski, H et al. Lower-limb salvage in a patient with recalcitrant venous ulcerations. *J Reconstr Microsurg* 1997; 13(6):431–7

105. Weinzweig, N, Schuler, J, Vitello, J. Simultaneous reconstruction of extensive soft-tissue defects of both lower limbs with free hemiflaps harvested from the omentum. *Plast Reconstr Surg* 1997; 99(3):757–62

106. Weinzweig, N, Schuler, J. Free tissue transfer in treatment of the recalcitrant chronic venous ulcer. *Ann Plast Surg* 1997; 38(6):611–9

Venous Reconstruction: Evidence-based Analysis of Results

14

Robert L. Kistner, Bo Eklof, Danian Yang and Elna M. Masuda

Introduction

The purpose of this chapter is to analyze evidence in the literature for the validity of reconstruction in the deep venous system. This must begin with the recognition that there are no large or small randomized studies of different treatments in this field that would satisfy the criteria for Level I or Level II clinical evidence for therapy as defined by Sackett.[1] In all of the venous reconstruction literature there is only one trial that is nonrandomized with concurrent controls[2] (Level III evidence) while all of the rest of the reports are case series with no controls (Level V evidence). For these reasons, evidence in this subject can only be examined in light of the reliability of the original diagnosis, the types of testing used in the pre- and post-treatment analyses, the size of the various published series and the comparative results of different authors using similar treatment in similar patients.

In deep venous reconstruction, the very nature of an invasive and sometimes complicated surgical procedure creates the need for specific diagnosis of the whole venous tree in the extremity as a prerequisite to the procedure. Objective studies of the problem and its anatomic extent are crucial to decision-making before the very first surgical procedure is done in these patients. For this reason, data in publications about venous reconstruction begin from a base of thorough diagnosis of the entire extremity. This precision in pre-operative diagnosis provides a reliable base for evaluation of post-treatment results. This fact has created a qualitative improvement in data that has accumulated in publications about deep venous reconstructive surgery compared to non-surgical treatment and to surgical procedures on the superficial veins where the demands for precision in diagnosis of the entire venous tree are less compelling and seldom done.

Clinical diagnosis alone can be very misleading in advanced chronic venous insufficiency (CVI) and cannot be utilized for reliable evidence because similar external appearances and histories are found in extremities with very different pathologic findings. As an example, the six extremities in Figure 14.1 all show pigmentation and other skin changes that appear pre-ulcerative or actually are ulcerative. By clinical inspection all of these appear to be examples of the post-thrombotic extremity, but five of the six extremities were not postthrombotic upon detailed investigation of the veins.

Diagnostic Testing Methods in CVD

Testing methods used in chronic venous disease have been the subject of a recent consensus

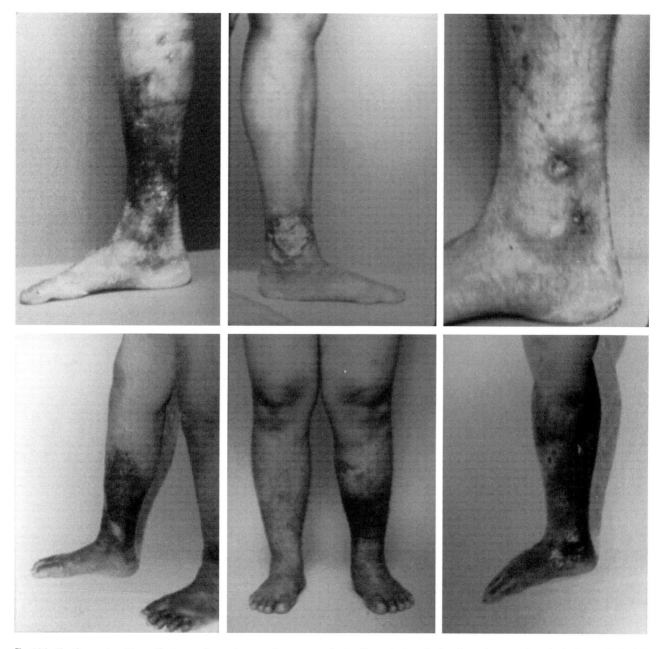

Fig. 14.1. The three extremities on the top row have primary saphenous or perforator disease in the veins but do not have postthrombotic disease. On the left bottom the venous disease is primary reflux of saphenous, perforator and deep veins. The left middle illustration is a postthrombotic extremity with disease of the saphenous, deep and perforator veins. The right bottom case had normal veins and the skin changes are due to repeated bruising in a diabetic patient.

conference in Paris.[3] The requirements that have been outlined for evaluating a diagnostic test itself are discussed in the article by Raskob on "Evidenced-Based Recommendations for the Diagnosis and Treatment of Thromboembolic Disease: Rules of Evidence for Assessing the Literature".[4] The rudiments of these requirements for a given test are:

- The test should be evaluated against a gold standard
- In a broad spectrum of patients, both with and without disease
- Both the test in question and the gold standard should be interpreted independently
- In a sufficient number of patients to satisfy 95% confidence intervals

- And errors of both workup and interpretative bias should be avoided.
- The test should be examined for the validity of a negative result.

In this paper, the methods of testing for chronic venous disease will be categorized as follows:

Level 1. Clinical, including history, physical examination, and C-W Doppler examination.
Level 2. Laboratory, including plethysmography and venous pressure.
Level 3. Imaging, including duplex scanning and venography.

In the literature on non-surgical management of chronic venous problems the majority of diagnoses are based upon clinical syndromes such as varicose veins, "venous ulcer," lipodermatosclerosis and stasis changes. These clinical syndromes cannot be accepted as definitive tests because they fail the test of diagnosis against a gold standard, are subject to interpretive bias, and not, examined for validity of a negative result. In advanced disease as seen in cases that undergo deep venous reconstruction, level 1 testing methods cannot be relied upon for any definitive diagnosis.

The level 2 testing methods of plethysmography and venous pressure in the vascular laboratory are recognized to be non-specific tests of abnormal venous physiology and they do satisfy the requirements for reliable tests. Although they are associated with clinical syndromes, they are not diagnostic in themselves of a given clinical or anatomical state. Their validity is that of a confirmatory test of the presence of venous disease without being definitive about the exact diagnosis of the problem.

The level 3 testing methods of duplex scanning and venography are specific tests of abnormal anatomy and function which do satisfy the requirements for reliable testing methods. These are the highest levels of testing evidence for pre- and post-operative data.

Diagnosis of Chronic Venous Disease

In chronic venous disease the definitive diagnosis of the entire venous system in the lower extremity has seldom been practiced because it was not practical to do so prior to the availability of duplex scanning. Elements needed for a complete diagnosis are those required to fulfill the CEAP classification[2,5] of chronic venous disease:

1. The clinical state itself, including varicose veins, swelling, pain, skin changes and ulceration.
2. The etiology of the venous state, be it primary, secondary or congenital.
3. The anatomy of the involved portions of the venous tree, whether superficial, perforator or deep.
4. The pathophysiology of the condition, whether it is reflux or obstruction, or a combination of the two, and which anatomic segments are affected.

The literature on varicose veins, for example, lacks definitive data about the status of other segments of the venous tree because such data is not needed for diagnosis of the clinical condition and it hasn't been thought to be necessary unless it would change the recommendations for treatment. Without this data, however, it is not possible to analyze poor results or late recurrences when other attributes of venous disease become more obvious in later follow-up, such as large incompetent perforators, or post-thrombotic deep veins, or extensive deep vein reflux that was never identified or ruled out. With the advent of easy access to duplex scanning some of this information is now becoming available for analysis.

After clinical examination, the diagnostic workup for deep venous reconstruction always requires imaging of the extremity veins by duplex scanning, and venography is needed to plan the procedure. In addition, variable types of physiologic testing including plethysmographic and pressure methods are used to identify severity of the venous malfunction. Before the surgical procedure, every segment of the lower extremity veins should have been analyzed for both obstruction and reflux, and the distribution of primary and secondary changes should have been detailed. Since this same level of diagnosis is not needed for non-surgical treatment in the veins, there are no series of cases in the literature whose diagnoses are comparable to those treated by surgery because the diagnostics have not been done to identify similar patients in the non-reconstructed population. For this reason, there are no reliable historic non-operated controls that would be useful for Level IV evidence (nonrandomized studies with historic controls) in the analysis of venous reconstruction.

Analysis of the Literature on Venous Reconstruction

The tables contain references to the major publications on venous reconstruction and provide a listing of the numbers of cases and the quality of the data presented in each case. The validity of the testing data published in these peer-reviewed journals is accepted as being as reliable as the reported standards for the same tests that are accepted in the literature without requiring the individual author to report his own validity studies in his testing facilities. Any weakness incurred by this approach is common to the literature on CVD.

Judgment of the reliability of data in each quoted reported is shown in the tables and has been made by analyzing the report according to this schema:

A. Direct imaging. This includes duplex scan and venographic data.

B. Indirect testing. This includes laboratory evaluations of any form of plethysmography (APG, PPG, SPG) or pressure determination (ambulatory venous pressure, arm-foot, femoral, or Valsalva techniques)

C. Clinical examination. This includes history, physical examination, C-W Doppler in the office.

D. Non-patient contact. Questionnaires, telephone interviews.

Level D information is the least reliable and A is the most reliable. For each article that was analyzed, one of these letters is noted in the tables to provide an estimation of the reliability of the data. The main factor that argues for validity in these reports is that of objectivity gained from the imaging studies which exists in greater measure in these series than it does in other methods of treatment for CVD. Deficiencies in the data are multiple and include factors such as:

- the sample size of most of the reports is too small to fulfill the criteria for evidence-based reliability,
- the individual laboratory's credentials are not established for each test
- there are no controls except for one report on valvuloplasty.[2]
- there are no randomized trials.

Deep venous reconstruction is broadly divided into procedures for bypass of obstructed segments and procedures for correction of reflux in the deep veins. Saphenous and perforator procedures are not considered reconstructive and are not included in these tables. Although surgery on the saphenous and perforator veins is an important part of caring for the patients with deep vein reconstruction, it has not been singled out for separate consideration in enough reports to make it an analyzable entity now.

Surgery for Venous Obstruction

The first attempts to perform surgery to correct deep venous problems were for bypass of superficial femoral and later of iliac vein occlusions, while the later ones have focused much more on correction of venous reflux states. The first report was by Warren and Thayer in 1954[6] and involved the use of the greater saphenous vein to bypass the obstructed post-thrombotic superficial femoral vein but this did not achieve wide acceptance and it wasn't until the 1970s that Frileux[7] in France and Husni[8] in the United States published further reports on this operation with concurrent and subsequent reports by May[9] in Austria.

A more popular bypass procedure has been that of Palma[10] from Ecuador for the occluded iliac vein by use of the saphenous vein placed trans-pubically from the normal leg to the occluded side. This was taken up with much more enthusiasm and reported by Halliday in Australia,[11] Dale[12] and Husni[8] in the United States, and Frileux[7] and Vollmar[13] and Gruss[14] in Europe. AbuRhama in the United States reported a larger series of bypasses in 1991 with objective follow-up and late venography.[15]

Gruss[14] in Germany reported an optimistic experience with cross femoral and femoral-iliac synthetic bypass using PTFE in 32 cases, followed by other reports from Europe,[16] the United States[15,17] and Japan[18] who have reported smaller series of this procedure.

Saphenopopliteal Bypass

Table 14.1 presents 7 series of saphenopopliteal bypass procedures that were reported from 1972 to 1997, comprising 126 cases in all. The largest series was 30 cases, smallest 6 cases, so none of the series

Table 14.1. Results of saphenopopliteal bypass

Grade	Author	Year reported	No. patients	FU months	Clinical success (%)	Patency (%)
C	Frileux[7]	1972	23	12–36	31	67
A	Husni[8]	1978	26	6–120	69	63
A	Dale[12]	1982	6	NR	50	50
C	May[9]	1985	30	NR	30	97
A	Abu Rahma[15]	1991	19	66	58	56
C	Danza[16]	1991	8	NR	75	NR
C	Gruss[14]	1997	14	60	50	NR

NR = not reported.
Grade = A, imaging testing; B, physiologic testing; C, office examination only.
Tables 14.1 through 14.6 adapted from: Eklof B, Kistner RL, Masuda EM. Venous bypass and valve reconstruction: long-term efficacy. Vasc Med in press.

achieved statistical validity in numbers of cases. About 40% of the cases had either no follow-up reported or less than 12 months of follow-up and 60% were evaluated only by clinical (C) criteria. There is a maximum of 51 cases that may have had objective late follow-up by imaging techniques. The most objective long-term follow-up was by Abu Rhama[15] of 19 cases with venography, and this report showed 56% cumulative 8-year patency. May[9] of Austria concluded after a long experience with this procedure that it is too prone to long-term failure in his hands to justify its continued use. Abu Rhama[15] concluded that it can help in the highly selected case with low outflow in the leg, mild reflux, and especially in those with venous claudication. The summary evaluation of saphenopopliteal bypass:

- 7 reports, total of 126 cases.
- 4 of 7 series < 20 cases, none over 30 cases.
- 60% of cases reported with level C data, 40% with level A data.

Conclusion:

- Unreliable data for validity of procedure.
- Durability of good result is highly questionable.
- Procedure remains experimental/developmental

Cross-Femoral Autogenous Vein Bypass (Palma Procedure)

Table 14.2 presents 12 series of autogenous femorofemoral bypass procedures reported from 1960 to

Table 14.2. Results of autogenous femorofemoral vein bypass

Grade	Author	Year reported	No. patients	FU months	Clinical success (%)	Patency (%)	Adjunct AVF (%)
C	Palma[10]	1960	8	NR	87	NR	0
C	Frileux[7]	1972	12	NR	25	NR	25
C	Vollmar[13]	1979	20	6–78	69	44	69
A	Husni[8]	1981	78	7–144	74	73	10
C	Dale[12]	1982	50	NR	78	NR	0
A	Halliday[11]	1985	50	60	89	75	10
C	May[9]	1985	100	NR	60–90	NR	
A	Raju[32]	1986	8	27	25	37	100
A	O'Donnell[17]	1987	6	24	100	100	66
A	Abu Rahma[15]	1991	24	66	88	75	0
C	Danza[16]	1991	27	NR	81	NR	
B	Gruss[14]	1997	20	60	71	NR	100

NR = not reported.
Grade = A, imaging testing; B, physiologic testing; C, office examination only.

1997 comprising 403 patients. The series varied from 6 cases to 100 cases. In over half of the cases the follow-up was limited to clinical or to indirect laboratory examination, and a maximum of 166 cases were found to have late follow-up by imaging. Of those with late imaging, 4 of the 5 series, comprising 158 of the 166 cases, demonstrated high patency rates of 73%, 75%, 75%, and 100%; a single series reported the low figure of 37% (for 8 cases).

The indications for surgery in these series contained significant variables, one of which was the amount of obstructive disease in the bypassed extremity. Excellent results can be achieved with this procedure in cases where the obstruction is limited to the iliac vein itself and the femoral-popliteal veins are normal, but less optimistic results are likely when the entire extremity is affected by post-thrombotic occluded veins.[15] There is doubt that the isolated iliac vein obstruction requires a bypass in most instances and it may be inappropriate to do this as an early procedure when the distal veins and valves are not affected. This aspect of the natural history of post-thrombotic disease remains to be worked out. A different point of view is expressed by Halliday[11] who believes that the cross-femoral bypass may protect the extremity from developing post-thrombotic irreversible damage in the calf. Abu Rhama found 75% 7-year cumulative patency rate and a low risk to the procedure and cites a good outcome in patients with low outflow who have only mild reflux and venous claudication. With all of this, the scientific proof of the validity of this procedure remains weak.

Summary evaluation of cross-femoral autogenous bypass:

- 12 series comprising 403 cases
- Sizes of series from 6–100 cases. 6 of the series were 20 cases or less. 3 series were 50 or more cases, but 150/200 cases in these series were evaluated only by clinical testing without imaging.
- 217/403 (54%) were evaluated by level C data (clinical examination alone), 166/403 (41%) by level A data (direct imaging).
- 40% or less were followed for > 5 years
- High patency rates of 75% or greater were reported in 4/5 series (164 cases) with level A data (direct imaging).

Conclusion:

- Poor quality of data in over half of reported cases.
- Patency rates at 5 years are not reported in one half of the cases.
- Reported results are widely variable between authors.

Synthetic Grafts in Iliac Vein Occlusion

Table 14.3 presents 10 series of synthetic grafts for iliac vein obstruction reported from 1979 to 1997 comprising 116 patients. The series varied from 4 to 32 cases, follow-up was over 12 months in the vast majority and two thirds were followed up with postoperative imaging studies. In the nine studies reporting patency there were 2 below 50% (20% and

Table 14.3. Synthetic grafts for iliac vein obstruction

Grade	Author	Year reported	No. patients	FU months	Clinical success (%)	Patency (%)	Adjunct AVF (%)
C	Vollmar[13]	1979	6	5–60	67	67	100
A	Ijima[33]	1985	5	22–36	60	60	100
A	Yamamoto[34]	1986	5	1–18	60	60	20
A	Raju[32]	1986	8	20	25	25	100
A	Okadome[35]	1989	4	12–48	100	100	100
A	Eklof[36]	1989	10	2–108	20	20	100
B	Gruss[14]	1997	32	60	85	NR	100
A	Gloviczki[37]	1997	13	60	62	62	100
A	Juhan[38]	1997	8	10–45	88	88	100
A	Sottiurai[39]	1997	25	18–123	92	92	100

NR = not reported.
Grade = A, imaging testing; B, physiologic testing; C, office examination only.

25%), while the rest were above 60% and 3 (37 cases) were above 85%. Adjunctive AVF's (arteriovenous fistulas) were used in nearly all of these cases and are the standard of care.

The reasons to use synthetic bypass for iliac vein obstruction are several. Often, the saphenous vein is a very small conduit to substitute for the large iliac vein, and sometimes it isn't even available. Also, it may be undesirable to invade the normal leg for a good saphenous vein in patients who are prone to have recurrent episodes of DVT. The appeal of the larger conduit and its ready availability make the use of ringed PTFE for bypass an attractive alternative if it can be demonstrated to have a reasonable long-term patency. The accumulated results demonstrated in this table fall short of a convincing argument in favor of liberal use of this procedure but they do support further exploration of the operation in highly selected cases.

Summary evaluation of Synthetic grafts in iliac vein occlusion:

- 10 series comprising 116 cases
- Size of series from 4–32 cases, 7 series were 10 cases or less, only 2 series over 20 cases,
- Level A data in 78 cases, B in 32 cases, and C level in 6 cases
- < 50% were followed for 5 years
- Patency rates of > 60% in 7/10 series (66/116 cases), or 52%

Conclusion:

- Small series, poor follow-up, unconvincing follow-up data
- Durability of patency may approach 60% at 5 years.
- The method appears to deserve a well designed protocol with objective follow-up.

Summary of reconstruction for venous obstruction in the lower extremity.

The series presented here represent the majority of information available in the Western world on deep venous bypass surgery and taken together do not present a convincing scientific case for venous bypass. When there is little in the way of alternative choice for the afflicted patient except limitation of the way of life, these procedures deserve consideration. They are relatively safe operations that can be done with an acceptable hospital stay. When they are successful the patient may benefit greatly, and when they fail there is little harm to be done to

most of these patients so the cost-benefit ratio may tilt in favor of an aggressive stance in the active, productive patient. But the scientific data to support its validity has not been published.

Surgery for Venous Reflux

It has become recognized that the most frequent condition leading to the severe sequelae of CVD is reflux and surgical methods have been developed to reverse deep reflux in many instances. These procedures vary from repair of the floppy deep valve in primary reflux to valve substitution methods for post-thrombotic valvular destruction. Valve repair is performed inside the vein by several different but comparable techniques. Other techniques are used to narrow the vein externally at valve sites and thereby accomplish an external form of valve repair. In post-thrombotic veins where the valve itself is destroyed and cannot be repaired it is possible to anastomose adjacent vein segments and utilize the proximal valve of one segment, such as the profunda femoris vein (PFV), to provide competence for other segments such as the SFV (superficial femoral vein). This is the technique of transposition. Another technique is transplantation of a vein segment that contains a competent valve from one site to another, such as from the axillary vein to the SFV or to the popliteal vein.

Direct Valve Repair (Valvuloplasty) for Primary Valve Incompetence

Table 14.4 presents six series of valvuloplasty surgery for primary deep valve incompetence, comprising 537 cases. In each series and in nearly all cases late post-operative imaging studies were performed. The size of the series range from 27 to 211 cases. Follow-up has been from 6 months to over 20 years and has been longer than 8 years in a significant number of cases in several series.[19–22] Good to excellent clinical results are reported from each series in the range of 62–75% over the very long term (>8 years). Competence of the repaired valve by late imaging study has correlated best with a favorable late clinical result.[19,20] Late imaging

Table 14.4. Results of internal valvuloplasty

Grade	Author	Year reported	No. limbs	FU months	Good results (%)	Competent valve
A/B	Eriksson[21]	1990	27	6–108	70	19/27 = 70% 4 years
A	Kistner[20]	1994	32	48–252	73	24/31 = 77% 4–15 years
A	Lurie[23]	1997	49	36–108		58/68 = 85% 5 years
A	Perrin[27]	1997	75	24–96		23/27 = 85% >12 months
A	Raju[19]	1996	68	12–144	62	52/68 = 76% 2–10 years
A	Sottiurai[22]	1997	143	9–168	75	107/143 = 75% 87 months

Grade = A, imaging testing; B, physiologic testing; C, office examination only.

studies extracted from the six series of valvuloplasty showed 189/262 (72%) of internal valvuloplasty repairs were still competent in follow-up of 1–8 years, and longer in some reports.

These results have appeared spontaneously from totally independent sites in the United States and Europe and represent the most consistent results in all of the deep reconstruction literature. The evidence here is that of patients studied objectively pre- and post-operatively with long-term follow-up sufficient to unmask bad results, with studies performed completely independently by non-related investigators.

There is one series that qualifies as Level III evidence in the internal valve repair literature,[23] reported from a large collection of CVD cases from the Sverdlovsk Vascular Center in Russia. In this study 127 limbs in 119 patients with severe venous insufficiency due entirely to primary reflux were evaluated. All 119 patients had surgical repair of the saphenous and perforator abnormalities. 49 of the patients also underwent internal valvuloplasty to repair the incompetent valve while 70 patients did not have valve repair and served as a control group. Objective follow-up by duplex imaging was carried out annually for 5 years. This study describes an original concept of grading reflux by comparing volume reflux with volume outflow in a given vein and correlates this measurement with pre- and post-operative clinical status in all of the cases. The result was that the addition of valve repair to saphenous and perforator surgery significantly improved the long-term results in cases that showed high volume reflux pre-operatively, but in those with lower volume reflux the valve repair did not add to the long-term results. This is a well-conceived study with long-term follow-up and objective endpoints.

Summary of internal valvuloplasty literature:

- Six series with 369 limbs
- Series ranged from 27–143 cases
- Level A data for all cases
- Follow-up from 6–252 months, approximately 40% or more >60 months
- Competent valve >87 months in >75%
- All six series showed similar results of valve competency, good clinical results, and ulcer-free interval.

Conclusion:

Consistent results reported from all investigators, long-term objective follow-up, and ample numbers of cases provide reasonable certainty about the validity of this procedure.

The literature on internal valvuloplasty is the strongest body of literature on the subject of venous reconstruction, and there is at least one study with control patients that elevated the evidence level to grade III. In addition to showing the statistical results of valve repair, these studies also demonstrate that long-term good clinical results correlate with late valve competence.

Transplantation of a Vein-Valve Segment

Table 14.5 presents seven series treated by transplantation of a vein-valve segment. There were 282 limbs treated with series size ranging from 15 to 102 cases, and follow-up from 18 months to 6 years. There is a wide variability in results from these series with clinical success as low as 31%[24] and as high as 90%.[25, 26] In five of the seven series the long-term results were below 50%,[19,24,27] and in some

Table 14.5. Results of vein–valve transplantation

Grade	Author	Year reported	No. limbs	FU months	Cinical success (%)	Ulcer recurrence (%)
A	Eriksson[24]	1990	35	60	31	?
A	Nash[25]	1988	23	18	90+	18
A	Raju[19]	1996	44	24	36	54
A	O'Donnell[17]	1997	15	64	92	21
A	Perrin[27]	1997	30	60	48	67
A	Sottiurai[22]	1997	33	74	39	?
A	Taheri[28]	1997	102	60	45	?

Grade = A, imaging testing; B, physiologic testing; C, office examination only.

series this low number occurred within the first two years. In one large series the 5-year results were favorable in 75% but fell to 45% in the later 5–10 year analysis.[28] There are several authors who are deeply discouraged by their experience with this procedure[24,27] while two[25,26] are highly encouraged. Actual recurrence of ulceration was reported in 18–67% in these series.

Summary of transplantation of vein-valve segment:

- Seven series with 282 cases
- Size of series from 15 to 102 limbs, only one series <20 cases
- Level A data in all series and nearly all cases
- Follow-up of >60 months in >65% (180+/282 cases)
- Clinical success widely variable >3–5 years: Two series with total 38 cases had 90%+ good clinical results, while five of seven series had less than 50% success, and three had <39% success. Overall, clinical success was about 53%.
- Ulcer recurrence found in 18–67% of cases, and >50% in two series.

Conclusion:
Variable results suggest differences in technique or patient selection may exist in this series of reports. The management of associated disease in these series may also be quite different. The findings do not establish validity to date, but it is possible that further study will show methods of selection and management that will be more consistent and favorable.

Transposition

Table 14.6 presents the results of the transposition operation in four series, comprising a total of 70 cases with follow-up ranging from 18 months to 10 years. In these small experiences there were 25–54% good clinical results, equivalent to the results in some of the transplanted vein-valve experience. This procedure is utilized in post-thrombotic cases where long-term results are less favorable than in the primary reflux cases in the experience of most investigators. The approximate results in terms of late valve competence is in the range of 40–50%.

Table 14.6. Results of vein transposition

Grade	Author	Year reported	No. limbs	FU months	Good results (%)	Competence
C	Johnson[40]	1981	12	18	25	NR
A	Kistner[20]	1994	14	120	40	10–14 partial competence
A	Perrin[27]	1997	13	60	54	5/12 competent 49 months
A	Sottiurai[22]	1997	31	89	39	12/31 competent

NR = not reported.
Grade = A, imaging testing; B, physiologic testing; C, office examination only.

Summary of Transposition experience:

- Four series with a total of 70 limbs.
- Size of series 12–31 cases.
- Follow-up 18–120 months and all with Level A testing except one series with 12 cases.

Conclusion:
Small total cases with majority of cases followed less than 5 years. Inadequate total number of cases to establish validity, but consistent findings that recurrence will be in the range of 50–60%. The validity of this procedure remains unproven. It is reserved for the postthrombotic case where there is a competent valve in a segment adjacent to the diseased refluxing vein, e.g., a competent PFV valve, or a GSV valve, adjacent to a refluxing SFV segment. It is surprising that this operation with a single anastomosis has not shown better statistics in follow-up, but it may be that the cases have not been well selected or the diagnosis of competence in the valve may not be reliable in post-thrombotic disease.

Other Procedures to Restore Valve Competence

Other techniques for repair of valvular reflux include variations of external narrowing of the vein and angioscopic repair of the valve itself. The simplicity of external repair makes it a highly desirable approach because it minimizes the amount of dissection of the vein needed to repair the valve, avoids the necessity to open the vein and thereby obviates the need for anticoagulation, and minimizes the likelihood of injuring the vein during the attempt to repair it. With the external suture technique[29] it is usually possible to obtain a competent valve in primary disease at the time of surgery, and since the technique is simple it can be done on multiple valves at a single sitting. There is a serious problem with the external method which is that it is not an anatomical repair of the elongated valve cusp and for this reason it doesn't repair the anatomic problem that causes the reflux in the floppy valve state. To date, the indication is that external repairs will have a lower long-term competence and will be followed by a higher recurrence rate of clinical findings. Since there is not a definitive series that tests the external repair in the literature, it is too early to know its long-term efficacy.

Another form of external repair is the external cuff which may be made of Dacron or any other material which is simply wrapped around the vein at the valve site to narrow the vein near the valve, and to prevent postoperative dilation of the valve. There are not enough of these reported and followed to know the results. Raju has used this approach in 22 cases where the vein that had shown reflux by pre-operative study was found to be competent when exposed at surgery, and the wrap was merely intended to maintain the same circumference. This is a special category of cases which has been encountered by all who have operated on venous valve reflux. His finding that 16 of 22 (72%) remained competent is encouraging and supportive of this approach. These cases should not be mixed with the rest of the primary cases where surgical exposure itself does not restore competence.

The angioscopic repair was introduced in 1990[30] but it hasn't been reported in sufficient numbers or adequate follow-up to permit a definitive opinion. It has found enthusiastic usage by several surgeons[18,26,30] and will be available for analysis in the future.

A recent report from Raju[19] reports the follow-up results in patients who had surgical repair of secondary disease to be similar to those who had valvuloplasty for primary disease. This report is more enthusiastic for surgical treatment of secondary disease than most others. Part of the experience he reports is a reflection of cases who have a repairable proximal valve in the presence of distal postthrombotic disease and this is a well recognized segment of the CVD population who have been classified by others as having proximal primary and distal postthrombotic disease. This was the pathology of the first patient in 1968 to ever have a valve surgically repaired.[31] Although it is not clear from the manuscript[19] it appears Raju has found other cases in the secondary group to be repairable by external repair techniques and, if so, this finding requires more specific study by him and others. It is clear, however, that in those whose valve is destroyed by postthrombotic disease a valve substitution procedure is needed to achieve surgical correction.

Summation

This review of the literature on venous reconstruction provides an analysis of 1366 limbs reported in 46 series with 47% representing bypass surgery for

Table 14.7. Summary table of venous reconstruction series in the literature

Operation	No. series	No. cases	Size of series	Length of FU	Data level A–B–C (%)	Patency	Competence	Clinical success (%)
Saphenopopliteal bypass	7	126	6–30 limbs 4/7:< 20 cases	50%/5 years	40-0-60	♠60%	NA	♠50
Cross femoral	12	403	6–100 limbs 6/12:< 21 cases	Good >5 years	39-7-54	Variable 37–75% /5 years	NA	25–75
Synthetic for iliac occlusion	10	116	4–32 limbs 7/10:< 11 cases	<50%/5 years	67-27-6	♠50%/5 years	NA	20–80
Valvuloplasty	6	369	27–143 limbs One series with controls	♠50%/5 years ♠20%>8 years	100-0-0	NA	75%/4 years consistent in all series	70
Vein valve transplant	7	282	15–102 limbs	65%/5 years	100-0-0	NA	Variable 35–90%	40–90
Transposition	4	70	12–32 limbs	18–120 months	83-0-17	NA	Variable 40–50% /5 years	40

obstructive problems and 53% representing repair or substitution surgery for reflux disease. The literature on bypass procedures is for the most part older, the series are smaller, and the level of testing is less reliable than in the reflux reports. The results for all operations are variable except for internal valvuloplasty for primary valve reflux where the data is consistent from all authors, the follow-up is significant, and the testing methods are at the highest level of reliability. The only series with controls and some element of randomization is one by Lurie on valvuloplasty; the rest are case series with no controls. The use of historic controls is not possible since there is no data in existence other than the surgical literature where the diagnostic workups satisfy the CEAP criteria for clinical, etiologic, anatomic, and pathophysiologic diagnoses for all of the cases.

The evidence for validity of deep venous reconstruction resides at the weakest level of evidence-based analysis, Class V, with the sole exception of one report on valvuloplasty that qualifies for Level III Evidence. It remains for the future to design meaningful trials, at least with concurrent controls, to test most of these procedures. In the meantime, it need be recognized that this body of literature represents the first attempts to deal with the ravages of advanced venous insufficiency by correcting the specific functional abnormalities that are uncovered by detailed diagnostic evaluations. The return to health of 75%, 50%, or even 35% of these patients for periods of 5–15 years, clearly demonstrated in these series, is a new milestone in the management

of chronic venous disease and it represents a new addition to the ancient principles of wrapping and elevation of the ulcerated extremity. Whether these same results can be achieved in this population of patients by simpler operations, or whether these operations need to be used more liberally in earlier cases, remains to be studied in the future.

References

1. Sackett DL Rules of evidence and clinical recommendations on the use of antithrombotic agents. Chest. 1989; 95 (Feb Suppl):2s–4s.
2. The consensus group. Classification and grading of chronic venous disease in the lower limb. A consensus statement. Vasc Surg. 1996; 30:5–11.
3. The investigation of chronic venous disorders of the lower limb. A Consensus Statement. Abbaye des Vaux de Cernay, France, March 5–9, 1997.
4. Raskob GE. Evidence-based recommendations for the diagnosis and treatment of thromboembolic disease: Rules of evidence for assessing the literature. In: Hull R, Pineo GF, eds. *Disorders of Thrombosis*. Philadephia: WB Saunders Co, 1996:1–6.
5. Classification and grading of chronic venous disease. A consensus statement. J Vasc Surg. 1995; 21:635–645.
6. Warren R, Thayer TR. Transplantation of the saphenous vein for postphlebitic stasis. Surg. 1954; 35:867–876.
7. Frileux C, Pillot-Bienayme P, Gillot C. Bypass of segmental obliterations of ilio-femoral venous axis by transposition of saphenous vein. J Cardiovasc Surg. 1972; 13:409–414.
8. Husni EA. Clinical experience with femoropopliteal venous reconstruction. In: Bergan JJ, Yao JST, eds. Venous Problems. Chicago: Yearbook Medical Publishers, Inc, 1978:485–491.
9. May R. The femoral bypass. Inter Angio. 1985; 4:435–440.
10. Palma EC, Esperon R. Vein transplants and grafts in surgical treatment of the postphlebitic syndrome. J Cardiovasc Surg. 1960; 1:94–107.

11. Halliday P. Harris J, May J. Femoro-femoral crossover grafts (Palma operation): A long-term follow-up study. In: Bergan JJ, Yao JST, eds. Surgery of the Veins. New York: Grune and Stratton, Inc, 1985: 241–254.

12. Dale A. Reconstructive venous surgery. In: Veith FJ, ed. *Critical Problems in Vascular Surgery*. New York: Appleton-Century-Crofts, 1982:199–213.

13. Hutschenreiter S, Vollmar J, Loeprecht H, et al. Rekonstructive Eingriffe am Venensystem; Spatergebnisse unter kritischer Bewertung funktioneller und gefassmorphologischer Kriterien. Chirurg. 1979; 50:555–563.

14. Gruss JD, Heimer W. Bypass procedures for venous obstruction: Palma and May-Husni bypasses, Raju perforator bypass, prosthetic bypasses, primary and adjunctive arteriovenous fistulae. In: Raju S, Villavicencio JL, eds. *Surgical Management of Venous Disease*. Baltimore: Williams and Wilkins, 1997:289–305.

15. Abu Rahma AF, Robinson PA, Boland JP. Clinical, hemodynamic and anatomic predictors of long-term outcome of lower extremity venovenous bypasses. J Vasc Surg. 1991; 14:635–644.

16. Danza R, Navarro T, Baldizan J. Reconstructive surgery in chronic venous obstruction of the lower limbs. J Cardiovasc Surg. 1991; 32:98–103.

17. O'Donnel TF, Mackey WC, Shepard AD, Callow AD. Clinical, hemodynamic and anatomic follow-up of direct venous reconstruction. Arch Surg. 1987; 122:474–482.

18. Hoshino S, Satokawa H, Takase S, Midorikawa H, Igari T, Iwaya F. External valvuloplasty for primary valvular incompetence of the lower limbs using angioscopy. Inter J Angio. 1997; 6:137–141.

19. Raju S, Fredericks RK, Neglen PN, Bass JD. Durability of venous valve reconstruction techniques for "primary" and postthrombotic reflux. J Vasc Surg. 1996; 23:357–367.

20. Masuda E, Kistner RL. Long-term results of venous valve reconstruction: A 14- to 21-year follow-up. J Vasc Surg. 1994; 19:391–403.

21. Eriksson I. Reconstructive surgery for deep vein valve incompetence in the lower limb. Eur J Vasc Surg. 1990; 4:211–218.

22. Sottiurai VS. Results of deep-vein reconstruction. Vasc Surg. 1997; 31:276–278.

23. Lurie F. Results of Deep-Vein Reconstruction. Vasc Surg. 1997; 31:275–276.

24. Eriksson I. Vein valve surgery for deep valvular incompetence. In: Eklof B, Gjores JE, Thulesius O, Bergqvist D, eds. *Controversies in the Management of Venous Disorders*. London: Butterworths, 1989:267–279.

25. Nash T. Long-term results of vein valve transplants placed in the popliteal vein for intractable post-phlebitic venous ulcers and pre-ulcer skin changes. J Cardiovasc Surg. 1988; 29:712–716.

26. Iafrati M, O'Donnell TF. Surgical reconstruction for deep venous insufficiency. J Mal Vas. 1997; 22:193–197.

27. Perrin MR. Results of deep-vein reconstruction. Vasc Surg. 1997; 31:273–275.

28. Taheri SA. Vein valve transplantation. Vasc Surg. 1997; 31:278–281.

29. Kistner RL. Surgical technique of external venous valve repair. The Straub Foundation Proceedings. 1990; 55:15–16.

30. Gloviczki P, Merrell SW, Bower TC. Femoral vein valve repair under direct vision without venotomy: A modified technique with angioscopy. J Vasc Surg. 1991; 14:645–648.

31. Kistner RL. Surgical repair of a venous valve. Straub Clinic Proceedings. 1968; 34:41–43.

32. Raju S. New approaches to the diagnosis and treatment of venous obstruction. J Vasc Surg. 1986; 4:42–54.

33. Ijima H, Kodama M, Hori M. Temporary arteriovenous fistula for venous reconstruction using synthetic grafts: A clinical and experimental investigation. J Cardiovasc Surg. 1985; 26:131–136.

34. Yamamoto N, Takaba T, Hori G, et al. Reconstruction with insertion of expanded polytetrafluoroethylene (ePTFE) for iliac venous obstruction. J Cardovasc Surg. 1986; 27:697–702.

35. Okadome K, Muto Y, Eguchi H, et al. Venous reconstruction for iliofemoral venous occlusion facilitated by temporary arteriovenous shunt. Arch Surg. 1989; 124:957–960.

36. Eklof B. Temporary arteriovenous fistula in reconstruction of iliac vein obstruction using PTFE grafts. In: Eklof B, Gjores JE, Thulesius O, Bergqvist D, eds. *Controversies in the Management of Venous Disorders*. London: Butterworths, 1989:280–290.

37. Gloviczki P. Chronic venous obstruction of lower extremities: The case for aggressive treatment. Vasc Surg. 1997; 31:319–320.

38. Alimi YS, DiMauro P, Fabre D, Juhan C. Iliac vein reconstruction to treat acute and chronic venous occlusive disease. J Vasc Surg. 1997; 25:673–681.

39. Sottiurai VS. Current surgical approaches to venous hypertension and valvular reflux. Inter J Angio. 1996; 5:49–54.

40. Johnson ND, Queral LA, Flinn WR, et al. Late objective assessment of venous valve surgery. Arch Surg. 1981; 116:1461–1466.

Editors' Commentary

Until recently, treatment options appeared quite limited for those patients afflicted with severe chronic venous insufficiency. However, knowledge regarding the role of valvular incompetence and venous reflux has led to a number of promising therapeutic approaches.

Macrosclerotherapy, as described by Guex, can be used with success for more severe forms of chronic venous insufficiency. Guex represents the point of view of an angiologist trained in phlebology. His experience from France nicely complements the presentation of Sladen from Canada. Their observations indicate that sclerotherapy can play a major role in the treatment of CVI. This approach for treatment of proximal and distal venous pathophysiology is advantageous from a cost viewpoint. Minimal invasion leads to a low rate of complications. However, now that noninvasive ultrasound imaging is available worldwide, validation of this method of treatment will be requisite before it is accepted as standard.

Subfascial endoscopic perforator surgery has revitalized surgical interest in treating chronic venous insufficiency. This technique has emerged rapidly over the past few years, and Dr Gloviczki's chapter provides thorough evidence for this phenomenon. Venous hemodynamics after perforator interruption sometimes demonstrates improved calf muscle pump function and decreased venous reflux. However, since an inflammatory process associated with leukocyte infiltration and activation is fundamental to the causation of CVI, it would not be expected that hemodynamic improvement would occur in every limb. Although we use a single-scope, single-port approach, our experience parallels that of Dr Gloviczki's group. We too have been impressed with acceleration of wound healing and lack of serious complications; the most serious of which continues to be wound infection. As indicated above, the Mayo group has championed a two-port technique but we, with others principally from Europe, have worked toward development of a single-port, open-scope approach. Descriptions of the various subfascial endoscopic perforator surgery techniques emphasize the importance of perforator interruption, which can be achieved by a variety of alternative methods.

Despite the above techniques, some ulcers will require more advanced treatment. Dr Dunn and colleagues discuss skin grafting techniques and describe the difference between nonexcisional grafting and excisional grafting. Local or microsurgical free flaps may be required for more extensive reconstructions. Recalcitrant ulceration may require skin grafting and free flaps to achieve healing within an acceptable period of time. However, simple ulcer coverage without attention to the venous pathophysiology is doomed to failure. Experience teaches that full-thickness excision of the ulcer down to and including fascia must be an integral part of the grafting procedure.

The final chapter in this section summarizes all available data concerning reconstruction of the deep venous system. Dr Kistner and colleagues provide evidence-based analysis for a variety of techniques used for deep venous reconstruction. This remarkable compilation of data will serve as the benchmark for future data comparison. Reconstructive vein surgery has dominated discussions of treatment of CVI in the recent past. However, it is clear that knowledge that superficial reflux and perforator outflow are important to causation of venous ulceration has relegated direct venous reconstruction to a position in which valve reconstruction is considered only after these two elements are eliminated.

Section D

THROMBOSIS AND THROMBOLYSIS

Disorders Predisposing to Venous Thromboembolism

15

Graham F. Pineo and Russell D. Hull

Introduction

Pulmonary embolism is responsible for approximately 150,000 to 200,000 deaths per year in the United States. Venous thromboembolism (VTE) (deep-vein thrombosis (DVT) and/or pulmonary embolism (PE)) usually occurs as a complication in patients who are sick and hospitalized but it may also affect ambulatory and otherwise healthy individuals. In addition to a significant mortality rate, VTE causes considerable morbidity including the development of the post-thrombotic syndrome. In order to provide more effective prophylaxis and treatment of VTE a knowledge of risk factors predisposing to thrombosis is essential. This chapter will review these risk factors with particular reference to congenital or acquired deficiency states predisposing to thrombosis, the hypercoagulable states.

Pathophysiology of Venous Thrombosis

More than 100 years ago, Virchow defined factors predisposing to venous thrombosis; decreased blood flow, abnormalities of the blood and damage to the vessel wall.[1] In modern terms, these translate into stasis, the prothrombotic state of blood and damage to the endothelium. Decreased blood flow results from immobility caused by various medical and surgical conditions, but is also influenced by blood rheology. Thus factors that increase blood viscosity decrease blood flow and predispose to the deposition of platelet fibrin thrombi in valve pockets where venous thrombosis is thought to commence. Factors influencing blood viscosity include an increase in red cell mass or increased proteins such as fibrinogen and other acute phase reactants which rise following trauma, surgery and in cancer.

The role of the coagulation system (Fig. 15.1) in the initiation of thrombosis has been an area of intense study over the past 20 years. This is because evidence has demonstrated that various deficiencies of inhibitors of the coagulation system play a major role in the generation of thrombosis. Generation of the serine protease enzyme thrombin in sites of venous stasis or endothelial cell damage is thought to be the main stimulus of thrombogenesis.[2,3] Thrombin may be generated through the intrinsic or extrinsic pathway.[4] In the intrinsic pathway, Factor XI is activated (XI_a) by activated Factor XII (XII_a) or thrombin and XI_a in turn activates Factor IX (IX_a) which then becomes part of the "tenase complex" consisting of activated Factors VIII, IX and X.[5] The complex is assembled on the surface of platelets which also possess some of these coagulation factors as well as provide phospholipids for the

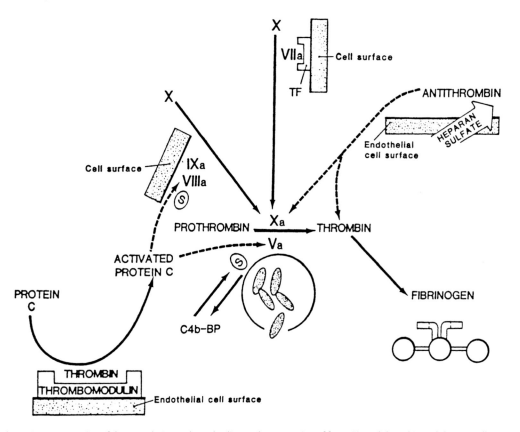

Fig. 15.1. The schematic representation of the coagulation pathway leading to the generation of factor Xa and thrombin and the naturally occurring inhibitors anti-thrombin and Protein C and S. Adapted from Millenson and Bauer (1996, in Hull RD & Pineo GF (eds) Disorders of Thrombosis. Philadelphia, PA: Saunders with permission)

reaction. Thus, an increase in platelet count, as may occur following trauma or infection, or as a primary disorder as in essential thrombocytosis may play a minor role in enhancing venous thrombosis.

Factor X may also be activated through the extrinsic pathway in which tissue factor activates Factor VII (VII$_a$) which in turn activates Factor X via the tenase complex. In addition, VII$_a$ activates Factor IX through the tissue factor pathway.[2,6] The extrinsic system appears to play a major role in the initiation of the coagulation system with the intrinsic system being more responsible for ongoing generation of thrombin.

Activated Factor X (X$_a$) becomes part of the pro-thrombinase complex with activated Factor V and prothrombin attached to platelet membranes. This complex leads to the generation of thrombin. In addition to converting fibrinogen to fibrin, thrombin further activates Factors VIII, IX and XI, stimulates platelet aggregation and converts Factor XIII to activated Factor XIII (XIII$_a$) which stabilizes fibrin making it insoluble to fibrinolysis. Thrombin

also activates the fibrinolytic system by converting plasminogen to plasmin and activates the protein C pathway by activating thrombomodulin which activates protein C and protein S.[2,7]

Thrombin, X$_a$ and the majority of the coagulation enzymes are serine proteases. The exceptions are activated V and VIII (V$_a$ and VIII$_a$) which are cofactors which interact with serine proteases. Antithrombin (previously known as antithrombin III) is a potent serine protease inhibitor, whereas activated protein C and activated protein S are inhibitors of VIII$_a$ and V$_a$.[2,3] Deficiencies of these inhibitors therefore predispose to thrombosis, particularly in the venous circulation.

The fibrinolytic system is activated by generation of thrombin. Tissue plasminogen activator (TPA) is converted to the serine protease enzyme, plasmin, which in turn is neutralized by a$_2$ antiplasmin.[8] Plasmin generation is also inhibited by plasminogen activator inhibitor-1 (PAI-1). Decreased a$_2$ antiplasmin or increased PAI-1 predisposes to thrombosis. Congenital or acquired abnormalities of fibrinogen may predispose to thrombosis by the generation of fibrin which is insoluble by plasmin.[2,3]

The third component of Virchow's triangle is abnormalities of blood vessels, which in practical terms refers to endothelial cell damage. Damage to the endothelium may occur during surgical procedures or mechanical trauma. Endothelial cells are metabolically active and release a number of substances active in the coagulation system.[9] Endothelium plays a significant role in the generation of certain activators and inhibitors of the coagulation system as well as being a site for activation of coagulation if damaged. Exposure of subendothelial connective tissue leads to platelet adhesion and aggregation thereby initiating the development of a thrombus particularly at damaged valve pockets.

The relatively simple theories of Professor Virchow have become more complicated with identification of all of these activators and inhibitors of the coagulation system. However, some knowledge of these factors is essential to the understanding of coagulopathies predisposing to thrombosis.

Clinical Factors Predisposing to the Development of Venous Thromboembolism

Epidemiological studies, particularly in hospitalized patients have identified a number of clinical factors that predispose to venous thromboembolism. Known risk factors for venous thromboembolism are demonstrated in Table 15.1. There are intrinsic problems in the interpretation of thrombosis rates in hospital-based studies, as many patients in such studies had multiple risk factors.[10] Thus, many patients had surgical procedures involving the use of anesthesia and prolonged immobility and they received a variety of medications while in hospital. Many of these patients also had multiple comorbid factors such as advanced age, the presence of cancer or previous venous thromboembolism.[10-12] In designing clinical trials for the prevention of venous thromboembolism these various risk factors are taken into account. However, in many cases, high risk patients are excluded, making results somewhat

Table 15.1. Clinical risk factors predisposing to the development of venous thromboembolism

Surgical and nonsurgical trauma
Previous venous thromboembolism
Immobilization
Malignant disease
Heart disease
Leg paralysis
Age (> 40)
Obesity
Estrogens
Parturition

less generalizable. Even so, effective prophylactic measures have been identified for patients undergoing total hip or total knee replacement, various kinds of surgery including cancer surgery, general surgery, urologic and gynecologic surgery, and medical conditions such as cardiac disease and stroke. Two conditions of particular interest since the identification of various natural inhibitors predisposing to thrombosis are pregnancy and use of the oral contraceptive pill. Although venous thrombosis is relatively uncommon in users of oral contraceptive pills or in pregnant patients, it is now clear that presence of an inhibitor deficiency increases the likelihood of a thrombotic disorder. Thus, identification of inhibitor deficiencies is particularly important for such patients at risk.[13-17]

Coagulopathies Predisposing to Venous Thromboembolism

Known inhibitor deficiencies predisposing to thrombosis include protein C deficiency, protein S deficiency, activated protein C resistance, antithrombin deficiency, the prothrombin mutant and decreased fibrinolytic activity. Homocysteinemia (sometimes referred to as hyperhomocysteinemia) predisposes to both venous and arterial thrombosis. Abnormalities in the fibrinolytic system or dysfibrinogenemia may also predispose to thrombosis.

In reviewing these various prothrombotic states, an attempt will be made to identify incidence of the defect in the population, the ethnic distribution, the link to venous thrombosis particularly in pregnancy, high risk surgery and cancer, and recommendations regarding prophylaxis and treatment of venous thrombosis.

Protein C Deficiency

Protein C is a vitamin-K-dependent glycoprotein requiring gamma-carboxylation for its activity. Thus, its biological activity is decreased by oral anticoagulants. Protein C is activated by the binding of thrombin to thrombomodulin, a transmembrane protein receptor on endothelial cells, to become activated protein C (APC). Activated protein C inactivates Factor V_a and Factor VIII_a.[18] This inactivation is markedly enhanced by the formation of a complex of APC and protein S. Activated protein C also activates fibrinolysis and has anti-inflammatory effects.[3,19]

Protein C deficiency is a heterogeneous disorder. Type I is characterized by a concordant reduction of biological activity and antigen level whereas Type II is associated with reduced activity but normal protein C antigen. There are a total of 160 different mutations reported for protein C deficiency and there are clinically recessive and dominant forms.[3,20,21]

The prevalence of protein C deficiency in healthy donors is 0.2–0.4%, in consecutive patients with a first episode of deep vein thrombosis 3.0% and in thrombophilic patients from 1.0 to 9.0%.[22–26] There does not appear to be an ethnic distribution of protein C deficiency.

There is an increased thrombotic tendency in patients with the heterozygous form of protein C deficiency regardless of the type of defect.[24,25,27–29] The increased risk of thrombosis is about eight- to tenfold[27,28] with a relative risk estimate of seven.[24] Patients with heterozygous protein C deficiency have a higher risk of thrombosis in pregnancy although the risk is much less than with antithrombin deficiency.[13,14] Coumadin-induced skin necrosis has been associated with protein C deficiency (as well as protein S deficiency). The rare finding of homozygous protein C deficiency has been frequently associated with purpura fulminans.[30] The combination of protein C deficiency and APC resistance increases the incidence of thrombosis.

Protein S Deficiency

Protein S is a vitamin-K-dependent glycoprotein requiring g-carboxylation and as with protein C, its activity is decreased by oral anticoagulants. Protein S circulates free (40%) and bound to complement (C_4b, 60%). Only free protein S has protein C cofactor activity. Protein S deficiency is a heterogeneous group of disorders with three separate types: Type I, decreased biological and antigen activity; Type II functional but normal antigen; and Type III, decreased biological activity, decreased free protein S antigen, but normal total antigen.[3,31–33] Genetic abnormalities have been more difficult to sort out than with either protein C or antithrombin deficiency states.[3] The prevalence of protein S deficiency in the general population has been difficult to estimate. In patients presenting with a first episode of deep vein thrombosis the incidence is 1.0–2.0% and for patients with thrombophilia a 1.0–13.0% incidence has been found.[3,22,24] Protein S deficiency does predispose to thrombosis, particularly in the presence of the Factor V Leiden defect, but data are less firm than with protein C.[22,24,34] The rare patient with homozygous protein S deficiency has a major thrombotic tendency similar to homozygous protein C deficiency.[33] As with other deficiencies of inhibitors, incidence of thrombotic episodes during pregnancy is increased by the presence of protein S deficiency.[13,14] Patients with protein S deficiency who have had a previous thrombotic episode require heparin prophylaxis throughout pregnancy and in the postpartum period.[34]

Protein S levels vary with the level of complement C_4b.[33] Protein S decreases during pregnancy making it difficult to accurately measure levels. Levels of protein S are also decreased in diabetes mellitus and in a variety of seriously ill patients including the acquired immunodeficiency syndrome. It is unclear whether these decreased levels of protein S have any impact on thrombotic tendency.

Activated Protein C Resistance

Since the early observations that APC resistance predisposed to venous thrombosis,[15,16] an enormous amount of information has been generated. Activated protein C resistance is the most common genetic defect predisposing to thrombosis. Activated protein C inactivates Factor V_a and Factor VIII_a by proteolytic degradation.[18] The most common mutation leading to APC resistance is the Factor V Leiden resulting in a transposition of arginine to glutamine at the 506 site.[35-39] Approximately 90% of patients who have the biological assay positive for APC resistance also have the Factor V Leiden mutation, indicating that there are other genetic defects responsible for APC resistance.[40] The Factor V Leiden mutation has been identified in 3.0–7.0% of normal individuals of Caucasian origin, but numerous studies have shown a much lower incidence in non European populations such as African, Asian and native North Americans.[35,41-43] In a number of studies of patients presenting with a first episode of idiopathic or a secondary deep vein thrombosis the incidence of APC resistance is around 20%. However, the incidence is around 52% in patients with recurrent venous thromboembolism. Relative risk of thrombosis with APC resistance is 7.0 compared with normal controls.[44-47] Also it has been estimated that by age 50, 25% of individuals with APC resistance will have had thrombosis.[24,35] However, in numerous family studies, many individuals are found to have the Factor V Leiden mutation and no evidence of thrombosis throughout life.[29,48] These data indicate that Factor V Leiden alone is a moderate risk factor but when combined with other risks such as advancing age,[44] oral contraceptive pills,[17] pregnancy,[15,16] or in the presence of another deficiency state, such as protein S or antithrombin deficiency, the likelihood of thrombosis is much greater.[22,49,50]

In two studies of patients undergoing total hip replacement the incidence of postoperative venous thrombosis was not higher in individuals with Factor V Leiden defect as compared to normal controls.[51,52] Also, in a series of patients with positive antibody tests for heparin-induced thrombocytopenia, the incidence of thrombosis was no higher in those who were positive for Factor V Leiden compared with those who were negative.[53] Most studies have shown a higher incidence of recurrent venous thrombosis in patients with the Factor V Leiden defect,[54] whereas one similar study showed no higher incidence of recurrent thrombosis in Factor V Leiden positive patients.[55]

With some of these conflicting data, it is difficult to make firm recommendations regarding individuals who are found to have the Factor V Leiden defect. Those patients with APC resistance who have had previous thrombotic episodes or who have combined defects require special attention at times of risk of venous thrombosis such as surgery or pregnancy. In addition, they require more extended treatment for recurrent thrombosis. For patients with the Factor V Leiden defect who have never had thrombosis (even at times of risk), treatment for an initial episode of deep vein thrombosis or pulmonary embolism is the same as for those who do not have the defect.[34] Caution should be taken in the use of oral contraceptive pills, and possibly hormone replacement therapy, in patients with the APC resistance, but at this time, it would not be warranted to screen all patients for APC resistance before going on the oral contraceptive pill, before becoming pregnant or before undergoing high risk surgery.[34]

Antithrombin

There are two forms of antithrombin deficiency (Type I and Type II). Antithrombin deficiency is, clearly, a heterogeneous disorder. Type I is associated with both a functional and an immunological reduction of antithrombin.[3,56,57] Recent reports indicate that there are eighty distinct antithrombin point mutations and 12 major gene deletions causing Type I antithrombin deficiency. Type II deficiency is associated with defects in the reactive site and the heparin binding sites of antithrombin as well as multiple functional defects.[3,34,56-58] Type II antithrombin deficiency is associated with reduced functional but normal immunological levels of antithrombin. There are 12 distinct mutants for the reactive site, 12 for the heparin binding site and 11 for the multiple functional defect sites.[56]

Estimates of the prevalence of Type I antithrombin deficiency vary from 0.2% of healthy individuals to 1.0% of consecutive patients with a first deep vein thrombosis and 0.5–7.0% of patients with thrombophilia (inherited thrombotic tendencies).[3,22,59,60] In one study, prevalence of Type II antithrombin deficiency in healthy blood donors was 1.45 per thousand.[60] There is no reliable information on ethnic distribution of Type I and Type II antithrombin deficiency.

Type I antithrombin deficiency is clearly associated with an increased risk of thrombosis occasionally occurring in adolescence, but usually occurring between puberty and middle age with a median age of onset of 26 years.[3,61,62] Type II antithrombin deficiency is associated with a lower risk of thrombosis when compared with Type I. Approximately half the patients with thrombosis associated with antithrombin deficiency have idiopathic deep vein thrombosis whereas the rest have thrombosis associated with conditions of increased risk such as surgery or pregnancy. Pregnancy presents a significant management problem particularly in antithrombin-deficient patients who have had previous deep vein thrombosis.[13,14,63] Heparin prophylaxis is required throughout pregnancy with antithrombin concentrates being needed at the time of delivery or for acute thrombotic events.[63] Similarly, for antithrombin-deficient patients requiring major surgical procedures, antithrombin concentrates from human blood products may be given during the risk period, together with prophylactic heparin.[34,63] Combined Factor V Leiden and Type I or Type II antithrombin deficiency has been identified in families. The combined defects predisposed individuals to thrombotic episodes at an earlier age (16 years) compared with antithrombin deficiency alone (median age of onset 26 years).[50]

Prothrombin 20210A Mutant

A mutation of prothrombin consisting of a transition of glutamine to arginine at the nucleotide position 20210 has recently been shown to be a risk factor for venous and arterial thrombosis. The defect results in elevated levels of prothrombin, which may represent a further predisposition to thrombosis.[64] Incidence of the prothrombin mutant in the general population is quite similar to that of APC resistance. Thus, in Europeans the incidence ranges from 0.7 to 4.0%, being higher in southern Europe than northern Europe (3.0 versus 1.7%),[65] to 5.5% in the UK[66] and 4.6% in France.[67] The defect has been found to be rare in people of Asian or African descent.[65] Incidence of the defect in patients presenting with a first episode of venous thrombosis ranges from 19[68] to 28%.[69] When the prothrombin mutant is com-

bined with other defects such as the Factor V Leiden defect, or protein C or protein S deficiency, incidence of venous thrombosis significantly increases.[70]

Although less is known about the risk of thrombosis in patients with the prothrombin mutant than with APC resistance, incidence of this defect is very similar in the general population and in patients presenting with a first episode of deep vein thrombosis. Therefore, at this time it would be reasonable to apply the same recommendations for prophylaxis and treatment to the prothrombin mutant as are applied to those who have APC resistance.

Homocysteinemia

It has been known for many years that congenital homocysteinuria is associated with the early onset of arterial thrombosis and atherosclerosis. More recently, studies have shown that milder forms of hyperhomocysteinemia are associated with an increased incidence of both arterial and venous thrombotic disease. This section will deal only with homocysteinemia as a cause of venous thrombosis.

Homocysteine metabolism is rather complicated and is interrelated with the metabolism of vitamins B_6 and B_{12} and folic acid. Homocysteine is a sulfur-containing amino acid which is involved in two metabolic pathways: remethylation and transsulfuration.[71-73] In remethylation, a methyl group is acquired by homocysteine from methyltetrahydrofolate, a reaction which requires vitamin B_{12}. Adenosyl homocysteine, which is generated from these reactions, is eventually converted back to homocysteine. Abnormalities in the remethylation pathway lead to elevated levels of plasma homocysteine either as a result of inadequate folate or vitamin B_{12}, or to a defect in the gene encoding for methylenetetrahydrofolate reductase (*MTHFR*).[72,73]

The other pathway in which homocysteine is involved is a transsulfuration pathway which requires vitamin B_6 for the breakdown of homocysteine. An impairment of this pathway will lead to a mild increase in fasting levels of homocysteine which increase after a methionine loading test or following a meal.[71,73-75]

Tests most commonly carried out to detect homocysteinemia are plasma levels of homocysteine or an assay to detect a mutation in *MTHFR*.[76,77] Abnormalities of *MTHFR* are quite common in the general population and it is still unclear how much of a risk for venous thrombosis is caused by this mutation.

Studies linking elevated levels of plasma homocysteine and venous thrombosis have shown an odds ratio of between 1.9 and 13.2 for venous thrombosis, representing strong evidence for the association.[75-81] The presence of APC resistance or deficiencies of antithrombin, protein C and protein S increases the risk of venous thrombosis.[82] The finding of the homozygous mutant for *MTHFR* is associated with elevated levels of plasma levels of homocysteine and, at least in some studies, represents a risk factor for the development of venous thrombosis.[76] Ethnic distribution of the homozygous form of the mutant *MTHFR* shows a relatively high incidence in Caucasians, Asians and Native Americans (7.8–20.0%) and a low incidence in those of African descent.[65,66,77]

Decreased Fibrinolytic Activity

Impaired fibrinolysis can predispose to thrombosis if there is decreased generation of plasmin because of plasminogen deficiency,[83] defective synthesis or release of tissue plasminogen activator (TPA) or increased levels of the inhibitor of plasminogen activator inhibitor (PAI-1).[3] Also, dysfibrinogenemia can lead to the production of fibrin, which is only partially soluble by plasmin, and this also predisposes to thrombosis.[84]

Conclusion

Venous thromboembolism continues to be a challenging disorder despite advances in prevention and treatment. Recent advances in our understanding of the pathogenesis of venous thrombosis, with detection of a number of abnormalities in the coagulation system that predispose patients to venous thromboembolism has heightened our awareness of the need for more intense prophylaxis and extended

treatment in many of these at-risk patients. Much more work is required to define the exact role of screening for these disorders prior to exposure to situations known to predispose to thrombosis such as major surgery, pregnancy or the use of the oral contraceptive pill. Furthermore, the need for extended anticoagulation following an episode of venous thromboembolism in patients who are heterozygous for deficiencies of protein C or protein S or antithrombin, or who have APC resistance, the prothrombin mutation, or hereditary or acquired abnormalities resulting in elevated levels of homocysteine, requires further study. Finally, despite all of these recent advances in our understanding of the hypercoagulable states, a large number of families with a predisposition to thrombosis have no detectable defect, suggesting that there are more genetic or acquired defects to be found.

References

1. Virchow, R. Phlogose und thrombose in GefaBsystem. In Virchow R (ed) Gesammelte Abhandlugen zur Wissenschaftlichen Medicin. von Meidinger Sohn, Frankfurt, 1856: 458
2. Millenson MM, Bauer KA. Pathogenesis of venous thromboembolism. In: Hull RD and Pineo GF (eds) Disorders of thrombosis, Chap. 15. WB Saunders Co, Philadelphia, PA, 1996
3. Lane DA, Mannucci PM, Bauer KA et al. Inherited thrombophilia: Part 1. Thromb Haemost 1996a; 76:651–2
4. Jesty J, Spencer AK, Nemerson Y. The mechanism of activation of factor X: kinetic control of alternative pathways leading to the formation of activated factor X. J Biol Chem 1974; 249:5614–22
5. Galiani D, Broze GJ. Factor XI activation in a revised model of blood coagulation. Science. 1991; 253:909–12
6. Novotny WF, Girard TJ, Miletich JP et al. Purification and characterization of the lipoprotein-associated inhibitor from human plasma. J Biol Chem 1989; 264:18,832–7
7. Dittman WA. Thrombomodulin: biology and potential cardiovascular applications. Trends Cardiovasc Med 1991; 1:331–6
8. Aoki N. Natural inhibitors of fibrinolysis. Prog Cardiovasc Dis 1979; 21:267–86
9. Jaffe EA. Endothelial cells and the biology of factor VIII. N Engl J Med 1977; 296:377–83
10. Anderson FA, Wheeler HB, Goldberg RJ et al. A population-based perspective of the hospital incidence and case-fatality rates of deep vein thrombosis within a defined urban population. The Worcester DVT study. J Intern Med 1992b; 232:155–60
11. Anderson FA, Jr., Wheeler HB, Goldberg RJ et al. Prevalence of risk factors for venous thromboembolism among hospital patients. Arch Intern Med 1992a; 152:1660–4
12. Nordström M, Lindblad B, Bergqvist D et al. A prospective study of the incidence of deep-vein thrombosis within a defined urban population. J Intern Med 1992; 232:155–60
13. Conard J, Horellou MH, Van Dreden P et al. Thrombosis and pregnancy in congenital deficiencies in AT III, protein C or protein S: study of 78 women. Thromb Haemost 1990; 63:319–20
14. Pabinger I, Schneider B and the GTH Study Group on Natural Inhibitors. Thrombotic risk of women with hereditary antithrombin

III-, protein C- and protein S-deficiency taking oral contraceptive medication. Thromb Haemost 1994; 71:548–52

15. Hirsch DR, Mikkola KM, Marks PW et al. Pulmonary embolism and deep venous thrombosis during pregnancy or oral contraceptive use: prevalence of factor V Leiden. Am Heart J 1996; 131:1145–8

16. Bokarewa MI, Bremme K, Blomback M. Arg[506]-Gln mutation in factor V and risk of thrombosis during pregnancy. Br J Haematol 1996; 92:473–8

17. Rintelen C, Mannhalter C, Ireland H et al. Oral contraceptives enhance the risk of clinical manifestation of venous thrombosis at a young age in females homozygous for factor V Leiden. Br J Haematol 1996; 93:487–90

18. Kalafatis M, Rand MD, Mann KG. The mechanism of inactivation of human factor V and human factor Va by activated protein C. J Biol Chem 1994; 269: 31,869–80

19. Dahlback B. The protein C anticoagulant system: inherited defects as basis for venous thrombosis. Thromb Res 1995; 77:1–43

20. Griffin JH, Evatt B, Zimmerman TS et al. Deficiency of protein C in congenital thrombotic disease. J Clin Invest 1981; 68:1370–3

21. Aiach M, Gandrille S, Emmerich J. A review of mutations causing deficiencies of antithrombin, protein C, and protein S. Thromb Haemost 1995; 74:81–9

22. Heijboer H, Brandjes DPM, Buller HR et al. Deficiencies of coagulation-inhibiting and fibrinolytic proteins in outpatients with deep-vein thrombosis. N Engl J Med 1990; 323:1512–16

23. Tait RC, Walker ID, Reitsma PH et al. Prevalence of protein C deficiency in the healthy population. Thromb Haemost 1995; 73:87–93

24. Koster T, Rosendaal FR, Briet E et al. Protein C deficiency in a controlled series of unselected outpatients: an infrequent but clear risk factor for venous thrombosis (Leiden Thrombophilia Study). Blood 1995; 85:2756–61

25. Miletich J, Sherman L, Broze G Jr. Absence of thrombosis in subjects with heterozygous protein C deficiency. N Engl J Med 1987; 317:991–6

26. Reitsma PH. Protein C deficiency: from gene defects to disease. Thromb Haemost 1997; 78:344–50

27. Bovill EG, Bauer KA, Dickerman JD et al. The clinical spectrum of heterozygous protein C deficiency in a large New England kindred. Blood 1989; 73:712–17

28. Allaart CF, Poort SR, Rosendaal FR et al. Increased risk of venous thrombosis in carriers of hereditary protein C deficiency defect. Lancet 1993; 341:134–8

29. McColl M, Tait RC, Walker ID et al. Low thrombosis rate seen in blood donors and their relatives with inherited deficiencies of antithrombin and protein C: correlation with type of defect, family history, and absence of the factor V Leiden mutation. Blood Coag Fibrinol. 1996; 7:689–94

30. Branson HE, Katz J, Marble R et al. Inherited protein C deficiency and coumarin-responsive chronic relapsing purpura fulminans in a newborn infant. Lancet 1983; 2:1165–8

31. Comp PC. Laboratory evaluation of protein S status. Semin Thromb Haemost 1990; 16:177–81

32. Koppelman SJ, Hackeng TM, Sixma JJ, et al. Inhibition of the intrinsic factor X activating complex by protein S: Evidence for specific binding of protein S to factor VIII. Blood 1995; 86:1062–71

33. Zoller B, Garcia de Frutos P, Dahlback B. Evaluation of the relationship between protein S and C4b-binding protein isoforms in hereditary protein S deficiency demonstrating type I and type III deficiencies to be phenotypic variants of the same genetic disease. Blood. 1995; 85:3524–31

34. Lane DA, Mannucci PM, Bauer KA et al. Inherited thrombophilia: Part 2. Thromb Haemost 1996b; 76:824–34

35. Svensson PJ, Dahlback B. Resistance to activated protein C as a basis for venous thrombosis. N Engl J Med 1994; 330:517–22

36. Bertina RM, Koeleman BP, Koster T et al. Mutation in blood coagulation factor V associated with resistance to activated protein C. Nature. 1994; 369:64–7

37. Griffin JH, Heeb MJ, Kojima Y et al. Activated protein C resistance: molecular mechanisms. Thromb Haemost 1995; 74:444–8

38. Shen L, Dahlback B. Factor V and protein S as synergistic cofactors to activated protein C in degradation of factor VIIIa. J Biol Chem 1994; 269:18,735–8

39. Sinclair GD, Low S, Poon MC. A hemi-nested, allele specific, whole blood PCR assay for the detection of the factor V Leiden mutation. Thromb Haemost 1997; 77:1154–5

40. Bernardi F, Faioni EM, Castoldi E et al. A factor V genetic component differing from factor V R506Q contributes to the activated protein C resistance phenotype. Blood 1997; 90:1552–7

41. Ridker PM, Glynn RJ, Miletich JP et al. Age-specific incidence rates of venous thromboembolism among heterozygous carriers of factor V Leiden mutation. Ann Intern Med 1997; 126:528–31

42. Pepe G, Rickards O, Vanegas OC et al. Prevalence of factor V Leiden mutation in non European populations. Thromb Haemost 1997; 77:329–31

43. Rees DC, Cox M, Clegg JB. World distribution of factor V Leiden. Lancet 1995; 346:1133–4

44. Greengard JS, Eichinger S, Griffin JH et al. Brief report: variability of thrombosis among homozygous siblings with resistance to activated protein C due to an Arg → Gln mutation in the gene for factor V. N Engl J Med 1994; 331:1559–62

45. Gillespie DL, Carrington LR, Griffin JH et al. Resistance to activated protein C: a common inherited cause of venous thrombosis. Ann Vasc Surg 1996; 10:174–7

46. Price DT, Ridker PM. Factor V Leiden mutation and the risks for thromboembolic disease: a clinical perspective. Ann Intern Med 1997; 127:895–903

47. Emmerich J, Alhenc-Gelas M, Ailaud MF et al. Clinical features in 36 patients homozygous for the ARG 506–GLN factor V mutation. Thromb Haemost 1997; 77:620–3

48. Middeldorp S, Henkens CMA, Koopman MMW. The incidence of venous thromboembolism in family members of patients with factor V Leiden mutation and venous thrombosis. Ann Intern Med 1998; 128:15–20

49. van der Meer FJ, Koster T, Vandenbroucke JP et al. The Leiden thrombophilia study (LETS). Thromb Haemost 1997; 78:631–5

50. van Boven HH, Reitsma PH, Rosendaal FR et al. Factor V Leiden (FV R506Q) in families with inherited antithrombin deficiency. Thromb Haemost 1996; 75:417–21

51. Woolson ST, Zehnder JL, Maloney WJ. Factor V Leiden and the risk of proximal venous thrombosis after total hip arthroplasty. J Arthrop 1998; 13:207–10

52. Ryan DH, Crowther MA, Ginsberg JS et al. Relation of factor V Leiden genotype to risk for acute deep venous thrombosis after joint replacement surgery. Ann Intern Med 1998; 128:270–276.

53. Lee DH, Warkentin TE, Denomme GA et al. Factor V Leiden and thrombotic complications in heparin-induced thrombocytopenia. Thromb Haemost 1998; 79:50–3

54. Simioni P, Prandoni P, Lensing, A et al. The risk of recurrent venous thromboembolism in patients with an Arg[506] → Gln mutation in the gene for factor V (factor V Leiden). N Engl J Med 1997; 336:399–403

55. Eichinger S, PabingerI, Stumpflen A et al. The risk of recurrent venous thromboembolism in patients with and without factor V Leiden. Thromb Haemost 1997; 77:624–8

56. Bayston TA, Lane DA. Antithrombin: molecular basis of deficiency. Thromb Haemost 1997; 78:339–43

57. Blajchman M, Austin R, Fernandez-Rachubinski F. Molecular basis of inherited antithrombin deficiency. Blood 1992; 80:2159–71

58. Lane DA, Olds RJ, Thein, SL. Antithrombin III: summary of first database update. Nucleic Acids Res 1994;22:3556–9

59. Rodeghiero F, Tosetto A. The epidemiology of inherited thrombophilia: the VITA project. Thromb Haemost 1997; 78:636–40

60. Tait RC, Walker ID, Perry DJ et al. Prevalence of antithrombin III deficiency subtypes in 4000 healthy blood donors. Thromb Haemost 1991; 65:839

61. Finazzi G, Caccia R, Barbui T. Different prevalence of thromboembolism in the subtypes of congenital antithrombin III deficiency: review of 404 cases. Thromb Haemost 1987; 58:1094

62. Hirsh J, Piovella F, Pini M. Congenital antithrombin III deficiency. Incidence and clinical features. Am J Med 1989; 87:34S–38S

63. Schulman S, Tengborn L. Treatment of venous thrombombolism in patients with congenital deficiency of antithrombin III. Thromb Haemost 1992; 68:634–6

64. Poort SR, Rosendall FR, Reitsma PH et al. A common genetic variation in the 3′-untranslated region of the prothrombin gene is asso-

ciated with elevated plasma prothrombin levels and an increase in venous thrombosis. Blood 1996; 88:3698–703

65. Rosendaal FR, Doggen CJ, Zivelin A et al. Geographic distribution of the 20210 G to A prothrombin variant. Thromb Haemost 1998; 79:706–8

66. Cumming AM, Keeney S, Salden A et al. The prothrombin gene variant: prevalence in a U.K. anticoagulant clinic population. Br J Haematol 1997; 98:353–5

67. Leroyer C, Mercier B, Oger E et al. Prevalence of 20210 A allele of the prothrombin gene in venous thromboembolism patients. Thromb Haemost 1998; 80:49–51

68. Kapur Rk, Mills LA, Spitzer SG et al. A prothrombin gene mutation is significantly associated with venous thrombosis. Arterioscl Thromb Vasc Biol 1997; 17:2875–9

69. Hillarp A, Zöller B, Svensson PJ et al. The 20210 A allele of the pro-thrombin gene is a common risk factor among Swedish outpatients with verified deep venous thrombosis. Thromb Haemost 1997; 78:990–2

70. Makris M, Preston FE, Beauchamp NJ et al. Co-inheritance of the 20210A allele of the prothrombin gene increases the risk of throm-bosis in subjects with familial thrombophilia. Thromb Haemost 1997; 78:1426–9

71. D'Angelo A, Selhub J. Homocysteine and thrombotic disease. Blood 1997; 90:1–11

72. D'Angelo A, Mazzola G, Crippa L et al. Advances in basic, labora-tory and clinical aspects of thromboembolic diseases: hyperhomo-cysteinemia and venous thromboembolic disease. Haematologica 1997; 82:211–19

73. Boers GHJ. Hyperhomocysteinemia as a risk factor for arterial and venous disease. A review of evidence and relevance. Thromb Haemost 1997; 78:520–2

74. Kluijtmans LA, van den Heuvel, Boers GH et al. Molecular genetic analysis in mild hyperhomocysteinemia: a common mutation in the methylenetetrahydrofolate reductase gene is a genetic risk factor of cardiovascular disease. Am J Human Genet 1996; 58:35–41

75. Kluijtmans LAJ, den Heijer M, Reitsma PH et al. Thermolabile Methylenetetrahydrofolate reductase and factor V Leiden in the risk of deep-vein thrombosis. Thromb Haemost 1998; 79:254–8

76. Arruda VR, von Zuben PM, Chiaparini LC et al. The mutation Ala677 Val in the methylene tetrahydofolate reductase gene: a risk factor for arterial disease and venous thrombosis. Thromb Haemost 1997; 77:818–21

77. Franco RF, Araújo AG, Guerreiro JF et al. Analysis of the 677 C T mutation of the methylenetetrahydrofolate reductase gene in dif-ferent ethnic groups. Thromb Haemost 1998; 79:119–21

78. Amundsen T, Ueland PM, Waage A. Plasma homocysteine levels in patients with deep venous thrombosis. Arterioscl, Thromb Vasc Biol 1995; 15:1321–23

79. den Heijer M, Blom HJ, Gerrits WBJ et al. Is hyperhomocys-teinaemia a risk factor for recurrent venous thrombosis? N Engl J Med 1995; 345:882–5

80. den Heijer M, Koster T, Blom HK et al. Hyperhomocysteinemia as a risk factor for deep-vein thrombosis. N Engl J Med 1996; 334:759–62

81. Simioni P, Prandoni P, Burlina A et al. Hyperhomocysteinemia and deep-vein thrombosis; a case–control study. Thromb Haemost 1996; 76:883–6

82. Mandel H, Brenner B, Berant M et al. Coexistence of hereditary homocystinuria and factor V Leiden – effect on thrombosis. N Engl J Med 1996; 334:763–8

83. Dolan G, Preston FE. Familial plasminogen deficiency and throm-boembolism. Fibrinolysis 1988; 2:26S–34S

84. Haverkate F, Samama M. Familial dysfibrinogenemia and throm-bophilia. Report on a study of the SSC subcommittee on fibrino-gen. Thromb Haemost 1995; 73:151–61

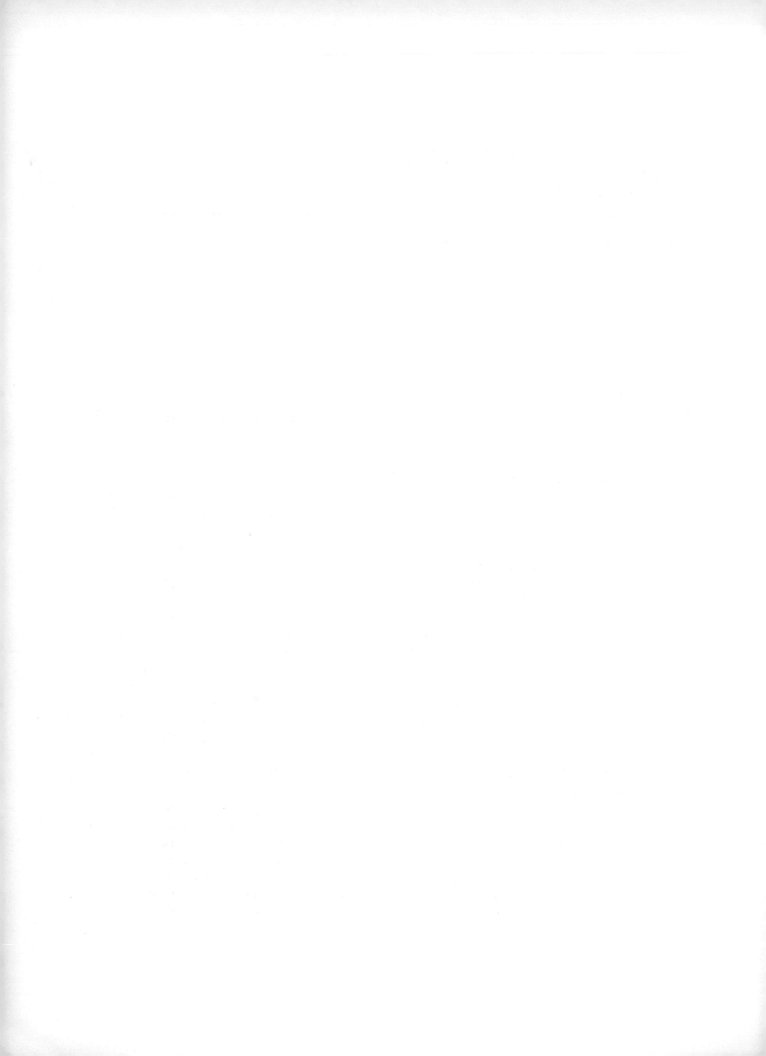

Thrombolysis, Angioplasty, and Stenting

16

Michael D. Dake and Suresh Vedantham

As seen in the preceding chapters, modern improvements in the management of venous disease have originated through medical, rehabilitative and surgical innovations. From a radiological perspective, emergence of duplex ultrasound as a reliable method of evaluating the structure and function of the venous system has significantly enhanced our understanding of the pathophysiology of chronic venous insufficiency (CVI). Simultaneous advances in the interventional radiological management of arterial occlusive disease have created the theoretical foundation and technology supportive of a new approach to the prevention and treatment of venous disease: combined endovascular therapy using regional thrombolysis, balloon venoplasty and endovascular stent placement. While the results of long-term, controlled trials are not yet available, it has become increasingly clear that these percutaneous techniques have the potential to translate recent pathophysiological revelations into tangible clinical benefits.

The goals of this chapter are threefold: (1) to reinforce the concept that acute deep venous thrombosis (DVT) and chronic venous thrombosis represent entities upon one major pathway to chronic venous insufficiency; (2) to demonstrate the ability of aggressive endovascular intervention to interrupt this progression; (3) to highlight the clinical situations in which combined endovascular therapy can be expected to produce optimal clinical results.

DVT: Rationale for Endovascular Management

Major clinical sequelae of deep venous thrombosis include pulmonary thromboembolism and chronic venous insufficiency. Treatment of acute lower extremity DVT has traditionally been directed at the prevention of pulmonary embolism, considered the most devastating complication of venous thrombosis. Typically, such patients are treated with anticoagulation therapy, consisting of intravenous heparin (maintaining partial thromboplastin time 60–100 s) followed by oral warfarin (maintaining an international normalized ratio (INR) 2–3) for 6 months.[1] Patients having contraindications to, or failing, anticoagulation therapy (defined as pulmonary embolism or significant thrombus propagation despite therapeutic anticoagulation) are considered candidates for inferior vena cava filter placement. In this fashion, the mortality from pulmonary embolism has been drastically reduced in patients with recognized deep venous thrombosis.[2]

While streptokinase, the first thrombolytic agent, underwent intensive clinical investigation as a systemic treatment for DVT in the 1970s, only recently have innovations in interventional radiology sparked a rejuvenation in enthusiasm for this form of therapy using a catheter-directed regional infusion. The logical basis for using thrombolytic agents for DVT has of late emerged through several clinical and pathophysiological revelations having their origins in extensive studies of DVT patients using duplex ultrasound:

1. Most DVT patients treated with anticoagulation experience symptoms of chronic venous insufficiency, particularly those with iliofemoral venous thrombosis. This resulting disability has significant clinical and socioeconomic consequences.

The postphlebitic syndrome is characterized clinically by chronic leg edema, venous claudication, hyperpigmentation and venous ulceration in advanced cases. Despite adequate anticoagulation, symptoms of postphlebitic syndrome are experienced within three years by more than two-thirds of patients having an episode of lower extremity DVT, including lower extremity pain, measurable edema (60%), pigmentation (25%) and venous ulceration (5%).[3] For iliofemoral venous thrombosis, long-term studies have demonstrated that nearly all patients develop some degree of chronic leg edema, with 50% experiencing venous claudication and more than 85% showing venous ulceration within 10 years of the initial DVT.[4] These patients have significant job disability and increased health care utilization related to care of their chronic venous disease, with an average of eight clinic visits per year and five DVT-related hospitalizations over this 10 year period. It has, therefore, become clear that chronic venous insufficiency prevention should represent a fundamental goal of modern DVT therapy.

2. The postphlebitic syndrome results from ambulatory venous hypertension caused by two important factors: valvular insufficiency and chronic venous obstruction. The rate of spontaneous venous recanalization seen in deep venous thrombosis patients receiving anticoagulation therapy is not sufficient to prevent valvular damage and subsequent reflux in most patients.

The pathophysiology of the postphlebitic syndrome has been subject of intensive investigation over the last 20 years. While valvular insufficiency and chronic venous obstruction have long been recognized as critical determinants of long-term outcome, only recently has the emergence of duplex sonography as a highly reliable method of assessing venous integrity enabled investigators to conduct scientifically rigorous studies of venous patency and valvular function. Results of this work are heavily relied upon in this discussion, as they provide the fundamental rationale for application of aggressive endovascular techniques to DVT.

The primary determinant of long-term clinical outcome in DVT patients is the state of the valvular system, with chronic obstruction representing an important but secondary factor. Extensive longitudinal study of the timing of endogenous clot lysis, vessel recanalization, development of valvular insufficiency and symptom onset in a large number of DVT patients has been required to draw this conclusion; this is because most patients with postphlebitic syndrome demonstrate evidence of both reflux and obstruction within the first year of the initial DVT episode. Ultrasound studies have demonstrated that for femoropopliteal DVT, approximately half of anticoagulated patients will have a patent (recanalized) axial venous system within 3 months, 75% of venous segments will spontaneously recanalize within 6 months, and nearly all infrainguinal venous segments will recanalize within one year.[5,6] In other words, while clot propagation and rethrombosis do exist in balance with gradual clot lysis in DVT patients, eventual recanalization is the rule rather than the exception in anticoagulated patients with DVT limited to the femoropopliteal region.

Unfortunately, the gradual re-establishment of a patent venous system does not imply clinical welfare for the involved extremity. In fact, ultrasound-documented venous valvular insufficiency develops in almost 40% of patients within 1 month of the initial episode of DVT, and in two-thirds of patients within 1 year.[6] Typically, this is manifested by the development of or increase in leg edema several months after the initial episode. Reflux occurs with the highest frequency in those venous segments that have previously contained thrombus, but also develops with time in patent veins below occluded proximal segments.[7] Longitudinal sonographic studies have clearly demonstrated that the development of valvular reflux precedes or coincides with complete clot lysis, but almost never occurs after a patent venous system is re-established. Hence, it can be concluded that the valvular damage that causes chronic symptomatology in patients with femoropopliteal venous thrombosis occurs almost exclusively within the first few months, before venous recanalization has occurred.

To summarize, acute thrombosis causes valvular damage in involved venous segments and also contributes to peripheral valvular reflux by increasing venous pressures peripheral to the obstruction. While spontaneous recanalization is part of the natural history of femoropopliteal DVT treated with heparin, it occurs too late to prevent valvular damage, reflux and chronic symptomatology in the majority of patients. In this regard, it is important to remember that heparin, an antithrombin III cofactor, acts to prevent clot propagation, allowing the body to spontaneously lyse thrombus, but has no active thrombolytic effect. This biochemical truism is empirically confirmed by the presence of thrombus propagation in a significant number of patients (30%) during treatment with heparin.[9] It should therefore not be surprising that the rate of clot lysis in DVT patients treated with heparin is only sufficient to prevent valvular damage and chronic symptoms in a minority of patients. On the positive side, for patients with femoropopliteal DVT, further valvular damage is likely to progress at a much slower pace as the obstructive component is eventually removed. As will be discussed, the logical corollary is that endovascular approaches to chronic femoropopliteal DVT are less likely to have significant clinical impact as the vast majority of the valvular damage has already been done.

In contrast, spontaneous recanalization only rarely occurs in patients with iliofemoral (defined as common femoral vein and above) venous thrombosis. Continuing valvular damage occurs over a period of years with the progressive development of valvular reflux (95% of patients) and chronic symptoms (nearly all patients) because of the resulting chronically elevated venous pressures. These symptoms are often of greater severity than in patients with thrombus limited to the femoropopliteal venous system.[10,11] Endovascular therapy, therefore, represents the only nonsurgical method of removing chronic iliac vein thrombus. This, in turn, helps to reduce ambulatory venous pressure, and thereby prevent valvular damage and episodes of recurrent venous thrombosis.

3. *The best long-term outcomes are observed in DVT patients in whom re-establishment of antero-grade venous flow and elimination of thrombus are achieved early.*

Early spontaneous clot lysis is a consistent finding in the minority of patients who experience long-term complete symptom resolution after an episode of lower extremity DVT. This finding is true both for patients with iliofemoral venous thrombosis (although it rarely occurs in this setting) and

femoropopliteal thrombosis.[10,12] As noted earlier, it is known that valvular reflux almost never develops after complete clot lysis is achieved, and that only 15–20% of DVT patients show evidence of valvular reflux 1 week after initial symptom onset.[6] These findings suggest the existence of an early window period when venous recanalization might prevent valvular damage and long-term symptoms, providing strong justification for aggressive endovascular treatment of acute DVT. It can therefore be stated that the goal of modern DVT therapy should be redefined to include establishment of a patent axial iliofemoral venous system with expedient elimination of as much thrombus as possible.

Thrombolytic Agents

Thrombolytic agents have been available since 1947, and have in recent decades revolutionized clinical approaches to myocardial infarction, acute limb ischemia and massive pulmonary embolism. These agents are currently being investigated in many other clinical settings, including that of deep vein thrombosis. A brief discussion of those first- and second-generation thrombolytic agents that have been applied to DVT is provided.[13]

Streptokinase (SK)

Streptokinase (Astra, Westboro, MA) is a 47 kDa protein synthesized by group C b-hemolytic streptococci. When streptokinase forms a complex with human plasminogen, a conformational change occurs in plasminogen, exposing its active site and permitting conversion of a second plasminogen molecule to plasmin, which degrades fibrin clots, fibrinogen, and multiple coagulation factors. Effective SK therapy causes a plasminolytic state that includes decreases in plasma plasminogen, whole blood clotting time and fibrinogen; and an increase in fibrin degradation products. Disadvantages of SK compared with other agents include its rapid clearance from the bloodstream (half-life 10–20 min), lower efficiency due to the need for two plasminogen molecules per SK molecule for activity, and the systemic fibrinolytic state it induces (with increased hemorrhagic complications in some clinical settings). The bacterial origin of SK permits easy production and results in lower cost, but renders the compound extremely antigenic, with significantly increased incidence of fever (30%) and mild allergic reactions (12%). Incidence of anaphylaxis has been reported to be approximately 0.1%. Use of a loading dose is generally necessary to override the presence of anti-SK antibodies, which are present in the serum of many patients. Development of anti-SK antibodies after therapy precludes repeat use of SK within at least 6 months of the initial administration.

Urokinase (UK)

Urokinase (Abbott Laboratories, Abbott Park, IL) is an endogenous, 57 kDa enzyme initially discovered in urine, subsequently, mass produced from human fetal kidney cultures and now synthesized by recombinant genetic techniques. UK is capable of directly causing the conversion of plasminogen to plasmin, and theoretically has a greater affinity for fibrin-bound plasminogen. UK is thought to cause slightly less systemic fibrinolysis than SK, and is not associated with a significant incidence of allergic reactions. Because antibodies are not formed against UK, a loading dose is not required. UK is primarily cleared by the liver (half-life 10–20 min), and moderate degrees of hepatic failure can therefore prolong its effects. While UK is technically more expensive than SK, most investigators in the United States prefer UK for peripheral applications because its predictability and comparatively low complication rate have translated into superior overall cost-effectiveness compared with SK.[14]

Tissue Plasminogen Activator (TPA)

Tissue plasminogen activator (Genentech, San Francisco, CA) is an endogenous, 68 kDa serine protease secreted by vascular endothelium and rapidly degraded by the liver (half life 2–6 min).[15] TPA is currently synthesized using recombinant DNA technology, resulting in its much higher cost compared with urokinase. TPA is relatively clot specific, in that its activity is strongly enhanced by the presence of fibrin; while serum laboratory studies indicate less systemic fibrinolysis with TPA, significant advantages with respect to bleeding complications have not been clearly demonstrated in clinical trials.

Systemic Thrombolysis for Deep Venous Thrombosis

Numerous randomized clinical trials have found intravenous thrombolysis to be significantly more effective than heparin alone in causing lysis of acute thrombi in the deep venous system, and have been summarized in several meta-analytic studies.[16,17] Several factors have been found to play an important role in determining ultimate outcome of lytic therapy: (1) duration of symptoms (i.e., degree of clot organization); (2) involvement of the iliofemoral venous system; and (3) ability to continue infusion to completion. For patients with acute venous thrombosis (defined as less than 2 weeks from symptom onset), systemic thrombolysis can be expected to produce complete clot lysis in 45% of patients, compared with less than 5% of patients treated with heparin alone. Some degree of clot lysis is observed in more than 60% of patients treated with thrombolytic agents compared with 15–20% for heparin alone. For older thrombi, results are variable but much less impressive; in one cohort successful lysis was noted in only 14% of patients with symptoms for more than 4 weeks.[18] In the iliac venous system, clinical results with heparin alone for even acute thrombi are dismal, with only 20–30% showing significant clot lysis.[19] This is likely due to larger clot burden, complete lack of flow in the axial iliofemoral venous system, and the inability of blood-borne plasminogen activators to access large portions of thrombus. Concerning salvage of valvular function, long-term follow-up studies have demonstrated significantly less chronic venous insufficiency in DVT patients treated with urokinase or streptokinase compared with those receiving heparin alone.[20] Doses of lytic agent required to achieve these results, however, have been relatively high, and meta-analysis studies have shown a threefold increase in major bleeding complications using thrombolytic agents compared with heparin alone (14% versus 4%). This finding has engendered a certain degree of reluctance in the medical community to prescribe thrombolytic agents for DVT. The concern being that, while critical disorders such as myocardial infarction and limb ischemia might justify assumption of the attendant risks of thrombolytic therapy, prevention of postphlebitic syndrome might not warrant such an aggressive approach.[21] Hence, despite the experience gained in the 1970s and 1980s, systemic thrombolysis for DVT has not gained widespread acceptance.

Catheter-Directed Thrombolysis

Rationale

Recently, endovascular techniques have been applied to more effectively utilize thrombolytic agents while simultaneously lowering the required dosage, duration of therapy and associated complication rate. Several theoretical advantages are gained by directly administering thrombolytic agents through catheter systems embedded within thrombus, and explain why this represents the most effective method of achieving thrombolysis in the arterial and venous systems.[22] While systemically administered thrombolytic agent is directed away from occluded venous segments by collateral channels, direct intrathrombic administration ensures delivery of high concentrations of the agent to a greater surface area of thrombus. This is especially important in treating patients with large clot burdens in long segments of iliofemoral vein. The mechanical effect of direct intrathrombus infusion may play a small additional role in clot dissolution. In this fashion, a complete (if diminutive) channel, permitting antegrade blood flow through the thrombosed segment, is rapidly established; this in turn enables mechanical and chemical contributions of flow to enhance thrombolysis. These factors combine to expedite lysis, with subsequent earlier termination of infusion, lower overall administered dose and lower rate of major complications.

As in the arterial system, long-term patency of a recanalized vessel is in large part determined by inflow and outflow considerations as well as by re-establishment of a flow channel in the occluded segment. Many DVT patients, particularly those with iliofemoral DVT, have underlying venous stenoses or other lesions which predispose them to

episodes of venous thrombosis, for which adequate treatment might be achieved through the application of specific endovascular techniques. Typically, regional thrombolysis is first used to remove obstructing thrombus, thereby unmasking outflow venous stenoses. Balloon venoplasty and/or endovascular stent placement can then be performed to treat the underlying stenosis and compress residual thrombus against the vein walls, removing intrinsic outflow obstruction and providing mechanical support to maintain lumen caliber against any extrinsic compression. These maneuvers usually result in instantaneous reduction of venous pressures and rapid symptom resolution. They also theoretically serve to prevent future DVT episodes. In this fashion, true potential of combined endovascular therapy is realized by simultaneously addressing the acute obstruction as well as its underlying cause.

Basic Protocol for Treating DVT

Candidates for thrombolytic therapy have symptomatic deep venous thrombosis documented by conventional contrast venography, color Doppler ultrasound or magnetic resonance venography. Patients must have no contraindication to anticoagulation or thrombolysis, including history of hemorrhagic stroke, ischemic stroke less than 1 year ago, intracranial or intraspinal malignancy or arteriovenous malformation, recent surgery, pregnancy or recent delivery, urokinase allergy or other reaction (rare), recent gastrointestinal (GI) bleeding, or other bleeding disorder. As with systemic thrombolysis, duration of symptoms and involvement of the iliofemoral venous system are key factors that influence the likelihood of success and the degree of clinical benefit achieved with endovascular therapy.

While the intricacies of endovascular therapy are beyond the scope of this text, a basic methodological understanding is essential in comprehending which patients are likely to succeed with endovascular approaches, and in monitoring the patient during therapy. In selecting an access vessel from which to initiate therapy, consideration must be given to the possibility of venoplasty or endovascular stent placement following thrombolysis, and a vessel of appropriate caliber chosen. While retrograde access via the internal jugular vein, brachial vein, and contralateral femoral vein has been described,[23,24] in our view antegrade access enables easier guidewire and catheter passage without impediment by the iliac or femoral venous valves, thereby facilitating endovascular stent placement and preventing further valvular disruption during catheter passage. Femoral vein approaches may be difficult to tolerate by some patients in whom prolonged infusion is required. In addition, introduction of larger sheaths into the common femoral vein carries the inherent risk of venous thrombosis in patients with an already-demonstrated proclivity to such, and may lead to unsatisfactory thrombolysis near the sheath entry site if an ipsilateral approach is used. The contralateral femoral vein approach presents a significant mechanical disadvantage to catheterization of the iliac vein to be treated, particularly if iliac vein thrombus extends into the inferior vena cava or is flush with its bifurcation; the over-the-horn approach is even less advantageous when endovascular stenting is contemplated.

For these reasons, many investigators currently favor the antegrade popliteal approach in the setting of lower extremity DVT.[25,26] The patient is placed prone on the angiography table and preliminary ultrasound of the popliteal fossa performed to try to define the lowest extent of thrombus, if possible. The site is prepped in sterile fashion and the popliteal vein (or posterior tibial vein) is accessed using ultrasound guidance, preferably below the distal-most extent of thrombus. Particular care is given to obtaining a single-wall puncture to avoid an arteriovenous fistula between the popliteal artery and vein and to prevent hematoma formation during thrombolytic agent infusion. In cases where the popliteal vein is difficult to access, alternative routes of antegrade access have been described, including the greater saphenous vein, lower posterior tibial vein or pedal veins.[27] Ascending venography is performed and a 5 or 6 French venous sheath placed. A hydrophilic guidewire is manipulated across the occluded segment and into the inferior vena cava; a 4 or 5 French multi-sidehole infusion catheter is embedded in the thrombus.

Urokinase (120,000–160,000 units/h) is administered via overnight infusion, with the dose usually split evenly between the infusion catheter and sheath sidearm. The use of urokinase dosages that are significantly higher than those required for arterial thrombolysis is empiric, but considered necessary due to greater thrombus volume in the capacious pelvic veins and decreased contribution of flow in the venous system. Administration of a portion of the urokinase dose through the sheath ensures optimal inflow to the groin level, an important factor that effects the ultimate patency of the iliofemoral venous system. Patients are systemically anticoagulated with heparin, maintaining a partial thromboplastin time 60–100 s. Fibrinogen determinations are obtained every 6 h and maintained at levels greater than 100 mg/dl through adjustments in urokinase dose. While some investigators utilize a temporary caval filter for pulmonary embolism prophylaxis during infusion,[28] we have not found this to be necessary. We only consider this measure when large, free-floating, iliac vein or caval thrombi are identified venographically. Because of the small risk of iatrogenic pulmonary embolism, we do not employ the pulse–spray technique of urokinase administration.

Venography is performed through the venous sheath the next day and adjunctive measures instituted depend on venographic findings:

1. If *complete lysis* is seen and there is *no* underlying venous stenosis, infusion is terminated and treatment considered successful.
2. If *complete lysis* is seen and an *iliac vein stenosis* is unmasked, venoplasty and endovascular stent placement are performed in most clinical situations (Figs 16.1, 16.2 and 16.3). It is important to obtain venographic images of common iliac vein stenoses with the patient in different positions, as the prone position does occasionally artificially accentuate the physiologic impression upon the left common iliac vein by the crossing right common iliac artery. While any stenosis seen in the setting of venous thrombosis is likely to be clinically significant, a venous pressure gradient of 3 mmHg or greater represents objective evidence of hemodynamic significance. This can be used along with venographic criteria to direct therapy in patients considered less optimal candidates for stent placement. We generally prefer larger diameter (10–12 mm for external iliac veins, 14–18 mm for common iliac veins) self-expandable Wallstents (Schneider, Inc., Plymouth, MN) for iliac vein stenoses, due to their flexibility and low profile for introduction and delivery. The occasional need to extend the lower end of the stent into the common femoral vein to ensure adequate inflow also favors the more flexible Wallstent. We currently

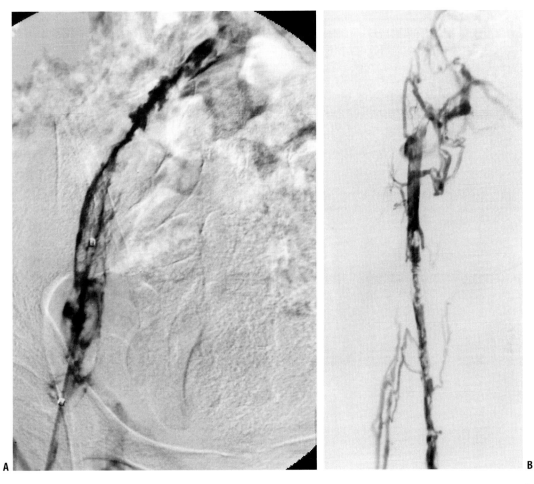

Fig. 16.1A, B. A 38-year-old woman with a chief complaint of 2 weeks' left lower extremity swelling and pain was evaluated with venography via the left popliteal vein. The examination demonstrates occlusive thrombus extending from the left common iliac vein **A** through the distal left superficial femoral vein. **B** A poorly-developed venous collateral network is demonstrated, consistent with subacute chronicity.

employ balloon-expandable Palmaz stents (Johnson and Johnson Interventional Systems, Warren, NJ) for select focal iliac vein stenoses when greater radial strength is desired, although the requirement for a larger sheath size renders introduction via popliteal vein access less suitable.

3. If *complete lysis* is seen and a *femoral venous stenosis* is uncovered, treatment with balloon venoplasty is performed. We do not generally advocate placement of venous stents below the common femoral vein, being guided by the poor patency achieved with infrainguinal arterial stents and by our own limited but disappointing experience with superficial femoral vein stents.

4. If *partial lysis* is achieved, the infusion catheter is repositioned within the residual thrombus and thrombolytic therapy continued for one

additional night. The patient is restudied the next day.

5. If *no clot lysis* is seen, treatment is considered unsuccessful and infusion terminated.

6. Whenever possible, patients are placed on warfarin therapy for at least 6 months after treatment. In addition, periodic (every 3 months initially) clinical and sonographic follow-up is instituted to evaluate for signs of restenosis or rethrombosis, and to evaluate for chronic venous insufficiency.

Endovascular Therapy for Acute DVT

Because some patients are unable to give an accurate historical account of the duration of symptoms, sonographic and venographic criteria may occasionally be employed to render an educated guess

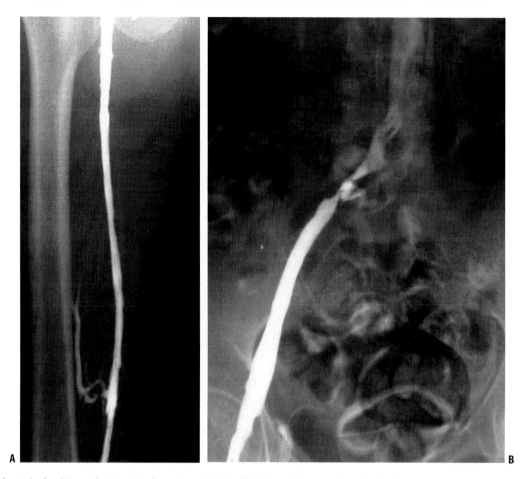

Fig. 16.2. A After 48 h of urokinase administration through a multi-sidehold infusion catheter, complete clot lysis has occurred. The degree of collateral vein flow is markedly reduced after the re-establishment of iliofemoral venous patency. **B** Successful thrombolysis has unmasked a causative focal left common iliac vein stenosis with the location and appearance typical of right common iliac artery commpression syndrome (May–Thurner syndrome). The patient's age, sex, and absence of other risk factors favored this diagnosis.

as to whether acute and/or chronic thrombus is present. While lack of flow, noncompressibility and loss of augmentation are sonographic features common to venous thrombosis of any age, the presence of diminutive venous channels, highly echogenic intraluminal material on ultrasound, irregular stringy venographic filling defects (corresponding to webs and synechiae) and abundant collateralization indicate the presence of chronic venous disease. In contrast, dilation of the involved vein and the presence of hypoechoic intraluminal material are typical sonographic features of acute thrombus. Venography generally depicts voluminous filling defects within dilated veins with a limited degree of collateralization. With this radiologic picture, the diagnosis of acute thrombus may often be made.

The preceding discussion on the technique of venous recanalization illustrates why patients with acute DVT respond better to thrombolytic therapy.

First, the axial venous system peripheral to an acutely thrombosed vein is usually dilated and quite easy to access under ultrasound guidance. Second, guidewire passage across the region of occlusion is nearly always possible in less organized ("soft") acute thrombus; such thrombi are also readily susceptible to chemical lysis with urokinase. Third, patients with acute DVT are often younger and healthier than those with chronic DVT, have a lower incidence of malignancy-related hypercoagulability and possess an intact peripheral venous system. These factors may lower the incidence of rethrombosis and reflux, favoring re-establishment of a normotensive venous system. Hence, aggressive endovascular approaches to DVT hold the promise of complete long-term recovery for this subset of patients.

Acute *iliofemoral* DVT represents the clinical situation in which endovascular therapy has so far

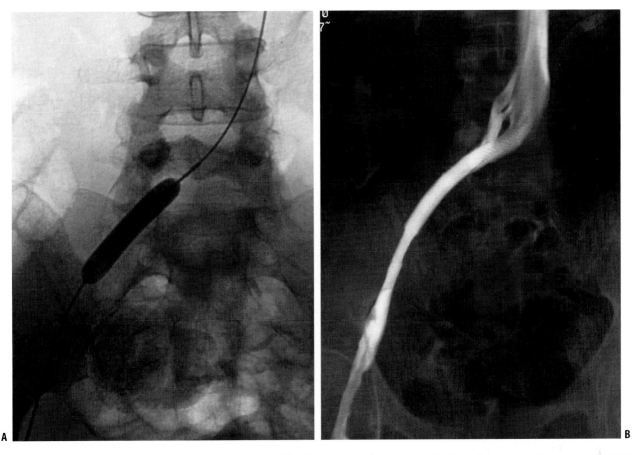

Fig. 16.3A, B. After balloon venoplasty and Wallstent placement, excellent flow into the inferior vena cava is observed through a widely patent, stented left common iliac vein. The woman's symptoms resolved completely after thrombolysis and stent placement.

been most commonly applied, presumably because of its discouraging natural history and therapeutic failures of anticoagulation and systemic thrombolysis. Iliofemoral DVT occurs more commonly in women and has a 3 : 1 left-sided predilection.[19] This finding is largely explained by the common venographic demonstration of left common iliac vein compression by the crossing right common iliac artery. This anatomic disturbance may cause elevated venous pressures and predispose to venous thrombosis in patients with other risk factors for DVT, or may in itself cause intimal injury, venous stenosis and subsequent thrombosis (May–Thurner syndrome).[29] The latter condition is thought by many investigators to be much more common than previously described, and may in large part explain the historically high rate of recurrent thrombosis and continued disability in patients with iliofemoral venous thrombosis treated by venous thrombectomy or bypass.[30] Other common causes of iliac vein stenosis include extrinsic compression by

tumor, postradiation injury, postoperative, or post-traumatic injury, catheter-related injury and retroperitoneal fibrosis.

Since the first report of a retrograde brachial vein entry to treat a patient with acute iliofemoral DVT in 1991,[23] two major studies of combined endovascular therapy, both employing thrombolysis in all patients and venoplasty and stenting in selected patients, have been presented.[25,26] Initial results have been concordant, with an 85–90% success rate in achieving clot lysis and rapid symptomatic improvement in patients with acute iliofemoral DVT who have no known malignancy. Patients with underlying malignant disorders appear to fare slightly worse initially (technical success approximately 80%). In the large University of Minnesota study, 2 year primary patency of the iliofemoral venous system was 75% in patients without malignancy and 40% in patients with cancer (60% overall). However, secondary patency for both groups was comparable (78%).[26] This difference was presumably due to underlying hypercoagulability and the poorer overall condition of cancer patients, but it is encouraging that repeated interventions were able to maintain patency. Primary patency rates have been somewhat higher in the Stanford experience (90% at 1 year). This variation may be due to a slightly younger and healthier patient population, lower number of cancer patients, differences in the use of adjunctive surgical techniques (favored by the Minnesota group) and the use of long-term antiplatelet therapy by the Stanford group. In any case, these results compare very favorably to those of anticoagulation therapy alone and systemic thrombolysis, although no direct comparative studies have yet been published. Lower overall average dose (5 million units) of urokinase and shorter average duration of therapy (30 h) required to achieve these results also favor catheter-directed thrombolysis over systemic infusion.

Phlegmasia cerulea dolens represents a grave condition at one extreme end of the spectrum of iliofemoral venous thrombosis. The mortality of this disorder untreated is 25–30% with a limb loss rate of 50%. Previous treatment approaches have included anticoagulation with leg elevation, systemic thrombolysis, and venous thrombectomy with or without arteriovenous fistula creation. However, none of these techniques have been particularly successful when venous gangrene was present (55% of patients).[31] Recently, catheter-directed thrombolysis has been applied to the treatment of this disorder with dramatic results.[24,32] While the relatively small number of such cases and dire patient condition preclude controlled studies, emergent endovascular therapy currently appears to offer the best hope of extremity salvage in this unfortunate subset of patients.

Results of endovascular stenting in the iliac venous system are still emerging, with the two centers with the largest experience reporting differing patency rates, perhaps due to the above mentioned protocol differences between the two studies. The University of Minnesota group[33] has reported 1 year primary patency and secondary rates of 50 and 81%, respectively, for iliofemoral venous stents, with no differences detected between patients in whom stenting was performed for isolated venous stenosis versus stenosis with thrombosis. In this series, approximately 40% of the patients had a known malignancy. Secondary patency of stented iliac veins was significantly lower in this subgroup

(64% 1 year secondary patency for cancer patients versus 94% for benign disease), possibly because cancer patients with stent thrombosis were less likely to undergo invasive attempts at recanalization. Patients requiring stent extension below the inguinal ligament had significantly lower patency rates, as expected, presumably due to the greater extent of thrombosis in these patients. Comparison with the Stanford experience, in which patients receiving iliac vein stents had a 1 year primary patency of greater than 90% when no associated malignancy was present and venous inflow was normal, is rendered even more difficult by the use of adjunctive, surgically placed arteriovenous fistulas in patients with slow flow after venous stenting in the University of Minnesota study. Interestingly, iliac vein stenting in this patient group was actually associated with lower primary patency. Hence, while there is no question that stenting of venous stenoses is essential to achieving symptom resolution, long-term controlled studies will ultimately be required to establish the degree of long-term benefit with regards to venous patency and prevention of chronic venous hypertension, reflux and episodes of rethrombosis.

Patients with isolated acute femoropopliteal DVT without iliac vein involvement represent a less studied group, but may also achieve benefit from lytic therapy provided treatment is instituted within several weeks of symptom onset, prior to the development of valvular reflux. As discussed previously, thrombolytic therapy will not reverse already sustained valvular damage which results in reflux and postphlebitic syndrome in a large number of these patients. Since the femoral veins uniformly spontaneously recanalize within 3–6 months, there is no need for lytic agents to re-establish a venous channel after this time. Because the frequency and severity of the postphlebitic syndrome are somewhat lower in this patient population than in those with iliofemoral DVT, thrombolytic therapy might be best reserved for younger, more active patients with longer life expectancy.

A venous registry has been established to track patients treated with catheter-directed thrombolysis to evaluate if the results achieved will exceed those of systemic thrombolysis and anticoagulation with regards to venous patency and prevention of recurrent venous thrombosis, valvular reflux and postphlebitic syndrome. Based on a preliminary tabulation of results, catheter-directed thrombolysis will likely become the treatment of choice for patients with acute iliofemoral DVT and for select patients with acute femoropopliteal DVT.

Endovascular Therapy for Chronic DVT

Chronic DVT (defined as symptom duration 4 weeks or greater) presents several challenges to catheter-directed therapy. First, guidewire passage through chronically occluded segments is often not successful due to the hard consistency of intraluminal material, the development of fibrotic web-like intraluminal septa and the smaller lumen caliber. Second, effective thrombolytic therapy is often impeded by the absence of forward flow to aid lysis, as well as by the chemical resistance of organized thrombus to lytic agents. Most importantly, irreversible valvular damage has already ensued in these patients. This may limit the clinical benefit derived even if successful clot lysis or mechanical endovascular recanalization is achieved.

Two important differences between iliofemoral and femoropopliteal venous thrombosis have a major impact upon the management of chronic venous thrombosis. First, the frequency of causative iliac vein stenoses appears to be greater than that of femoral vein stenoses. Furthermore, iliac vein stenoses are more amenable to successful endovascular treatment which might prevent future thrombotic episodes. Second, after an episode of femoropopliteal venous thrombosis, major axial veins recanalize spontaneously within a few months. CVI in these patients is due to venous hypertension caused by completed valvular damage and venous scarring, which endovascular techniques cannot reverse, as compared with the persistent chronic venous obstruction seen after an episode of iliofemoral venous thrombosis. Therefore, thrombolytic therapy more than 4–6 weeks after onset of symptoms offers little benefit with regard to ultimate clinical outcome in patients with femoropopliteal thrombosis. The exception may be those patients in whom symptom exacerbation is caused by superimposed acute thrombus upon a background of chronic DVT; in this situation a trial of thrombolytic therapy is certainly warranted.

For isolated chronic iliac vein occlusion, thrombolysis may have something to offer, not by salvaging valvular function but by facilitating removal of persistent chronic iliofemoral venous obstruction using other endovascular techniques. In these cases, thrombolytic agents are used not with the expectation of causing a significant reduction in clot burden, but as a method of softening the intraluminal material to facilitate balloon venoplasty and endovascular stenting (which crush and trap thrombus against the vein walls).[34] These techniques may also be used to treat underlying stenoses that are unmasked by antecedent thrombolytic therapy. In this manner, reduction of ambulatory venous pressure may be achieved, with subsequent prevention of ongoing valvular damage and episodes of rethrombosis. Reported experience with this approach is variable; we have found this method to offer significant clinical benefit in more than half of patients undergoing therapy, although nearly all patients continue to experience some degree of CVI. We do not generally advocate catheter-directed therapy in patients with extensive chronic thrombus extending from the calf veins to involve the entire popliteal, femoral and iliac veins. In this situation, extremely poor venous inflow to the iliac veins limits success of endovascular techniques. In the subset of patients with refractory, disabling symptoms, we have occasionally resorted to aggressive stent-based venous reconstruction to restore patency of the iliofemoral venous system, and have observed incremental mid-term improvements in quality of life in some of these patients. Because this approach is ultimately limited by poor venous inflow, these patients are counseled not to necessarily expect long-term primary patency, but understand that frequent clinical and sonographic follow-up will guide repeated assisted interventions (balloon venoplasty and re-stenting) to achieve long-term symptom palliation.

Complications of Endovascular Therapy

While various minor complications of thrombolytic therapy have been described (puncture site hematoma, contrast-related renal failure, mild allergic reactions), incidence of major complications has been extremely low. Pooled data of two major studies[25,26] using combined endovascular therapy for DVT indicate that major bleeding complications (defined as intracranial bleeding, GI bleeding or other transfusion-requiring bleeding event) occur in approximately 4% of patients. There have been no instances of intracranial hemorrhage or bleeding-related deaths. Half of these complications occurred during the initial experience with these methods and would now be considered preventable. Two patients had undergone recent arterial bypass surgery within 2 days of thrombolytic agent administration and one patient had brachial artery puncture for blood gas determination during TPA administration. Only one patient (less than 1%) has been suspected of having a pulmonary embolism during catheter-directed therapy. A few instances of balloon-stent slippage and dislodgement have been described, but successful deployment was achieved without clinical sequelae. These occurrences will likely be less frequent with the common use of self-expandable Wallstents. Hence, if careful patient selection criteria are adhered to and close monitoring of fibrinogen and partial thromboplastin time (PTT) parameters instituted, thrombolytic therapy is extremely well-tolerated and safe.

Conclusion

Deep venous thrombosis should be regarded as a treatable cause of chronic severe venous insufficiency, particularly within the first month of symptom onset. While anticoagulation therapy is sufficient for pulmonary embolism prophylaxis, it does not adequately address the problem of postphlebitic syndrome. Catheter-directed thrombolysis has demonstrated superior success rates in lysing acute venous thrombi when compared to systemic thrombolysis and anticoagulation alone. This emerging technique promises rapid symptom resolution in patients with even extensive iliofemoral thrombi and phlegmasia cerulea dolens at lower doses and duration of therapy. Thrombolytic agents are also useful as an adjunct to venoplasty and endovascular stenting for chronic iliofemoral venous occlusion. The ability to rapidly restore normal venous pressure by directly addressing causative venous stenoses should diminish the incidence of valvular insufficiency and recurrent episodes of DVT. Complications of thrombolytic therapy have been extremely infrequent and largely preventable, with no episodes of intracranial hemorrhage or major pulmonary embolism during therapy. Although these endovascular techniques appear very promising, results of prospective con-

trolled trials must demonstrate that the postphlebitic syndrome is prevented by early institution of regional thrombolytic therapy before it is generally accepted as the treatment of choice for most patients with acute iliofemoral DVT and for select patients with acute femoropopliteal DVT. In this manner, widespread use of combined endovascular therapy may ultimately impact upon the clinical and socioeconomic consequences of chronic severe venous insufficiency.

References

1. Goldhaber SZ. Venous thrombosis: prevention, treatment, and relationship to paradoxical embolism. Cardiol Clin 1994; 12:505–16
2. Barritt DW, Jordan SC. Anticoagulant drugs in the treatment of pulmonary embolism: a controlled clinical trial. Lancet 1960; 1:1309–12
3. Strandness DE, Langlois Y, Cramer M et al. Long-term sequelae of acute venous thrombosis. JAMA 1983; 250:1289–92
4. O'Donnell TF, Browse NL, Burnand KG et al. The socioeconomic effects of an iliofemoral venous thrombosis. J Surg Res 1977; 22:483–8
5. Van Ramshorst B, Van Bemmelen PS, Hoeneveld H, et al. Thrombus regression in deep venous thrombosis: quantification of spontaneous thrombolysis with duplex scanning. Circulation 1992; 86:414–19
6. Markel A, Manzo RA, Bergelin RO et al. Valvular reflux after deep vein thrombosis: incidence and time of occurrence. J Vasc Surg 1992; 15:377–84
7. Caps MT, Manzo RA, Bergelin RO et al. Venous valvular reflux in veins not involved at the time of acute deep vein thrombosis. J Vasc Surg 1995; 22:524–31
8. Meissner MH, Manzo RA, Bergelin RO et al. Deep venous insufficiency: the relationship between lysis and subsequent reflux. J Vasc Surg 1993; 18:596–608
9. Meissner MH, Caps MT, Bergelin RO et al. Propagation, rethrombosis, and new thrombus formation after acute deep venous thrombosis. J Vasc Surg 1995; 22:558–67
10. Sherry S. Thrombolytic therapy for deep vein thrombosis. Semin Intervent Radiol 1985; 4:331–7
11. Comerota AJ, Aldridge SC. Thrombolytic therapy for deep venous thrombosis: a clinical review. Can J Surg 1993; 36:359–64
12. Killewich LA, Bedford GR, Beach KW et al. Spontaneous lysis of deep venous thrombi: rate and outcome. J Vasc Surg 1989; 9:89–97
13. Comerota AJ, Cohen GS. Thrombolytic therapy in peripheral arterial occlusive disease: mechanisms of action and drugs available. Can J Surg 1993; 36:342–8
14. Graor RA, Young JR, Risius B et al. Comparison of cost-effectiveness of streptokinase and urokinase in the treatment of deep vein thrombosis. Ann Vasc Surg 1987; 1:524–8
15. Goldhaber SZ, Meyerovitz MF, Green D et al. Randomized controlled trial of tissue plasminogen activator in proximal deep vein thrombosis. Am J Med 1990; 88:235–40
16. Goldhaber SZ, Buring JE, Lipnick RJ et al. Pooled analyses of randomized trials of streptokinase and heparin in phlebographically documented acute deep vein thrombosis. Am J Med 1984; 76:393–7
17. Comerota AJ, Aldridge S. Thrombolytic therapy for acute deep vein thrombosis. Semin Vasc Surg 1992; 5:76–81
18. Theiss W, Wirtzfeld A, Fink U et al. The success rate of fibrinolytic therapy in fresh and old thrombosis of the iliac and femoral veins. Angiology 1983; 34:61–9

19. Hill SL, Mortin D, Evans P. Massive venous thrombosis of the extremities. Am J Surg 1989; 158:131–5

20. Arnesen H, Hoiseth A, Ly B. Streptokinase or heparin in the treatment of deep vein thrombosis. Acta Med Scand 1982; 211:65–8

21. O'Meara JJ, McNutt RA, Evans AT et al. A decision analysis of streptokinase plus heparin as compared with heparin alone for deep-vein thrombosis. N Engl J Med 1994; 330:1864–9

22. Becker GJ, Rabe FE, Richmond BD et al. Low-dose fibrinolytic therapy: results and new concepts. Radiology 1983; 148:663–70

23. Okrent D, Messersmith R, Buckman J. Transcatheter fibrinolytic therapy and angioplasty for left iliofemoral venous thrombosis. J Vasc Intervent Radiol 1991; 2:195–200

24. Molina JE, Hunter DW, Yedlicka JW. Thrombolytic therapy for iliofemoral venouos thrombosis. Vasc Surg 1992; 26:630–7

25. Semba CP, Dake MD. Iliofemoral deep venous thrombosis: aggressive therapy with catheter-directed thrombolysis. Radiology 1994; 191:487–94

26. Bjarnason H, Kruse JR, Asinger DA et al. Iliofemoral deep venous thrombosis: safety and efficacy outcome during 5 years of catheter-directed thrombolytic therapy. J Vasc Intervent Radiol 1997; 8:405–18

27. Cragg AH. Lower extremity deep venous thrombolysis: a new approach to obtaining access. J Vasc Intervent Radiol 1996; 7:283–8

28. Cope C, Baum RA, Duszak RA. Temporary use of a bird's nest filter during iliocaval thrombolysis. Radiology 1996; 198:765–7

29. Ferris EJ, Lim WN, Smith PL et al. May–Thurner syndrome. Radiology 1983; 147:29–31

30. Masuda EM, Kistner RL. Long-term results of venous valve reconstruction: a four- to twenty-one-year follow-up. J Vasc Surg 1994; 19:391–403

31. Weaver FA, Meacham PW, Adkins RB et al. Phlegmasia cerulea dolens: therapeutic considerations. South Med J 1988; 81:306–12

32. Robinson DL, Teitelbaum GP. Phlegmasia cerulea dolens: treatment by pulse-spray and infusion thrombolysis. Am J Radiol 1993; 160:1288–90

33. Nazarian GK, Bjarnason H, Dietz CA et al. Iliofemoral venous stenoses: effectiveness of treatment with metallic endovascular stents. Radiology 1996; 200:193–9

34. Marache P, Asseman P, Jabinet JL et al. Percutaneous transluminal venous angioplasty in occlusive iliac vein thrombus resistant to thrombolysis. Am Heart J 1993; 125:362–6

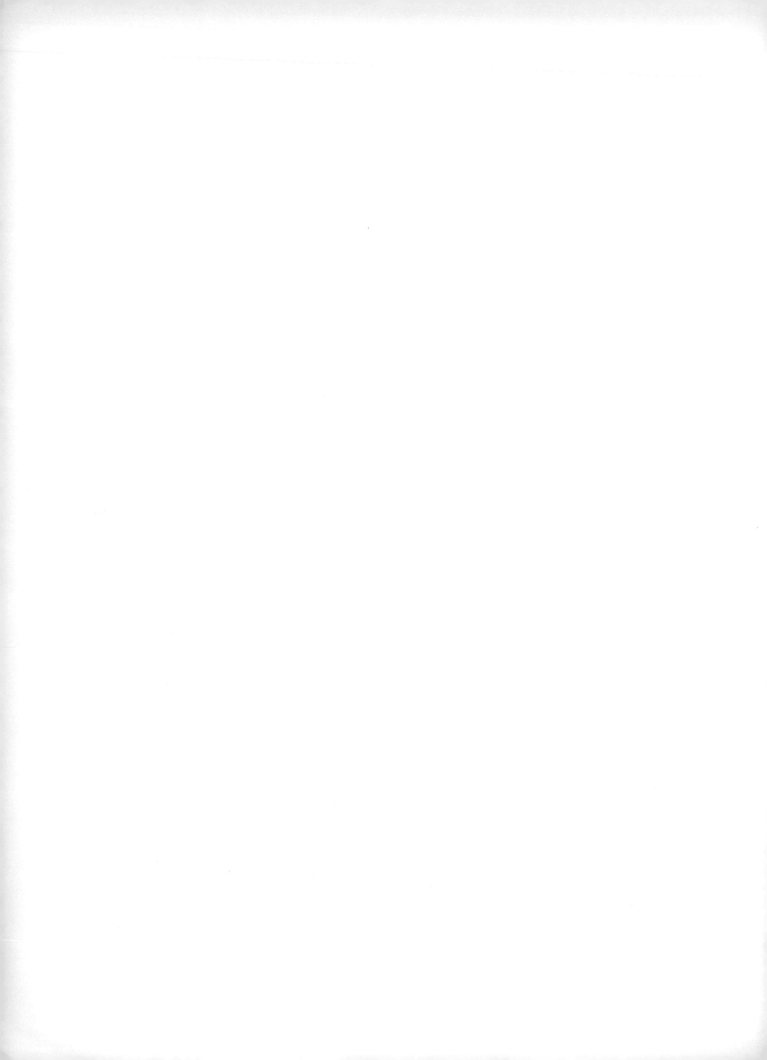

Endovascular Therapy for Chronic Venous Obstruction

17

Patricia E. Thorpe

Introduction

Severe chronic venous insufficiency (CVI) is characterized by reflux through the superficial venous system as well as the deep venous system. These phenomena are found in concert with perforating vein outflow. A sizable fraction of patients with chronic venous insufficiency has experienced deep venous thrombosis and some carry persistent venous occlusions. Reports from the Subfascial Perforating Vein Registry have emphasized the importance of such venous obstruction in failures of perforator vein surgery. Surgical approaches to correcting the pathophysiology of venous obstruction have been disappointing. Therefore, exploration of endovascular therapy for chronic venous obstruction has certain appeal.

For the most part, chronic venous obstruction begins with acute thrombosis. Acute deep venous thrombosis, diagnosed and treated with anticoagulation within 7 to 10 days, is less likely to result in the severe post-thrombotic sequelae than untreated thrombosis.[1] Patients with thrombus propagating into the popliteal vein and above are thought to have a 35% chance of developing mild post-thrombotic syndrome and a 40% chance of severe post-thrombotic syndrome within 6 years.[2] This and other studies indicates that between 45 and 80% of patients will develop post-thrombotic venous insufficiency after an episode of deep venous thrombosis.[3,4] Many will have mild edema and/or discomfort that can be treated only with compression. An additional 25–35% will be asymptomatic, which leaves a significant number of patients with severe chronic venous insufficiency. These patients may be disabled by persistent edema and an ever-present sensation of heaviness and/or aching that accompanies severe limitation of venous outflow. Some of these patients are unable to work or participate in normal everyday activities despite leg elevation and compression supports.

In seeing patients with acute thrombosis, a treatment dilemma arises from an inability to differentiate those who will do well with anticoagulation alone from those who will do poorly. It is the latter who will develop the post-thrombotic syndrome. If a true correlation between extent of thrombus and sequelae were true, it would be easy to predict which patients would fail to improve with standard therapy: heparin, leg elevation, and warfarin. However, this is not true. We lack the ability to identify patients who will recanalize thrombus and develop adequate collaterals. Those who remain symptomatic or will have recurrent thrombosis cannot be identified during the acute event.[5] Also, the ability to lyse thrombus autogenously varies among individuals. Two patients with the same extent of thrombosis may respond differently to heparin and bedrest.

Most immediate symptoms of venous thrombosis abate within 7 to 10 days. Therefore, physicians generally take a conservative approach to treatment of the acute event. This is usually adequate for nonocclusive, short-segment thrombosis. Combined iliac and superficial femoral vein thrombosis, in contrast, can overwhelm the body's fibrinolytic capacity. Recanalization may be inadequate to relieve outflow obstruction.[6,7] In addition, it is uncommon for extensive proximal axial vein occlusion to occur without thrombosis of distal tibial and popliteal veins.[8,9] Such extensive thrombosis, with organization of thrombus, limited development of collaterals, and associated valvular damage all contribute to the pathophysiology of severe post-thrombotic syndrome.

After the acute event, the pathologic processes described above appear to be progressive. Although some patients with extensive thrombosis improve over time, others do not. In their study of 130 legs in 67 patients, Browse et al. found a trend toward a higher incidence of post-thrombotic syndrome in limbs with axial vein thrombosis.[9] However, 42% of limbs with calf, femoral, and iliac thrombosis were without symptoms at $6\frac{1}{2}$ years. Even more confusing was Taylor's study of patients with calf vein thrombosis. At 7–10 years, hemodynamic evidence of venous insufficiency was present in nearly 80% of patients, many of whom were asymptomatic.[4]

These data demonstrate the complexity of chronic post-obstruction physiology. Hemodynamic tests may identify reflux but fail to uncover obstruction. Ultimately, what matters most to the patient with severe symptoms of venous hypertension is what therapy will alleviate the pain and edema and stop the progressive skin changes. Endovenous therapy, including flow- and catheter-directed thrombolysis, balloon dilatation, and stent placement should be considered for such patients. This therapy is designed to decrease obstruction and increase venous flow. How this can be accomplished with minimally invasive endovascular techniques, using digital imaging and duplex sonography, is the subject of this chapter.

Why Thrombolytic Therapy?

Use of a fibrinolytic agent to treat deep venous thrombosis was first reported in 1962.[10–12] Early clinical experience subsequently demonstrated an advantage of thrombolysis with heparin therapy.[13–16] However, prolonged systemic infusions of high thrombolytic doses led to concern for patient safety[17–20] which delayed acknowledgement of thrombolytic therapy as a practical treatment for DVT. Also, systemic therapy proved to have limited success in treatment of lower extremity DVT, because collateral pathways became preferred routes of venous flow and relatively little thrombolytic agent reached the obstructing thrombus.[21–25] Finally, signs and symptoms of DVT normally resolve upon development of collateral pathways and autogenous recanalization. These three facts diminished the impetus for using thrombolysis in treatment of DVT.

Experience in treating arterial obstructions revealed that lysis of thrombus was optimally achieved by using local delivery instead of systemic infusion.[26–28] This lesson was applied to venous occlusion. Bleeding complications using coaxial systems and multi-sidehole catheters in venous thrombolysis decreased complications encountered with systemic infusion.[29] Catheter-directed delivery of a thrombolytic agent was shown to lyse thrombi in subclavian and axillary veins.[30–32] Ultimately, the technique was effectively used to treat iliofemoral thrombosis as well.[33–37]

DVT in the lower extremity is frequently multi-segmental, affecting lengths of the superficial femoral, popliteal, or tibial veins. Worse yet, acute thrombus is often superimposed on chronic thrombus or synechiae from prior recanalization. Patients with recurrent DVT often have such residual obstruction in axial and distal veins. Catheter access to these area may be difficult or even impossible. Nevertheless, lysis of thrombus may be important to improve total venous flow.

Patient Selection

Essentially, there are two types of patients that can be considered candidates for endovascular treatment. The first is the patient with an acute episode of venous thrombosis who is progressing poorly on standard treatment with heparin. Such patients will have massive edema of the extremity, often with cyanosis and bursting pain. The second type of patient will be one with severe chronic venous insufficiency, unrelieved by standard surgical interventions, including ablation of superficial reflux and correction of perforating vein outflow. Experience has taught that, regardless of the age of the thrombus or the number of episodes of prior DVT, subjective and even objective improvement can be achieved and sustained with endovascular therapy. However, long-term success is dependent on the patient remaining anticoagulated. Therefore, an important factor to be considered in patient selection is ability of the patient to follow instructions with long-term anticoagulation. In such patients with intolerance to warfarin, Miradon (anisindione) can be used.

Contraindications for thrombolytic therapy are listed in Table 17.1. As indicated, renal failure is a relative contraindication to endovenous recanalization of chronic venous thrombosis. This is true because of the need for iodinated contrast media. Chronic venous occlusions require manipulation of catheters and guide wires. This requires fluoroscopic visualization of vessels and infusions of iodinated contrast media. This is not true of acute DVT where catheter placement and monitoring can be done with ultrasound. Unfortunately, carbon dioxide, which is useful in arterial occlusive disease, is not suitable for the slow flow imaging required for venous treatments.

Table 17.2 displays the characteristics of patients selected for lytic therapy. This shows that severe edema and lower extremity pain dominated the symptoms and that two-thirds of the patients were treated for chronic obstructive manifestations. The expected dominance of the left lower extremity over

the right was seen and the prevalence of multisegment distal obstructive disease was demonstrated. While there are contraindications to lytic therapy, we have performed prolonged infusions of lytic agents in patients within 14 days of major surgery without complications. Such infusions must be done carefully, but our experience includes patients 14 days after gastric bypass, 10 days after abdominal hysterectomy, and 5 days after total knee arthroplasty. One patient was treated 14 days after vaginal delivery, and incidental note is made of several women treated during their regular menstrual period, none of whom had increased bleeding.

Techniques for Thrombolytic Infusion

Philosophically, in treating patients with endovascular therapy for thrombotic occlusion, especially

Table 17.1. Selection criteria for thrombolytic therapy

Exclusion criteria
Contraindication to long-term anticoagulation
Unexplained contraindication to radiographic contrast; creatine > 2.5
Thrombocytopenia < 50,000
Diabetic retinopathy
Blunt head trauma < 90 days
Cerebrovascular accident < 6 months
Other known intracranial pathology
Active gastrointestinal bleeding
Eye surgery < 3 months (except cataract)
Major trauma < 2 weeks
Abdominal or cardiac surgery < 2 weeks
Severe hypertension (systolic pressure > 180 mmHg)
Relative exclusions
Pericarditis
Pregnancy
Systemic corticosteroid therapy
Poor prognosis (< 2 weeks expected survival)

Table 17.2. Patients selected for lytic therapy

		Number of limbs
Initial signs and symptoms	Lower extremity edema	91 (98%)
	Lower extremity pain	78 (84%)
	Phlegmasia	7 (8%)
	Non-healing ulcers	7 (8%)
Type of symptoms	Acute	30 (32%)
	Chronic	63 (68%)
Location of thrombus	Left lower extremity	63 (68%)
	Right lower extremity	30 (32%)
	IVC	9 (10%)
	Iliac	61 (66%)
	Femoral	91 (98%)
	Popliteal	78 (84%)
	Tibial	61 (66%)
Risk factors	Malignancy	13 (14%)
	May – Thurner Syndrome	29 (31%)
	Recurrent DVT	26 (28%)
	Oral contraceptives	3 (3%)
	Travel	5 (5%)
	Trauma	11 (12%)
	Post-op	19 (20%)
	Post partum	6 (6%)
	Hypercoagulability	12 (14%)
Duration of symptoms	Acute < 30 days	26 (28%)
	> 30 days	4 (4%)
	Chronic < 30 days	8 (9%)
	< 90 days	11 (12%)
	> 90 days	43 (47%)

those with a chronically occluded lower extremity, the leg is considered an "organ system." Specific sections cannot be treated in isolation from the rest of the system. For example, venous flow in the femoral segment depends on flow entering from the popliteal and infrapopliteal segments. If there is subacute and chronic DVT in the calf and thigh, treating the superficial femoral vein without addressing the occlusive thrombus in segments below will not produce an effective restoration of deep venous flow. If flow in the calf preferentially goes to the saphenous veins, the pattern will persist even when the superficial femoral vein is reopened. If there is too little infrapopliteal deep venous flow, the reopened superficial femoral vein will not be the preferred path of least resistance.

Clinical improvement can be limited by failure to treat hemodynamically significant tibial and popliteal obstructions. The interaction of all venous segments must be kept in mind in order to achieve optimal results in lytic therapy. Ultimately, a combination of catheter-directed and flow-directed therapy will be effective in treating multisegmental thrombosis. In calf veins tourniquets are required to direct urokinase into the path of most resistance – the thrombus, while catheters deliver local urokinase into the thrombosed axial veins. Thrombolytic infusions may be combined with balloon dilatation and stent placement. All of these techniques comprise the main components of endovenous therapy.

Catheter-Directed Therapy

Venous access for catheter placement to treat chronic iliofemoral and proximal superficial femoral thrombosis can be achieved through the contralateral femoral vein, the ipsilateral femoral vein, or through popliteal veins. The right internal jugular approach can be used but it is difficult to manipulate catheter tips from such a distance. The jugular approach works better for acute thrombosis.

Following placement of a vascular sheath, a multi-sidehole catheter is directed over a guide wire and positioned in the thrombosed vein. If initial guide wire traversal of the thrombosed segment is difficult, a 5F endhole catheter is positioned into the thrombus as far as possible for initial infusion of lytic therapy. When subsequent attempts to pass the guide wire are successful, the multi-sidehole catheter can be advanced and strategically posi-

tioned throughout the thrombosed segment. A variety of 4F and 5F multi-sidehole catheters can be used, including those with a predetermined infusion length (i.e., 10, 20, 30, 40, 50 cm), an adjustable infusion length, or a combination catheter-wire system. The length of the infusion catheter is selected according to the ability to position the catheter across the thrombosed area. A long, continuous segment of thrombus is treated with a single catheter when possible.

Extensive thrombus often requires serial advancement and repositioning of the catheter at the time of interval follow-up. An adjustable-length catheter can avoid need for multiple catheter exchanges if it is not possible to traverse the entire occlusion at the initial setting. A catheter may be safely advanced over a wire in both a retrograde or antegrade direction. Although it is easier to advance through venous valves from a distal approach, the popliteal vein may be obliterated or occluded. Using a more superficial vein to enter the deep system is an effective alternative.[38] Hydrophilic wires such as the Roadrunner™ wire (Cook, Inc., Bloomington, IN) and the angled Glide™ wire (Medi-Tech, Boston Scientific, Waterstown, MA) are suggested for passing venous valves in either direction. A 4F or 5F straight or 45° degree angle catheter can then be used in combination with these wires. Due to the resistance of organized thrombus and the tortuosity of the fenestrations, the wire will frequently advance much more easily than the catheter. A super stiff Amplatz exchange wire (Medi-Tech) is used alternatively with the hydrophilic probing wires to advance catheters. A coaxial system consisting of a 5F multi-sidehole Mewissen catheter (Cook, Inc.) in combination with a 0.035-in (0.889 mm) Katzen wire (Medi-Tech) can be useful. This system permits a split infusion at separate sites within the same venous system to achieve the most effective intrathrombus delivery of lytic agent. The slit-sidehole catheter (AngioDynamics, Inc., Queensbury, NY) has multiple infusion lengths and operates with an end-occluding wire. It works well with the automatic Pulse Spray™ pump which has been found to be very effective in both acute and chronic occlusions.

The coaxial Mewissen–Katzen system requires two infusion pumps with a divided dose of urokinase while the heparin infusion is piggybacked into the catheter. Urokinase (Abbokinase, Abbott Laboratories, Abbott Park, IL) is reconstituted by using 1,000,000 IU in 500 ml of 0.9% NaCl and is delivered in an infusion dose of 2000 IU cm^{-3} for 150,000–200,000 IU h^{-1}. Adjustments in concentration and volume can be made for patients with cardiac disease. When a flow-directed infusion from a pedal access site is required, the total dose can be divided between the two sites. The amount of infusion is determined by the initial flow rate seen fluoroscopically as well as the amount and distribution of thrombus. Laboratory monitoring every 4–6 h (using mini-samples of less than 2.5 ml) is done for determination of fibrinogen, partial thromboplastin time (PTT), hemoglobin, and platelet count. The fibrinogen level is maintained at greater than 25% of baseline, which is usually over 100 mg dl^{-1}. The PTT is maintained between 50 and 80 seconds.

Flow-Directed Therapy

A 22-gauge intercath is placed in a dorsal pedal vein for the purpose of performing initial or baseline venogram. It is also used for the flow-directed infusion. A single puncture in a pedal vein below the ankle is desirable. Since multiple punctures cannot be avoided in some patients, it is best to work from a distal-to-proximal direction. This avoids infusing urokinase into failed puncture sites. If the edema is tremendous, the foot and ankle are elevated above the heart and an Ace wrap is used to reduce swelling. Sitting the patient upright helps distend dependent pedal veins. Placing the dependent foot in a bucket of warm water can also make pedal veins visible. Use of 1% lidocaine without epinephrine can help patients tolerate the pedal cannulation. A direct cut-down is never indicated. A small, clear, plastic dressing is placed over the 22-gauge catheter to maintain visualization of the site throughout the procedure. It is important to loop the IV tubing to prevent inadvertent loss of the site. Infection and/or bleeding are not problems but care is taken to detect any extravasation of contrast during each injection.

A short, clear, plastic connecting tube with a three-way stopcock is used to facilitate interval injection of contrast in follow-up evaluation of progress of lytic therapy. A saline infusion is maintained through the pedal site if urokinase is not being infused. A velcro-type Tiger™ tourniquet (Cook, Inc. Bloomington, Indiana) is placed at the malleolar

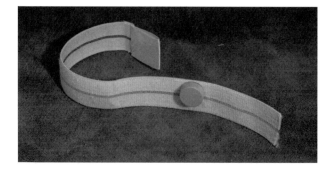

Fig. 17.1. Diagram of tourniquet position demonstrates redirection of venous flow from greater saphenous to the deep system via a perforator.

level (Fig. 17.1). A foam disk is positioned to provide focal compression of the saphenous vein against the medial malleolus (Fig. 17.2). Under fluoroscopic visualization, a small amount of contrast is injected to insure compression the saphenous vein and redirection of flow into the deep system (Fig. 17.3). The disk position as well as the upper and lower margins of the tourniquet are marked on the skin. This allows placement in the correct position after release of the tourniquet once every hour. A folded 4 × 4 gauze pad is placed under the disk to protect the skin from pressure. The pedal pulse is marked and monitored along with blood pressure. The tourniquet should provide adequate redirection of venous flow without any compromise of arterial flow. It is released for 10 min every hour and reapplied at the designated location to assure proper disk position and tightness.

Normally, blood flows preferentially from the superficial to the deep system. However, in the presence of proximal DVT, one may see contrast reflux through the perforating veins into the superficial system in the mid-calf or above. When this is recognized fluoroscopically, a second tourniquet is placed at the knee to compress the greater saphenous vein against the femoral condyle to promote flow into the tibiopopliteal veins.

Adjunctive Procedures

After 48–72 hrs of thrombolytic therapy, additional intervention may be performed to treat residual venous stenosis. Persistently narrowed venous channels should be dilated but rarely is the result hemodynamically optimal. Improvement does occur, and

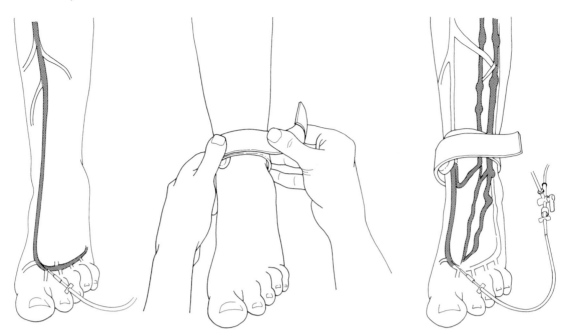

Fig. 17.2. The tourniquets used in venous procedures are wide-band elastic with long segments of Velcro suited for treating various ankle sizes. The movable disk can be positioned with fluoroscopy to effectively compress the saphenous vein and thereby redirect flow into the deep calf veins.

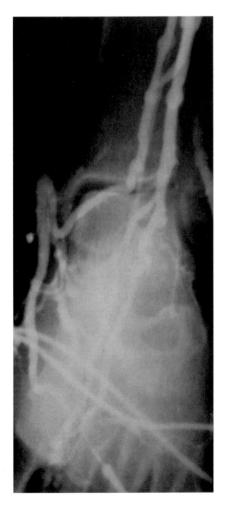

greater widening of the chronically occluded ileofemoral lumen, after overnight use of the Pulse Spray technique during lysis, as opposed to drip infusion, has been empirically noted. Significant residual luminal irregularity and per-sistent narrowing of the iliofemoral segments can be treated with one or more self-expanding metallic stents in order to augment flow. Pull-back pressures are always obtained before and after stent placement. In the supine position, greater than a 4 mmHg pressure gradient between the inferior vena cava and the external iliac vein is considered hemodynamically significant. Also the presence of transpelvic or pre-sacral collaterals seen on contrast infusion confirms outflow resistance. This is most likely greater in an upright position. The self-expanding metallic stents may be placed from the ipsilateral or contralateral approach after balloon dilatation. Duplex imaging is used to confirm stent patency at 24 h and to assess flow velocities at intervals of 1, 3, 6, and 12 months, and yearly thereafter.

Fig. 17.3. Radiograph (with ankle tourniquet in place) showing contrast being redirected via a perforator into the tibial veins.

Anticoagulation

Patients are systemically heparinized (PTT > 50 and < 80 s) throughout the period of thrombolysis and following angioplasty or stent procedures. Oral anticoagulation is tapered before therapy (2 days off Coumadin before admission) and restarted 1 day prior to stent placement. This allows removal of the sheath before the international normalized ratio (INR) is therapeutic. Upon completion of thrombolysis, heparinization is continued until oral anticoagulation is consistent (PT > 20 s, INR of 2.5 to 3.0). Oral anticoagulation is monitored cooperatively with the referring physician. Inadequate anticoagulation is the most frequent cause of early failure.

Younger patients with chronic conditions may have a hypercoagulable state, making warfarin titration challenging. We must emphasize the great importance of diligent monitoring of the PT and the INR. While a minimum of 6–12 months of warfarin is standard in acute DVT, patients with chronic disease and/or multiple stents are placed on indefinite anticoagulation. Compression stockings or leggings are prescribed and fitted for all patients before discharge. Patients are followed with clinic visits, duplex examinations, photoplethysmography, and air plethysmography as indicated above.

Measures of Success

Results of endovascular procedures are evaluated in terms of immediate and long-term technical success and clinical improvement. Technical success is defined as the ability to improve venous flow as measured by venographic clearance of contrast through the visualized deep venous system. It may be assessed by improved flow on duplex. In chronic thrombosis, quite often there is no pretreatment flow visualized in the femoral or iliac systems either by ultrasound or fluoroscopy. Restoration of any flow can represent relative improvement in a leg characterized by extreme stasis. Flow in any one segment is related to the overall flow pattern in the entire extremity. The physiology of increased flow volume cannot be separated from reflux.

Restoration of flow may uncover unsuspected reflux. As endovascular methods decrease venous obstruction, technical success can be inferred from normalization of flow patterns and increased rate of contrast clearance in addition to the improved phlebographic appearance of the veins after therapy.

In acute thrombosis, lytic results are generally classified as: (1) complete lysis when the occluded vein is reopened along its entire length with less than 10% residual thrombus; (2) partial lysis if significant change occurs in the venogram with increased outflow but incomplete removal of residual mural thrombus; and (3) minimal lysis if no change occurs in the venogram or rate of contrast clearance.

The standard determination of complete versus partial lysis, applicable in patients with acute thrombosis, is not applicable to chronic occlusions. Phlebographic improvement in chronic cases is measured by: (1) decrease in resistance when injecting contrast into the deep system from the pedal site; (2) decrease in stasis of contrast and more rapid clearance of contrast through the calf and thigh; (3) greater visualization of deep veins, particularly in the calf; and (4) continuity of flow between segments. These improvements are not totally captured on still films. Rather it is the real-time flow pattern through the entire limb that confirms the impression of greater flow capacity due to retrieval of deep veins that were not functioning before lytic therapy. This value of videophlebography has been recognized in the literature by Bjorgell.[39]

As flow in main venous channels improves, collaterals decrease and it is possible to advance wires and catheters in thrombosed femoral and iliac veins. Forward progress (catheter advancement) may be slow in cases of very chronic occlusion. It is important to continue urokinase, infusing the apparently occluded veins. Eventually, a wire can be advanced through a retrieved lumen. Once the probing wire and catheter reach the inferior vena cava, an Amplatz stiff exchange wire can be positioned to secure the access. Balloon dilatation and stent placement are then performed to reestablish antegrade flow in the axial veins.

Duplex imaging will provide some indication of flow improvement but not rate of contrast clearance. However, measurement of flow velocity in the femoral and iliac stent is an important predictor of success. Velocities less than 10–15 cm s^{-1} usually indicate too little inflow from the distal veins.

Stents with velocities more than 15 cm s^{-1} have a greater likelihood of long-term patency. As with arterial stents, abnormally high velocities may indicate stenosis from intimal hyperplasia. This is uncommon and not possible to predict. In our experience, it occurs in less than 20% of patients. Recognition and re-treatment with balloon dilatation or double stenting have been effective in correcting restenosis.

Results

Between 1988 and 1998, among the DVT patients treated at Creighton University, Omaha, NE with thrombolytic therapy, 84 had clinical and/or phlebographic evidence of post-thrombotic chronic venous insufficiency. A total of 28 patients (30 limbs) with chronic asymptomatic venous changes on phlebography had an acute clinical presentation without prior history of DVT. In contrast, 56 patients (63 limbs) presented with one or more documented episodes of DVT. All patients had multisegmental involvement. The location of the predominant thrombus included superficial femoral (98%) and popliteal (84%) venous segments. Thrombus was also found in tibial and iliac regions (66%) in over half of the patients.

The series included a spectrum of ages (12–83, mean 47.5 years) and were evenly divided among male (42) and female (42). The mean length of hospital stay was 7.4 days (range 2–27). The mean urokinase dose per treated extremity was 8.7 million units (range 2.2–11). Nine patients had bilateral lower extremity and inferior vena cava involvement. Two of these had already undergone below-knee amputation for severe venous stasis disease. Seven patients presented with nonhealing ulcers.

Demographic data and interventional results are listed in Tables 17.2 and 17.3. The majority of patients present with edema (98%) (Table 17.4). Fewer had advanced skin changes (39%). Minor skin changes were seen in 22%. Seven patients had ulcerated limbs (2 healed, 5 unhealed). Among patients in classes 5 and 6, only lytic therapy was used in three patients and a combination of lysis/ stent was used in four. All ulcers healed with a median healing time of 48 days. In three patients, the ulcer reopened due to noncompliance with compression. Further examination for contributing incompetent perforators revealed several present in each affected limb.

Arm/leg pressure differential pressures were obtained in some patients. The data are misleading

Table 17.3. Immediate late outcome in treated limbs

		Number of limbs
Thrombolysis		
Complete		18 (18%)
	No further intervention	14 (78%)
	Angioplasty, sent placement	4 (2%)
Partial		74 (80%)
	No further intervention	22 (30%)
	Angioplasty	7 (10%)
	Angioplasty, stent placement	45 (60%)
None		1 (1%)
	No further intervention	1 (1%)
	Angioplasty, stent placement	0 (0%)
Technical failure		
Unable to pass guidewire		
	Femoral	8 (9%)
	Iliac	1 (1%)
Clinical outcome		
	Can go without compression	30 (33%)
	Need compression for edema, no pain	47 (52%)
	Pain + edema still a factor but less	22 (24%)
	No improvement	1 (1%)

Table 17.4. Classification of treated limbs

Class 0:	Normal	0
Class 1:	Telangectasia	20 (22%)
Class 2:	Varicosities	6 (6%)
Class 3:	Edema	91 (98%)
Class 4:	Hyperpigmentation	34 (37%)
Class 5:	Healed ulcer	2 (2%)
Class 6:	Nonhealing ulcer	7 (8%)

when the patient is morbidly obese or when there is iliac occlusion with extensive collateralization.

Air plethysmography (APG) data were obtained before and after endovascular intervention. Presence of large collateral veins obscure the findings of common iliac obstruction.

Duplex imaging could document dramatic post-treatment changes in flow and velocity in the iliac and femoral segments. Patients with no demonstrable flow in the common femoral segment had as much as 20–40 cm s^{-1} flow after endovascular therapy.

Self-expanding metallic stents were placed in 49 patients (53%). The Wallstent™ (Schneider, USA, Plymouth, MN) was used in 98% of those stented. The most common iliac and femoral stents were 10 mm (70%) followed by 12 mm (20%), and in the distal femoral vein, 8 mm (9%). The average number of stents was 3.3 per patient with tandem interlocking deployment preceded and followed by balloon dilatation of target segments. Flow velocities were monitored in all of these.

Although the majority of the 93 limbs underwent successful treatment with a single procedure, reintervention was necessary 25 times in 18 patients to treat rethrombosis or previously unidentified inflow/outflow problems. Immediate success with thrombolysis was consistently achieved in patients with acute thrombus superimposed on chronic venous changes. Using both flow-directed and catheter-directed techniques, complete lysis of acute thrombus was accomplished in all of these patients. Residual chronic thrombus, which was commonly present, caused only 18% of patients to have total lysis. Partial lysis, therefore, was achieved in the majority of patients (80%), with only one patient experiencing no clinical improvement after onset of venous gangrene. Overall, in the 63 limbs with clinical presentation of recurrent DVT or chronic edema after the initial DVT episode, improvement was seen. However, in no instance did the phlebogram return to normal.

Phlebographic changes after urokinase are characterized by demonstration of numerous recanalized venous channels not seen on pretreatment studies. The rate of venous flow through the limb is increased in patients receiving iliofemoral and caval stents. Reintervention was required 15 times due to decreased flow in the stent (6), intimal hyperplasia (3), and untreated venous stenosis (6). Primary stent patency was 82% with long-term cumulative patency of 95% after reintervention.

Early rethrombosis (less than 30 days) occurred in nine limbs (10%) and late thrombotic occlusion (greater than 30 days) occurred 12 times. At least half of the thrombosis was due to inadequate oral anticoagulation.

Overall, the primary endovascular success rate was 77%. The secondary clinical success rate was 95% in surviving patients with a mean follow-up of 38.2 months (range 6 months to 10 years).

Complications included two deaths (less than 30 days). Both patients were systemically heparinized in addition to receiving urokinase. One 78-year-old male had a stroke 48 h after completion of lytic therapy. He had an occult history of cerebrovascular events. A 52-year-old female experienced retroperitoneal bleeding leading to multisystem organ failure despite aggressive resuscitation. The incidence of major and minor complications is listed in Table 17.5.

Subgroup Analysis

As indicated above, we have recognized three clinical patterns of chronic venous disease among patients presenting with symptomatic post-thrombotic

Table 17.5. Complications in endovenous procedures ($n = 118$)

Hematoma	12	(10%)
Transfusion	3	(2.5%)
Site infection	2	(1.6%)
CHF	3	(2.5%)
Compartment syndrome	2	(1.6%)
Transient femoral neuropathy	3	(2.5%)
Rethrombosis < 30 days	3	(2.5%)
Rethrombosis > 30 days	20	(17%)
↓ INR	16	(14%)
Intimal hyperplasia	4	(3.4%)
PE	0	(0%)
Death < 30 days	2	(1.6%)

CHF, congestive heart failure; PE; INR.

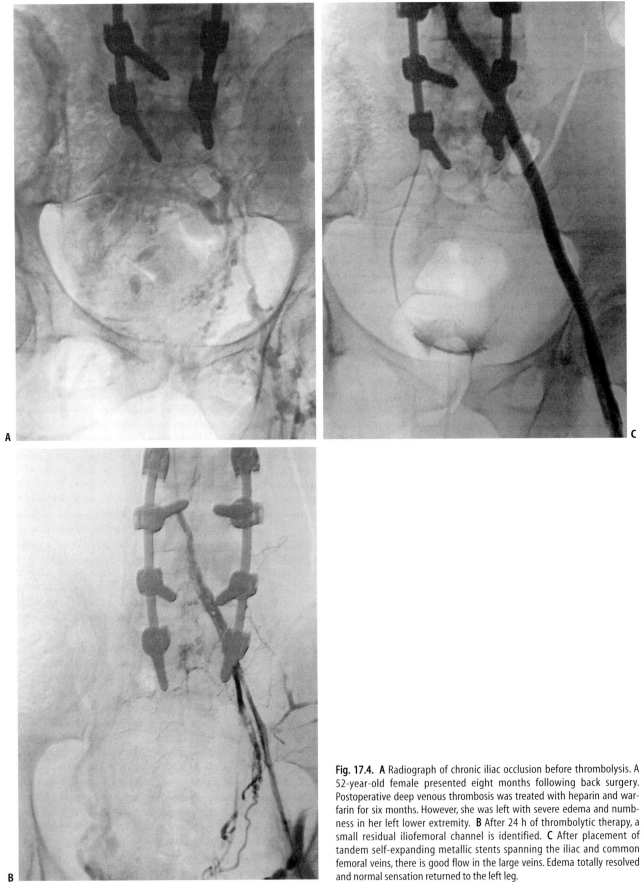

Fig. 17.4. A Radiograph of chronic iliac occlusion before thrombolysis. A 52-year-old female presented eight months following back surgery. Postoperative deep venous thrombosis was treated with heparin and warfarin for six months. However, she was left with severe edema and numbness in her left lower extremity. **B** After 24 h of thrombolytic therapy, a small residual iliofemoral channel is identified. **C** After placement of tandem self-expanding metallic stents spanning the iliac and common femoral veins, there is good flow in the large veins. Edema totally resolved and normal sensation returned to the left leg.

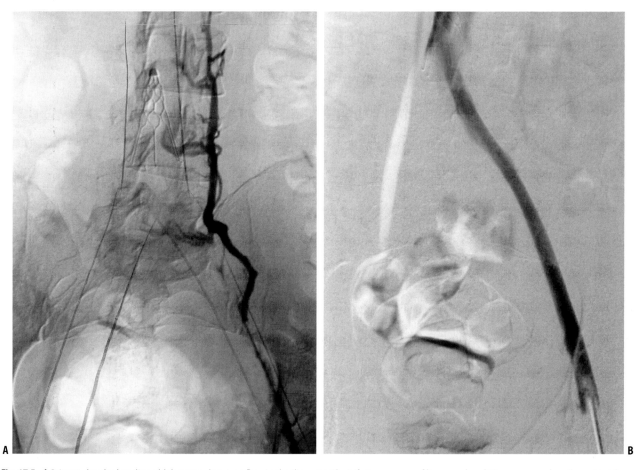

Fig. 17.5. A Prior to the, the baseline phlebogram shows no flow in the iliac vein. The inferior vena cava filter was placed 10 years ago when the patient (now aged 44) developed postpartum DVT. **B** Following 72 h of thrombolysis (12.8 million units of urokinase), a wire was advanced into the inferior vena cava and stents were placed to reconstruct the pelvic veins.

syndrome. One group presents with an acute episode of thrombosis and denies any history of DVT. However, phlebography reveals anatomical changes consistent with prior thrombosis of indeterminate age. This is an acute-on-chronic (AC) pattern.

A second subset of patients characteristically presents with multiple documented episodes of recurrent (R) thromboembolism. Many have been hospitalized more than once for pulmonary embolism and/or DVT. They are commonly readmitted for intravenous heparin therapy and further anticoagulation. Frequently, their recurrent DVT occurs shortly after discontinuing oral anticoagulation. As a relatively high percentage of this group has a family history of thrombosis, the question of an inherited hypercoagulability disorder is raised.

The third group of patients have a poor response to standard therapy and are considered conservative treatment failures (CTF). They present with varying degrees of unremitting pain and edema after the initial episode of anticoagulant-treated deep venous thrombosis. Invariably, these patients have sought and received timely diagnosis and treatment. They failed to respond to usual heparin and warfarin regimens. They have relatively symptomatic venous hypertension directly related to the extent of their thrombosis. They lack recanalization and so it is difficult to assess deep reflux. They are frequently disabled, cannot work, drive, or perform normal daily activities. Some have non healing ulcers. When the left limb is involved, there is commonly a chronic left common iliac vein obstruction.

All of these patients represent the consequences of deep venous thrombosis despite the apparent difference in timing of their clinical presentation. Evaluation of the subgroup demographics shows a few significant differences. The average age of acute/chronic patients is 52.2 years versus 41 years in the recurrent thrombosis group and 41.6 years in the conservative treatment failure group. Patients failing to respond to conservative therapy after surgery showed no tendency towards hypercoagulability or malignancy. Malignancy was equally common among the AC and CTF groups, but distinctly rare in patients with a pattern or multiple episodes of symptomatic DVT. Patients presenting with an acute episode of left leg DVT and occult chronic changes were twice as likely to have a May–Thurner compression syndrome than patients from the R or CTF groups.

Discussion

It has been frequently stated that venous thrombosis older than 14 days is not amenable to thrombolysis.[40,41] Such perception derives from early clinical experience with systemic infusion of streptokinase. This was much less effective than the current techniques of catheter-directed lytic therapy.[42] There is a current evolution in techniques and ideas about therapeutic intervention for both acute and chronic venous disorders. Surgical reconstruction for chronic obstruction is not widely practiced, and conservative management is commonly advocated as the initial therapy for venous obstruction following DVT.[43] There is a general belief that patients with acute venous thrombosis will not have severe long-term symptoms of post-thrombotic syndrome. This applies to single-segment subtotal occlusions. However, patients with extensive thrombosis extending from the calf to the pelvis will frequently develop post-thrombotic symptoms. Most reports do not stratify the extent and location of the initial thrombus load. Furthermore, age of thrombus with notation of mixed acute and chronic thrombus has rarely been described.[44]

The extent of thrombus and thrombus composition are important factors in determining clinical outcome after an episode of DVT. Furthermore, we presently lack both qualitative and quantitative predictors of intrinsic autolytic capacity that might allow identification of the patient who will adequately lyse the thrombus and avoid the sequelae of the post-thrombotic syndrome. We do know that early lysis preserves valvular integrity[45,46] and intrinsic ability to lyse thrombus differs between acute thrombus and old, organized thrombus.[47,48]

Why does thrombolysis work in chronic venous thrombosis? This seems to contradict almost everything previously taught. However, pathologic studies published by Sevitt describe thrombus recanalization and creation of small pockets of thrombus lysis.[6] Presumably, this is due to endothelial cell secretion of urokinase and tissue plasminogen activator. It is clear from the descriptions that thrombus is a dynamic substance undergoing constant remodeling. Although this may be largely undetectable on serial phlebograms, pathologic studies confirm that thrombus is an ever-changing state which produces different luminal configurations over time.

The Poiseuille equation teaches that flow through a cylindrical structure, such as a vein, is influenced by the width of the lumen (i.e., the radius). The work of French physician, Jean Leonard Marie Poiseuille (1799–1869) revealed that resistance to flow through a small glass tube depends on several factors, including the radius of the tube, the length of the tube, and the viscosity of the fluid.[49] These factors influence resistance to flow and, in the formal equation, flow is directly proportional to the fourth power of the radius. Therefore, a small increase or decrease in the internal diameter of a vein has a very large influence on resistance to flow. Decreasing the radius by half will increase the resistance by 16. Conversely, increasing the radius by half will logarithmically increase flow by lowering resistance. Therefore, opening totally occluded veins can dramatically augment venous flow despite the small increment of each individual radius (i.e., 0–2 mm).

Flow, as discussed, is regulated by changes in the vessel diameter since length and viscosity are not easily manipulated variables. If numerous unnamed small veins and the major veins are opened by urokinase, the physiologic change might be dramatic even though the phlebographic change is not impressive (Fig. 17.6). However, the overall resistance to flow can decrease because many small channels are slightly enlarged by the lytic process. Importantly, lysis of subacute thrombus superimposed on older layers adherent to the vessel wall changes the venous resistance in the entire limb.

If the composition of the thrombus is dynamic and reconfigured over time, and if peripheral pockets of autolysis are seen in chronic thrombus, why is it a surprise that purposeful local infusion of additional lytic agent will augment the natural response? Even though the balance between throm-

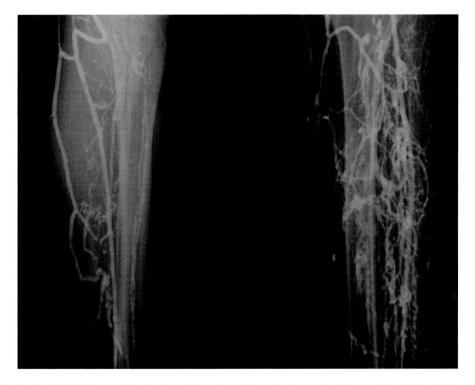

Fig. 17.6. Radiographs showing initial phlebogram 6 weeks after a fall causing a left patellar fracture in a 72-year-old female. Chronic changes are noted on both the baseline and the completion phlebograms. A significant increase in number of venous channels was achieved with flow-directed therapy.

bosis and thrombolysis is complex, the natural history of thrombus teaches that recanalization of chronic occlusion occurs. It is said that removal of old thrombus is not possible. This reflects a poor understanding that thrombus is composed of various layers and that the evolution of catheter techniques and observation of the improved flow patterns in the obstructed extremity provide proof of the effect of adjunctive lytic therapy.

The value of thrombolytic therapy is the removal of acute and subacute thrombus in order to restore the flow balance. The goal is not to remove all of the oldest thrombus but to restore an adequate system of venous conduits to accommodate venous blood at a rate that alleviates edema and pain.

Risk of complications must be weighed against the gain in quality of life. The most serious risks of endovascular therapy, particularly thrombolysis, are unwanted hemorrhage in a location not amenable to evacuation or surgical rescue. This includes intracranial bleeding and unrecognized retroperitoneal bleeding. Titration or cessation of the lytic agent and/or anticoagulation can control other sites of bleeding in less critical locations or from more readily identified sources. Although the incidence of major bleeding complications with peripheral vascular application of thrombolysis is reported less than 1%,[29] extreme diligence is required in monitoring all patients as well as prompt investigation of all complaints of pain and/or change in mental status.

The magnitude of chronic post-thrombotic venous disorders has undoubtedly been underestimated in many western societies.[50] Baker et al. suggested that prior thrombosis was most likely an unappreciated factor in a large percentage of patients with non healing ulcers.[51] On the other hand, despite timely diagnosis and the benefit of standard treatment, Porter and colleagues reported that a significant number of patients are left with post-thrombotic symptoms.[4,51,52] Moreover, patients without symptoms of venous insufficiency often have findings of asymptomatic deep vein reflux after DVT.[4] Further evaluation and treatment is often not offered due to lack of effective therapeutic interventions to treat chronic venous obstruction in the past.

A sense of hopeless resignation pervades treatment of chronic venous disorders. This is based on the lack of uniformly accepted therapy. Endovascular intervention is a new approach that may restore hope in patients and some physicians. It has been demonstrated that the degree of disability can decrease significantly after endovascular therapy for chronic occlusion.[53]

Our experience indicates that clinical improvement is sustained in the majority of patients followed long term. Reintervention is infrequent and well tolerated. It would appear thus far that extensive multisegmental thromboses have a high chance of causing hemodynamically significant residual post-thrombotic occlusion. Early lysis in these patients may prevent chronic post-thrombotic venous insufficiency.

References

1. Browse NL, Clemenson G, Lea Thomas M. Is the postphlebitic leg always postphlebitic? Relation between phlebographic appearance of deep venous thrombosis and late sequelae. Br Med J 1980; 282:1167
2. Cranley JJ, Krause RJ, Strasser ES. Chronic venous insufficiency of the lower extremity. Surgery 1961; 49:68
3. Beyth RJ, Cohen AM, Landefeld CS. Long-term outcomes of deep venous thrombosis. Arch Intern Med 1995; 155:1031–3
4. Lindner DJ, Edwards JM, Phinney ES et al. Long-term hemodynamic and clinical sequelae of lower extremity DVT. J Vasc Surg 1986; 4:436–2
5. Lagerstedt CI, Olsson CG, Fagher BO et al. Need for long-term anticoagulant treatment in symptomatic calf vein thrombosis. Lancet 1985; 2:515–18
6. Sevitt J. The mechanisms of canalization in deep venous thrombosis. J Pathol 1973; 110:153–65
7. Widmer LK, Zemp E, Widmer MT et al. Late results in deep vein thrombosis of the lower extremity. Vasa 1985;14(3):264–8
8. Bauer G. A venographic study on thromboembolic problems. Acta Chir Scand 1940; 84(61):1–75
9. Browse NL, Burnand KG, Thomas ML. The calf pump failure syndrome. In: Browse NL, Burnand KG, Thomas ML (eds) Diseases of the veins: pathology, diagnosis and treatment. Edward Arnold, London 1988: 301–23
10. Tsapogas MJ, Flute PT, Cotton LT, Milroy SD. Lysis of experimental thrombi by streptokinase. Br J Surg 1962; 50:334
11. Nilsson IM, Olow B. Fibrinolysis induced by streptokinase in man. Acta Chir Scand 1962; 123:247
12. Cotton LT, Flute PT, Tsapogas MJ. Popliteal artery thrombosis treated with streptokinase. Lancet 1962; 2:1081
13. Robertson BR, Nillson IM, Nylander G. Value of streptokinase and heparin in treatment of acute deep venous thrombosis. Acta Chir Scand 1968; 134:203–8
14. Kakkar VV, Flanc C, Howe CT et al. Treatment of deep venous thrombosis: a trial of heparin, streptokinase and arvin. Br Med J 1969; 1:806
15. Mavor GE, Bennett B, Galloway M, Karmody AM. Streptokinase in iliofemoral venous thrombosis. Br J Surg 1969; 56:564
16. Robertson BR, Nillson IM, Nylander G. Thrombolytic effect of streptokinase as evaluated by phlebography of deep venous thrombi of the leg. Acta Chir Scand 1970; 136:173
17. Sharma CVRK, O'Connell DJ, Belko JS, Sasahara AA. Thrombolytic therapy in deep vein thrombosis. Academic Press, London, 1977: 181–9
18. Nachbur BB, Beck EA, Jenn A. Can the results of treatment of deep venous thrombosis be improved by combining surgical thrombectomy with regional thrombolysis? J Cardiovasc Surg 1980; 21:347
19. Meissner AJ, Misiak A, Ziemski JM et al. Hazards of thrombolytic therapy in deep venous thrombosis. Br J Surg 1987; 74:991–3
20. Goldhaber SZ, Buring JE, Lipnick RJ, Hennekens CH. Pooled analyses of randomized trials of streptokinase and heparin in phlebographically documented acute deep venous thrombosis. Am J Med 1984; 76:393–7
21. LeVeen HH, Diaz CA. Venous and arterial occlusive disease treated by enzymatic clot lysis. Arch Surg 1972; 105:927
22. Tsapogas MJ, Peabody RA et al. Controlled study of thrombolytic therapy in deep venous thrombosis. Surgery 1973; 74(6):973–84
23. Dotter CT, Rosch J, Seaman AJ. Selective clot lysis with low-dose streptokinase. Radiology 1974; 111:31
24. Marder VJ, Soulen RL et al. Quantitative venographic assessment of deep venous thrombosis in the evaluation of streptokinase and heparin therapy. J Lab Clin Med 1977; 89(5):1018
25. Albrechtsson M, Anderson J, Einarsson E. Streptokinase treatment of deep venous thrombosis and the post-thrombotic syndrome. Arch Surg 1981; 116:33–7
26. Katzen BT, Edwards K, Arthur A, Van Breda A. Low-dose direct fibrinolysis in peripheral vascular disease. J Vasc Surg 1984; 1:718–22
27. McNamara TO, Fischer JR. Thrombolysis of arterial and graft occlusions: improved results using high-dose urokinase. Am J Radiol 1985; 144:769–5
28. LeBlang DS, Becker GJ, Benenati JF, Zemel G, Katzen BT, Sallee JS. Low-dose urokinase regimen for the treatment of lower extremity arterial and graft occlusions: Experience in 132 cases. J Vasc Intervent Radiol 1992; 3:474–83
29. McNamara TO. Complications in thrombolysis. Sem Int Rad 1994; 11:134–44
30. Becker LJ, Holden RW, Rabe FE et al. Local thrombolytic therapy for subclavian and axillary vein thrombosis. Radiology 1983; 149:419–23
31. Druy EM, Trout HH et al. Lytic therapy in the treatment of axillary and subclavian vein thrombosis. J Vasc Surg 1985; 2:821–27
32. Macheleder HI. Upper extremity venous thrombosis. Sem Vasc Surg 1990; 3:1–8
33. Thorpe PE, Siffring PA, Hunter DW. Direct lower extremity infusion of urokinase for the treatment of acute and subacute deep venous thrombosis. Radiology 1989; 173(P):621
34. Okrent D, Messersmith RO, Buckman J. Transcatheter fibrinolytic therapy and angioplasty for left iliofemoral venous thrombosis. J Vasc Intervent Radiol 1991; 2:195–200
35. Molina JE, Hunter DW, Yedlika JW. Thrombolytic therapy for iliofemoral venous thrombosis. J Vasc Surg 1992; 630–7
36. Semba CP, Dake MD. Catheter-directed venous thrombolysis. Semin Int Rad 1994; 11(4):388–95
37. Comerota AJ, Aldridge SC, Gohen G et al. A strategy of aggressive regional therapy for acute iliofemoral venous thrombosis with contemporary venous thrombectomy for catheter-directed thrombolysis. J Vasc Surg 1994; 20:244–54
38. Cragg AH. Lower extremity deep venous thrombolysis: a new approach to obtaining access. JVIR 1996; 7:283–8
39. Bjorgell O, Ekberg O, Akesson H, Olsson R. Videophlebography with foot venous pressure measurements: Description of a technique for diagnosing venous dysfunction. Phlebology 1997; 12:100–6
40. Hansen MCH, Wollersheim H, van Asten WNJC et al. The post-thrombotic syndrome: A review. Phlebology 1996; 11:86–94
41. Markel A, Manzo RA, Strandness DE Jr. The potential role of thrombolytic therapy in venous thrombosis. Arch Intern Med 1992; 152:1265–67
42. Semba CP, Dake MD. Iliofemoral deep venous thrombosis: aggressive therapy using catheter-directed thrombolysis. Radiology 1994; 191:487–94
43. Moneta GL. The case against aggressive treatment. Vasc Surg 1997; 31(3):320–21
44. Wells PS, Hirsh J, Anderson DR et al. Accuracy of clinical assessment of deep venous thrombosis. Lancet 1995; 345:1326–30

45. van Bemmelen PS, Bedford G, Beach K, Strandness DE Jr. Status of the valves in the superficial and deep venous system in chronic venous disease. Surgery 1991; 109:130–9

46. Meissner MH, Manzo RA, Bergelin RO et al. Deep venous insufficiency: the relationship between lysis and consequent reflux. J Vasc Surg 1993; 18:596–608

47. Killewich LA, Bedford GR, Beach KW, Strandness DE Jr. Spontaneous lysis of deep venous thrombi: Rate and outcome. J Vasc Surg 1989; 9:89–97

48. Mohrman DE, Heller LJ. Homeostasis and cardiovascular transport. In: Hefta J, Melvin S (eds) Cardiovascular physiology, 4th edn. McGraw-Hill Co., New York, 1997: 1–8

49. Van Den Oever R, Hepp B, Debbaut B, Simon I. Socioeconomic impact of chronic venous insufficiency: An underestimated public health problem. Int Angiol 1998; 17:161–7

50. Baker SR, Stacy AG, Jopp-McKay AG et al. Epidemiology of chronic venous ulcers. Br J Surg 1991; 78:864–7

51. Johnson BF, Manzo RA, Bergelin RO, Strandness DE Jr. Relationship between changes in the deep venous system and the development of the post-thrombotic syndrome after an acute episode of lower limb deep venous thrombosis: a one- to six-year follow-up. J Vasc Surg 1995; 21:307–13

52. Lagersted C, Olsson CG, Fagher B et al. Recurrence and late sequelae after first-time deep venous thrombosis: Relationship to initial lysis. Phlebology 1993; 8:62–7

53. Nazarian GK, Austin WR, Wegryn SA et al. Venous recanalization by metallic stents after failure of balloon angioplasty or surgery: four-year experience. Cardiovasc Intervent Radiol 1996; 19:227–33

Editors' Commentary

The pathophysiology of severe chronic venous insufficiency is dominated by the phenomenon of reflux. However, persistent venous occlusion in some patients remains an important component in the genesis of severe cutaneous changes. External venous compression, such as right iliac artery compression of the left common iliac vein, is linked to some forms of venous obstruction. However, it is thrombosis, with or without external compression that dominates in the case of venous occlusion.

Pineo and Hull have provided for this section a very clear and logical, stepwise explanation for the development of thrombosis. They have linked the theories of Virchow from 150 years ago to the research of present-day investigators. They have even included the most recently uncovered prothrombin mutant. Of practical importance, they have emphasized the prevalence of resistance to activated protein C and have shown that this important cause of thrombosis varies in its incidence in various patient populations. They have underscored the fact that a single procoagulant abnormality is less important than a combination of two factors such as resistance to protein C coupled with advancing age.

The pathology of venous thrombosis and its causes is directly linked to care of patients with severe chronic venous insufficiency. A sizable fraction has experienced venous thromboembolic events and must be protected as they proceed through surgical treatment. Fortunately, outpatient prophylaxis of venous thromboembolism is not only possible but also quite easy. Ready availability of fractionated heparins allows outpatient manipulations to be conducted in a safe fashion and even patients who are taking lifetime Coumadin anticoagulation can be protected by fractionated heparin while the Coumadin effect is reversed for the surgical intervention.

As persistent venous occlusion retards clinical care of patients with chronic venous insufficiency, methods of correcting the pathophysiology underlying this are important. Venous reconstruction by grafting and bypass has been replaced by the techniques of the interventional radiologist. Dake's group at Stanford has been a leader in exploration of disobliteration of venous occlusions. They have provided rationale for thromboembolic interventions and have re-emphasized the importance of restoring venous competence in prevention of chronic venous insufficiency. They have stressed the differentiation between systemic administration of thrombolytic agents and catheter-directed thrombolysis. Their emphasis on endovascular treatment for acute deep venous thrombosis provides guidelines for treatment of this important subset of patients and their introduction to the subject of treatment of chronic thrombosis-induced venous occlusion is most valuable.

As indicated above, it is chronic venous occlusion that vascular surgeons have approached with the bypass principle learned in arterial occlusive disease. Bypass techniques have proven disappointing and it is for this reason that venous angioplasty and stent placement is looked to with great interest by surgeons concerned with treatment of chronic venous insufficiency.

In the final chapter of this book, Thorpe describes the extensive Creighton University and Omaha experience in treatment of acute and chronic venous obstructions. Thorpe has clearly differentiated acute uncomplicated venous thrombosis from acute thrombosis superimposed on previous deep venous thrombosis. She has separated these two entities from the chronic occlusions seen in many patients with severe chronic venous insufficiency. The value of her report lies in the long-term follow-up of patients. She points out that early rethrombosis is related to inadequate anticoagulation and that long-term benefit is sustained in the majority of patients. It is remarkable that one-third of the treated patients discard external compression and over half use compression only to control mild edema. Thorpe's presentation makes a strong case for the use of endovascular therapy in treatment of chronic venous obstruction in patients with severe chronic venous insufficiency. This emphasizes again that all elements present in a given patient must be dealt with in order to achieve success. For example, venous stripping and phlebectomy should treat superficial reflux, incompetent perforator veins must be dealt with by direct techniques, and venous obstruction should be considered for venous lysis, angioplasty and stenting. Thus, we who are interested are presented with a variety of techniques for treatment of the pathophysiology of chronic venous insufficiency.

Index